Second Edition

MEDICAL ASSISTING
CLINICAL ASSISTING & PHARMACOLOGY—MODULE B

Material Selected from:

Essentials of Medical Assisting: Administrative and Clinical Competencies
by Bonnie F. Fremgen

Workbook
by Bonnie F. Fremgen and Kathleen Wallington
for *Essentials of Medical Assisting: Administrative and Clinical Competencies*
by Bonnie F. Fremgen

Medical Assistant Test Review Programmed Learner
by Bonnie F. Fremgen, Kathleen Wallington, and Mary King

Medical Terminology with Human Anatomy, Fourth Edition
by Jane Rice

Structure & Function of the Human Body
by Frederic H. Martini and Edwin F. Bartholomew

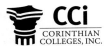

CCi
CORINTHIAN
COLLEGES, INC.

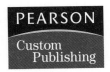

PEARSON

Custom
Publishing

Cover photograph courtesy of Taxi/Getty Images, Inc.

Material Selected from:

Essentials of Medical Assisting: Administrative and Clinical Competencies by Bonnie F. Fremgen
Copyright © 1998 by Prentice-Hall, Inc.
A Pearson Education Company
Upper Saddle River, New Jersey 07458

Workbook
by Bonnie F. Fremgen and Kathleen Wallington
for *Essentials of Medical Assisting: Administrative and Clinical Competencies* by Bonnie F. Fremgen
Copyright © 1998 by Prentice-Hall, Inc.

Medical Assistant Test Review Programmed Learner by Bonnie F. Fremgen, Kathleen Wallington, and Mary King
Copyright © 1999 Prentice-Hall, Inc.

Medical Terminology with Human Anatomy, Fourth Edition by Jane Rice
Copyright © 1999, 1995, 1991 by Appleton & Lange
Published by Prentice-Hall, Inc.

Structure & Function of the Human Body by Frederic H. Martini and Edwin F. Bartholomew
Copyright © 1999 by Frederic H. Martini, Inc.
Published by Prentice-Hall, Inc.

This special edition published in cooperation with Pearson Custom Publishing.

Printed in the United States of America

10 9 8 7 6 5 4 3 2 1

ISBN 0-536-84605-7

2004520023

EH/LD

Please visit our web site at *www.pearsoncustom.com*

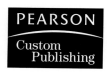

PEARSON CUSTOM PUBLISHING
75 Arlington Street, Suite 300, Boston, MA 02116
A Pearson Education Company

Credits and Acknowledgments

CCi Medical Assisting Program Series (Module A-G)

Publisher

Pearson Custom Publishing in cooperation with Corinthian Colleges, Inc.

Editor and Project Manager

Alicia Mata, BS, CMA, Medical Assisting Curriculum Project Manager, CCi

Kathy Case, MSN, RN, Program Manager Health Sciences

Donna Patterson, AA, CMA, Program Coordinator

Authors

Cheryl Niblett, CMA, BSC, Medical Assistant Program Chair

Kellie Stock, CMA, Medical Assistant Instructor

Ted Volkmann, BS, Mathematics

Shaun Holland, CMA, Lead Medical Assistant Instructor

Tanya Mercer, Medical Assistant Instructor

Irma Blanco, BS, Director of Education

Blanca Zepeda, AA, CMA, Medical Assistant Program Chair

Vince Dick, Medical Assistant Instructor

Claudia Chaparro, AA, CMA, Medical Assistant Instructor

Sally Stegmeier, CMA, Medical Assistant Instructor

Berta Williams, NRCMA, Director of Education

Brad Johnson, Medical Assistant Program Chair

Jennifer Montoya, Medical Assistant Instructor

Steve Dovalina, CMA, Medical Assistant Instructor

Gwen Schrader, Medical Assistant Program Chair

Christine Cusano, AA, CMA, Medical Assistant & Medical Administrative Assistant Instructor

Maria Leal, Allied Health Instructor

Rachael Washington, Placement Representative

Amanda Gaugler, BS, Director of Education

Niki Good, BA Education, School President

Jacqueline Ferguson, BA, Academic Dean

Joan Juang, BA, AA, CMA, Medical Program Director

John Etheridge, Medical Assistant Program Chair

Judith Enlow, CMA, Medical Assistant Instructor and Program Chair

Marchelle (Mickey) Weaver, BSBA, Director of Education

Kathryn Cremeans, Externship Coordinator

Sandra Shepherd, Medical Assistant Instructor

Dorit Soltanovich, MD, Medical Program Director

Dottie Fields, RMA, Education Chair, Medical Assistant and Medical Administrative Assistant Programs

CONTENTS

Material selected from: *Medical Assistant Test Review Programmed Learner*
by Bonnie F. Fremgen, Kathleen Wallington, and Mary King

Content Provided by Corinthian Colleges, Inc.

Material selected from: *Essentials of Medical Assisting: Administrative and Clinical Competencies*
by Bonnie F. Fremgen

Section One
MEDICAL TERMINOLOGY AND ANATOMY AND PHYSIOLOGY

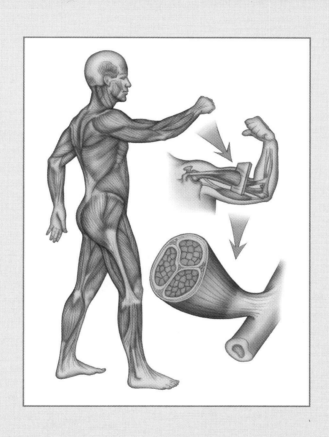

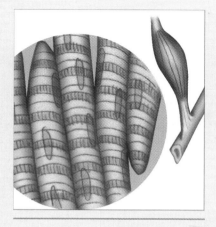

1

MEDICAL TERMINOLOGY OF THE MUSCULAR SYSTEM

OUTLINE

- Anatomy and Physiology Overview
- Types of Muscle Tissue
- Functions of Muscles
- Life Span Considerations
- Terminology with Surgical Procedures & Pathology
- Vocabulary Words
- Abbreviations
- Drug Highlights
- Diagnostic and Laboratory Tests
- Communication Enrichment
- Study and Review Section

  Learning Exercises

  Word Parts Study Sheet

  Review Questions

  Critical Thinking Activity

OBJECTIVES

On completion of this chapter, you should be able to:

- Describe the muscular system.
- Describe types of muscle tissue.
- Provide the functions of muscles.
- Describe muscular differences of the child and the older adult.
- Analyze, build, spell, and pronounce medical words that relate to surgical procedures and pathology.
- Identify and give the meaning of selected vocabulary words.
- Identify and define selected abbreviations.
- Review Drug Highlights presented in this chapter.
- Provide the description of diagnostic and laboratory tests related to the muscular system.
- Successfully complete the study and review section.

► ANATOMY AND PHYSIOLOGY OVERVIEW

The muscular system is composed of all the *muscles* in the body. This overview will describe the three basic types of muscles and some of their functions. The muscles are the primary tissues of the system. They make up approximately 42% of a person's body weight and are composed of long, slender cells known as *fibers*. Muscle fibers are of different lengths and shapes and vary in color from white to deep red. Each muscle consists of a group of fibers held together by connective tissue and enclosed in a fibrous sheath or *fascia*. See Figure 1–1. Each fiber within a muscle receives its own nerve impulses and has its own stored supply of glycogen, which it uses as fuel for energy. Muscle has to be supplied with proper nutrition and oxygen to perform properly; therefore, blood and lymphatic vessels permeate its tissues.

► TYPES OF MUSCLE TISSUE

Skeletal muscle, smooth muscle, and *cardiac muscle* are the three basic types of muscle tissue classed according to their functions and appearance (Fig. 1–2).

SKELETAL MUSCLE

Also known as *voluntary* or *striated* muscles, *skeletal muscles* are controlled by the conscious part of the brain and attach to the bones. There are 600 skeletal muscles that, through contractility, extensibility, and elasticity, are responsible for the movement of the body. These muscles have a cross-striped appearance and thus are known as striated muscles. They vary in size, shape, arrangement of fibers, and means of attachment to bones. Selected skeletal muscles are listed with their functions in Tables 1–1 and 1–2 and shown in Figures 1–3 and 1–4.

Skeletal muscles have two or more attachments. The more fixed attachment is known as the *origin,* and the point of attachment of a muscle to the part that it moves is the *insertion*. The means of attachment is called a *tendon,* which can vary in length from less than 1 inch to more than 1 foot. A wide, thin, sheet-like tendon is known as an *aponeurosis.*

A muscle has three distinguishable parts: the *body* or main portion, an *origin,* and an *insertion.* The skeletal muscles move body parts by pulling from one bone across its joint to another bone

THE MUSCULAR SYSTEM

ORGAN/STRUCTURE	PRIMARY FUNCTIONS
Muscles	Responsible for movement, help to maintain posture, and produce heat
Skeletal	Through contractility, extensibility, and elasticity, are responsible for the movement of the body
Smooth	Produce relatively slow contraction with greater degree of extensibility in the internal organs, especially organs of the digestive, respiratory, and urinary tract, plus certain muscles of the eye and skin, and walls of blood vessels
Cardiac	Muscle of the heart, controlled by the autonomic nervous system and specialized neuromuscular tissue located within the right atrium that is capable of causing cardiac muscle to contract rhythmically. The neuromuscular tissue of the heart comprises the sinoatrial node, the atrioventricular node, and the atrioventricular bundle
Tendons	A band of connective tissue serving for the attachment of muscles to bones

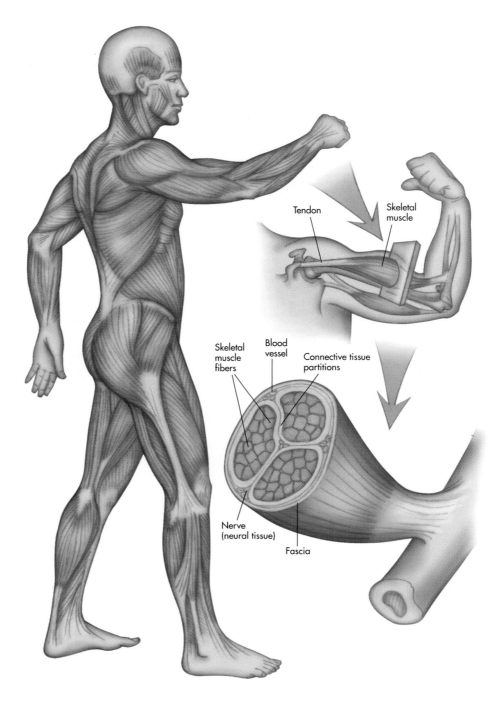

FIGURE 1–1

A skeletal muscle consists of a group of fibers held together by connective tissue. It is enclosed in a fibrous sheath (fascia).

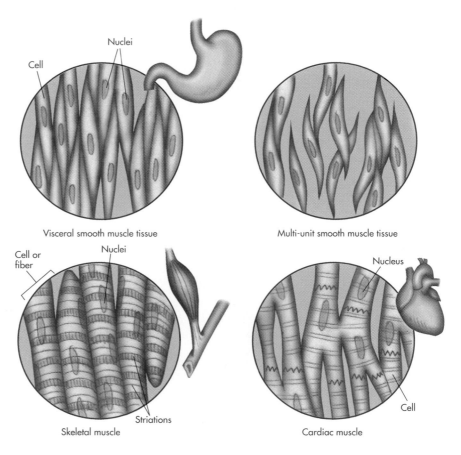

FIGURE 1–2

Types of muscle tissue.

TABLE 1–1   Selected Skeletal Muscles (Anterior View)

Muscle	Action
Sternocleidomastoid	Rotates and laterally flexes neck
Trapezius	Draws head back and to the side, rotates scapula
Deltoid	Raises and rotates arm
Rectus femoris	Extends leg and assists flexion of thigh
Sartorius	Flexes and rotates the thigh and leg
Tibialis anterior	Dorsiflexes foot and increases the arch in the beginning process of walking
Pectoralis major	Flexes, adducts, and rotates arm
Biceps brachii	Flexes arm and forearm and supinates forearm
Rectus abdominis	Compresses or flattens abdomen
Gastrocnemius	Plantar flexes foot and flexes knee
Soleus	Plantar flexes foot

TABLE 1–2   Selected Skeletal Muscles (Posterior View)

Muscle	Action
Trapezius	Draws head back and to the side, rotates scapula
Deltoid	Raises and rotates arm
Triceps	Extends forearm
Latissimus dorsi	Adducts, extends, and rotates arm. Used during swimming
Gluteus maximus	Extends and rotates thigh
Biceps femoris	Flexes knee and rotates it outward
Gastrocnemius	Plantar flexes foot and flexes knee
Semitendinosus	Flexes and rotates leg, extends thigh

with movement occurring at the diarthrotic joint. The types of body movement occurring at the diarthrotic joints are described in the chapter entitled The Skeletal System.

Muscles and nerves function together as a motor unit. For skeletal muscles to contract, it is necessary to have stimulation by impulses from motor nerves. Muscles perform in groups and are classified as:

- **Antagonist.** A muscle that counteracts the action of another muscle
- **Prime mover.** A muscle that is primary in a given movement. Its contraction produces the movement.
- **Synergist.** A muscle that acts with another muscle to produce movement

SMOOTH MUSCLE

Also called *involuntary, visceral,* or *unstriated, smooth muscles* are not controlled by the conscious part of the brain. They are under the control of the autonomic nervous system and, in most cases, produce relatively slow contraction with greater degree of extensibility. These muscles lack the cross-striped appearance of skeletal muscle and are smooth. Included in this type are the muscles of internal organs of the digestive, respiratory, and urinary tract, plus certain muscles of the eye and skin.

CARDIAC MUSCLE

The muscle of the heart *(myocardium)* is *involuntary* but *striated* in appearance. It is controlled by the autonomic nervous system and specialized neuromuscular tissue located within the right atrium.

▶ FUNCTIONS OF MUSCLES

The following is a list of the primary functions of muscles:

1. Muscles are responsible for movement. The types of movement are locomotion, propulsion of substances through tubes as in circulation and digestion, and changes in the size of openings as in the contraction and relaxation of the iris of the eye.
2. Muscles help to maintain posture through a continual partial contraction of skeletal muscles. This process is known as *tonicity.*
3. Muscles help to produce heat through the chemical changes involved in muscular action.

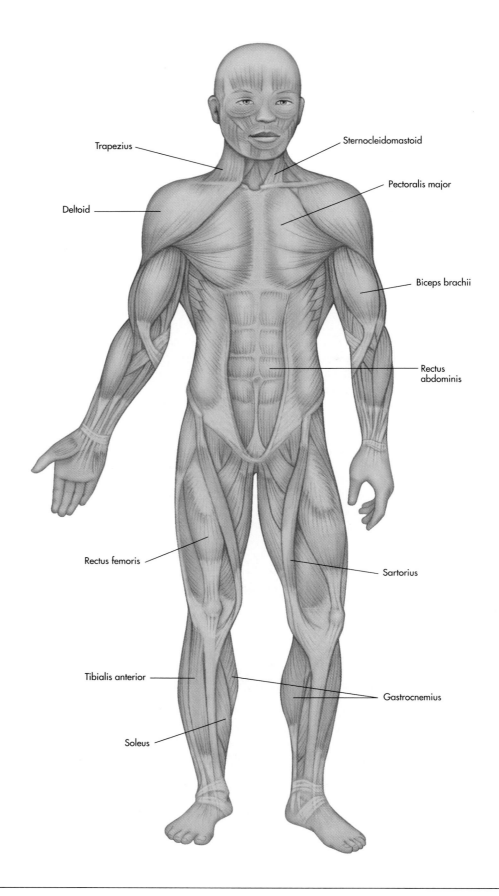

FIGURE 1–3

Selected skeletal muscles (anterior view).

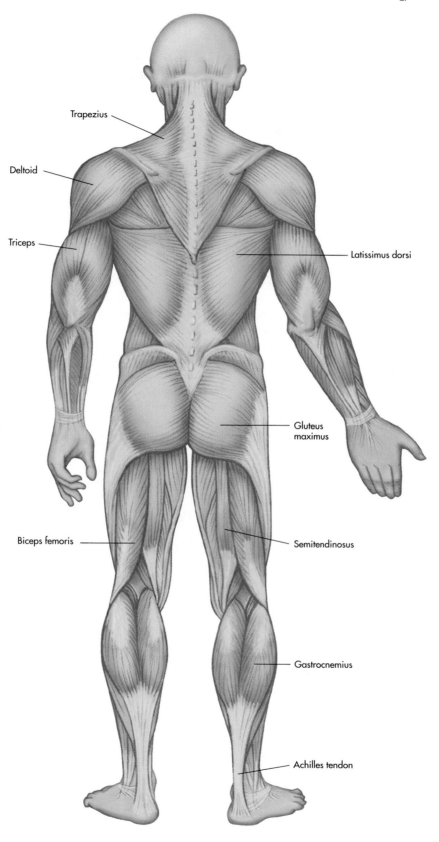

Trapezius

Deltoid

Triceps

Latissimus dorsi

Gluteus maximus

Biceps femoris

Semitendinosus

Gastrocnemius

Achilles tendon

FIGURE 1–4

Selected skeletal muscles and the Achilles tendon (posterior view).

Life Span Considerations

▶ THE CHILD

At about 6 weeks the size of the embryo is 12 mm (0.5 inch). The limb buds are extending and the skeletal and muscular systems are developing. At about 7 weeks the **diaphragm,** a partition of muscles and membranes that separates the chest cavity and the abdominal cavity, is completely developed. At the end of 8 weeks, the embryo is now known as the **fetus.** Fetal growth proceeds from head to tail **(cephalo** to **caudal),** with the head being larger in comparison to the rest of the body.

During fetal development the bones and muscles continue growing and developing. At about 32 weeks the developed skeletal system is soft and flexible. Muscle and fat accumulate and the fetus weighs approximately 2000 g (4 lb, 7 oz). At about 40 weeks the fetus is ready for birth and extra-uterine life.

The movements of the newborn are uncoordinated and random. Muscular development proceeds from head to foot and from the center of the body to the periphery. Head and neck muscles are the first ones that can be controlled by the baby. A baby can hold his head up before he can sit erect. The baby needs freedom of movement. The bath is an excellent time for the newborn to exercise.

▶ THE OLDER ADULT

With aging changes related to mobility are most significant. There is a decrease in muscle strength, endurance, range of motion, coordination and elasticity, and flexibility of connective tissue. There is an actual loss in the number of muscle fibers due to **myofibril atrophy** with fibrous tissue replacement, which begins in the fourth decade of life.

To prevent loss of strength, muscles need to be exercised. Regular exercise strengthens muscles and keeps joints, tendons, and ligaments more flexible, allowing active people to move freely and carry out routine activities easily. Exercises such as aerobic dance, brisk walking, and bicycling improve muscle tone and heart and lung function. To maintain aerobic fitness one needs to participate in such activities for 20 minutes or more at least three times a week and work at one's target heart rate. The target range declines with age and the following table shows the correct range during exercise for women between 45 and 65 years old.

AGE	TARGET HEART RATE (BEATS PER MINUTE)
45 years old	108 to 135
50 years old	102 to 127
55 years old	99 to 123
60 years old	96 to 120
65 years old	93 to 116

TERMINOLOGY

WITH SURGICAL PROCEDURES & PATHOLOGY

TERM	WORD PARTS			DEFINITION
abductor (ăb-dŭk′tōr)	ab	P	away from	A muscle that, on contraction, draws away from the middle
	duct	R	to lead	
	or	S	a doer	
adductor (ă-dŭk′tōr)	ad	P	toward	A muscle that draws a part toward the middle
	duct	R	to lead	
	or	S	a doer	
antagonist (ăn-tăg′ō-nĭst)	ant	P	against	A muscle that counteracts the action of another muscle
	agon	R	agony, a contest	
	ist	S	agent	
aponeurorrhaphy (ăp″ō-nū-ror′ă-fē)	apo	P	separation	Suture of an aponeurosis
	neuro	CF	nerve	
	rrhaphy	S	suture	
aponeurosis (ăp″ō-nū-rō′sĭs)	apo	P	separation	A fibrous sheet of connective tissue that serves to attach muscle to bone or to other tissues
	neur	R	nerve	
	osis	S	condition of	
ataxia (ă-tăks′ĭ-ă)	a	P	lack of	A lack of muscular coordination
	taxia	S	order	
atonic (ă-tŏn′ĭk)	a	P	lack of	Pertaining to a lack of normal tone or tension
	ton	R	tone, tension	
	ic	S	pertaining to	
atrophy (ăt′rō-fē)	a	P	lack of	A lack of nourishment; a wasting of muscular tissue that may be caused by lack of use
	trophy	S	nourishment, development	

☼ TERMINOLOGY SPOTLIGHT

Atrophy occurs with the disuse of muscles over a long period of time. Bedrest and immobility can cause loss of muscle mass and strength. When immobility is due to a treatment mode, such as casting or traction, one can decrease the effects of immobility by isometric exercise of the muscles of the immobilized part. Isometric exercise involves active muscular contraction performed against stable resistance, such as tightening the muscles of the thigh and/or tightening the muscles of the buttocks. Active exercise of uninjured parts of the body helps prevent muscle atrophy.

continued

Terminology - continued

TERM	WORD PARTS			DEFINITION

Other benefits of exercise:

- It may slow down the progression of osteoporosis.
- It reduces the levels of triglycerides and raises the "good" cholesterol (high-density lipoproteins).
- It can lower systolic and diastolic blood pressure.
- It may improve blood glucose levels in the diabetic person.
- Combined with a low-fat, low-calorie diet, it is effective in preventing obesity and helping individuals maintain a proper body weight.
- It can elevate one's mood and reduce anxiety and tension.

Lipoatrophy is atrophy of fat tissue. This condition may occur at the site of an insulin and/or corticosteroid injection. It is also known as lipodystrophy. See Figure 1–5.

TERM	WORD PARTS			DEFINITION
biceps (bī′ sĕps)	bi ceps	P S	two head	A muscle with two heads or points of origin
brachialgia (brā″ kĭ-ăl′ jĭ-ă)	brachi algia	CF S	arm pain	Pain in the arm
bradykinesia (brăd″ ĭ-kĭ-nē′ sĭ-ă)	brady kinesia	P S	slow motion	Slowness of motion or movement
clonic (klŏn′ ĭk)	clon ic	R S	turmoil pertaining to muscles	Pertaining to alternate contraction and relaxation of
contraction (kŏn-trăk′ shŭn)	con tract ion	P R S	with, together to draw process	The process of drawing up and thickening of a muscle fiber
dactylospasm (dăk′ tĭ-lō-spăzm)	dactylo spasm	CF S	finger or toe tension, spasm	Cramp of a finger or toe
diaphragm (dī′ ă-frăm)	dia phragm	P S	through a fence, partition	The partition, of muscles and membranes, that separates the chest cavity and the abdominal cavity
dystonia (dĭs′ tō′ nĭ-ă)	dys ton ia	P R S	difficult tone, tension condition	A condition of impaired muscle tone
dystrophy (dĭs′ trō-fē)	dys trophy	P S	difficult nourishment, development	Faulty muscular development caused by lack of nourishment

Terminology - continued

TERM	WORD PARTS			DEFINITION
fascia (făsh′ ĭ-ă)	fasc ia	R S	a band condition	A thin layer of connective tissue covering, supporting, or connecting the muscles or inner organs of the body
fasciectomy (făsh″ ĭ-ĕk′ tō-mē)	fasci ectomy	CF S	a band excision	Surgical excision of fascia
fasciodesis (făsh ĭ-ŏd′ ĕ-sĭs)	fascio desis	CF S	a band binding	Surgical binding of a fascia to a tendon or another fascia
fascioplasty (făsh′ ĭ-ō-plăs″ tē)	fascio plasty	CF S	a band surgical repair	Surgical repair of a fascia
fascitis (fă-sī′ tĭs)	fasc itis	R S	a band inflammation	Inflammation of a fascia
fibromyitis (fī″ brō-mī-ī′ tĭs)	fibro my itis	CF R S	fiber muscle inflammation	Inflammation of muscle and fibrous tissue
insertion (ĭn″ sûr′ shŭn)	in sert ion	P R S	into to gain process	The point of attachment of a muscle to the part that it moves
intramuscular (ĭn″ tră-mŭs′kū-lər)	intra muscul ar	P R S	within muscle pertaining to	Pertaining to within a muscle
isometric (ī″ sō-mĕt′ rĭk)	iso metr ic	CF R S	equal to measure pertaining to	Pertaining to having equal measure
isotonic (ī″ sō-tŏn′ ĭk)	iso ton ic	CF R S	equal tone, tension pertaining to	Pertaining to having the same tone or tension
levator (lē-vā′ tər	levat or	R S	lifter a doer	A muscle that raises or elevates a part
lordosis (lór-dō′ sĭs)	lord osis	R S	bending condition of	Abnormal anterior curve of the spine
myalgia (mī-ăl′ jĭ-ă)	my algia	R S	muscle pain	Pain in the muscle
myasthenia (mī-ăs-thē′ nĭ-ă)	my asthenia	R S	muscle weakness	Muscle weakness

continued

Terminology - continued

TERM	WORD PARTS			DEFINITION
myitis (mī-ī′ tĭs)	my itis	R S	muscle inflammation	Inflammation of a muscle
myoblast (mī′ ō blăst)	myo blast	CF S	muscle immature cell, germ cell	An embryonic cell that develops into a cell of muscle fiber
myofibroma (mī″ ō fĭ-brō′ mă)	myo fibr oma	CF R S	muscle fiber tumor	A tumor that contains muscle and fiber
myogenesis (mī″ō-jĕn′ ĕ-sĭs)	myo genesis	CF F	muscle formation, produce	Formation of muscle tissue
myograph (mī′ ō-grăf)	myo graph	CF S	muscle to write, record	An instrument used to record muscular contractions
myoid (mī′ oid)	my oid	R S	muscle resemble	Resembling muscle
myokinesis (mī″ ō-kĭn-ē′ sĭs)	myo kinesis	CF S	muscle motion	Muscular motion or activity
myology (mĭ-ōl ō-jē)	myo logy	CF S	muscle study of	The study of muscles
myolysis (mī-ŏl′ ĭ-sĭs)	myo lysis	CF S	muscle destruction	Destruction of muscle tissue
myoma (mī-ō′ mă)	my oma	R S	muscle tumor	A tumor containing muscle tissue
myomalacia (mī″ ō-mă-lā′ sĭ-ă)	myo malacia	CF S	muscle softening	Softening of muscle tissue
myomelanosis (mī″ ō-mĕl-ă-nō′ sĭs)	myo melan osis	CF R S	muscle black condition of	A condition of abnormal darkening of muscle tissue
myoparesis (mī″ ō-păr′ ĕ-sĭs)	myo paresis	CF S	muscle weakness	Weakness or slight paralysis of a muscle
myopathy (mī-ŏp′ ă-thē)	myo pathy	CF S	muscle disease	Muscle disease
myoplasty (mī′-ŏ-plăs″tē)	myo plasty	CF S	muscle surgical repair	Surgical repair of a muscle

Terminology - continued

TERM	WORD PARTS			DEFINITION
myorrhaphy (mī-ór′ ă-fē)	myo rrhaphy	CF S	muscle suture	Suture of a muscle wound
myorrhexis (mī-ór-ĕk′ sĭs)	myo rrhexis	CF S	muscle rupture	Rupture of a muscle
myosarcoma (mī″ ō-sar-kō′ mă)	myo sarc oma	CF R S	muscle flesh tumor	A malignant tumor derived from muscle tissue
myosclerosis (mī″ ō-sklĕr-ō′ sĭs)	myo scler osis	CF R S	muscle hardening condition of	A condition of hardening of muscle
myospasm (mī″ ō-spăzm)	myo spasm	CF S	muscle tension, spasm	Spasmodic contraction of a muscle
myotenositis (mī″ ō-tĕn″ ō-sī′ tĭs)	myo tenos itis	CF R S	muscle tendon inflammation	Inflammation of a muscle and its tendon
myotome (mī′ ō-tōm)	myo tome	CF S	muscle instrument to cut	An instrument used to cut muscle
myotomy (mī″ŏt′ ō-mē)	myo tomy	CF S	muscle incision	Incision into a muscle
myotrophy (mī″ŏt′ rō-fē)	myo trophy	CF S	muscle nourishment, development	Nourishment of muscle tissue
neuromuscular (nū″ rō-mŭs′ kū-lăr)	neuro muscul ar	CF R S	nerve muscle pertaining to	Pertaining to both nerves and muscles
neuromyopathic (nū″ rō-mī″ ō-păth′ ĭk)	neuro myo path ic	CF CF R S	nerve muscle disease pertaining to	Pertaining to disease of both nerves and muscles
neuromyositis (nū″ rō-mī″ ō-sī′ tĭs)	neuro myos itis	CF R S	nerve muscle inflammation	Inflammation of nerves and muscles
polymyoclonus (pŏl″ ē-mī ŏk′ lō-nŭs)	poly myo clon us	P CF R S	many muscle turmoil pertaining to	Pertaining to a shock-like muscular contraction occurring in various muscles at the same time

continued

Terminology - continued

TERM	WORD PARTS			DEFINITION
polyplegia (pŏl″ē-plē′jĭ-ă)	poly plegia	P S	many stroke, paralysis	Paralysis affecting many muscles
quadriceps (kwŏd′rĭ-sĕps)	quadri ceps	P S	four head	A muscle that has four heads or points of origin
relaxation (rē-lăk-sā′shŭn)	relaxat ion	R S	to loosen process	The process in which a muscle loosens and returns to a resting stage
rhabdomyoma (răb″dō-mī-ō′mă)	rhabdo my oma	CF R S	rod muscle tumor	A tumor of striated muscle tissue
rotation (rō-tā′shŭn)	rotat ion	R S	to turn process	The process of moving a body part around a central axis
sarcitis (sar-sī′tĭs)	sarc itis	R S	flesh inflammation	Inflammation of muscle tissue
sarcolemma (sar″kō-lĕm′ă)	sarco lemma	CF R	flesh a rind	A plasma membrane surrounding each striated muscle fiber
spasticity (spăs-tĭs′ĭ-tē)	spastic ity	R S	convulsive condition	A condition of increased muscular tone causing stiff and awkward movements
sternocleidomas-toid (stur″nō-klī″ dō-măs′toyd)	sterno cleido mast oid	CF CF R S	sternum clavicle breast resemble	Muscle arising from the sternum and clavicle with its insertion in the mastoid process
synergetic (sin″ĕr-jĕt′ĭk)	syn erget ic	P R S	with, together work pertaining to	Pertaining to certain muscles that work together
tenodesis (tĕn-ōd′ĕ-sĭs)	teno desis	CF S	tendon binding	Surgical binding of a tendon
tenodynia (tĕn″ō-dĭn-ĭ-ă)	teno dynia	CF S	tendon pain	Pain in a tendon
tenorrhaphy (tĕn-ōr′ă-fē)	teno rrhaphy	CF S	tendon suture	Suture of a tendon
tenotomy (tĕn-ŏt′ō-mē)	teno tomy	CF S	tendon incision	Surgical incision of a tendon

Terminology - continued

TERM	WORD PARTS			DEFINITION
tonic (tŏn′ ĭk)	ton ic	R S	tone, tension pertaining to	Pertaining to tone, especially muscular tension
torticollis (tŏr″ tĭ-kŏl′ ĭs)	torti collis	CF R	twisted neck muscles	Stiff neck caused by spasmodic contraction of the of the neck; wry neck
triceps (trī′ sĕps)	tri ceps	P S	three head	A muscle having three heads with a single insertion
voluntary (vŏl′ ŭn-tĕr″ ē)	volunt ary	R S	will pertaining to	Pertaining to under the control of one's will

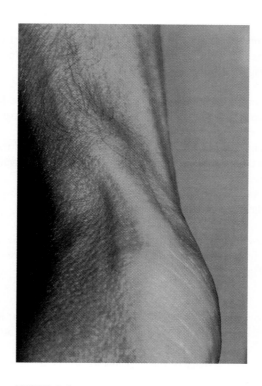

FIGURE 1–5

Lipoatrophy, wrist. *(Courtesy of Jason L. Smith, MD.)*

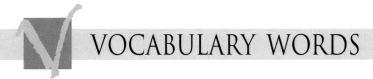

VOCABULARY WORDS

Vocabulary words are terms that have not been divided into component parts. They are common words or specialized terms associated with the subject of this chapter. These words are provided to enhance your medical vocabulary.

WORD	DEFINITION
amputation (ăm″ pū-tā′ shŭn)	Surgical excision of a limb, part, or other appendage
contracture (kŏn-trăk′ chūr)	A condition in which a muscle shortens and renders the muscle resistant to the normal stretching process
degeneration (dē-gĕn″ ĕ-rā′ shŭn)	The process of deteriorating; to change from a higher to a lower form
dermatomyositis (dĕr″ mă-tō-mī″ ō-sī′ tĭs)	Inflammation of the muscles and the skin; a connective tissue disease characterized by edema, dermatitis, and inflammation of the muscles. See Figure 1–6.
diathermy (dī′ ă-thĕr″ mē)	Treatment using high-frequency current to produce heat within a part of the body; used to increase blood flow and should not be used in acute stage of recovery from trauma. Types: **Microwave.** Electromagnetic radiation is directed to specified tissues **Short-wave.** High-frequency electric current (wavelength of 3–30 m) is directed to specified tissues **Ultrasound.** High-frequency sound waves (20,000–10 billion cycles/sec) are directed to specified tissues
Dupuytren's contracture (dū-pwē- tranz′ kŏn-trăk′ chŭr)	A slow, progressive contracture of the palmar fascia causing the ring and little fingers to bend into the palm so that they cannot be extended. See Figure 1–7.
dystrophin (dĭs-trŏf′ ĭn)	A protein found in muscle cells; when the gene that is responsible for this protein is defective and sufficient dystrophin is not produced, muscle wasting occurs
exercise (ĕk′ sĕr-sīz)	Performed activity of the muscles for improvement of health or correction of deformity. Types: **Active.** The patient contracts and relaxes his or her muscles **Assistive.** The patient contracts and relaxes his or her muscles with the assistance of a therapist **Isometric.** Active muscular contraction performed against stable resistance, thereby not shortening the muscle length **Passive.** Exercise is performed by another individual without the assistance of the patient

Vocabulary - continued

WORD	DEFINITION
	Range of Motion. Movement of each joint through its full range of motion. Used to prevent loss of motility or to regain usage after an injury or fracture **Relief of Tension.** Technique used to promote relaxation of the muscles and provide relief from tension
extrinsic (ĕks-trĭn′ sĭk)	Pertaining to external origin; a muscle or muscles partly attached to the trunk and partly to a limb
fatigue (fă-tēg′)	A state of tiredness or weariness occurring in a muscle as a result of repeated contractions
fibromyalgia (fī″ brō-mī-ăl′ jē-ă)	A condition with widespread muscular pain and debilitating fatigue; believed to have an organic or biochemical cause. Diagnosis may be made by testing for unusual tenderness at specific body points.
First Aid Treatment—RICE **Rest** **Ice** **Compression** **Elevation**	**Cryotherapy** (use of cold) is the treatment of choice for soft tissue injuries and muscle injuries. It causes vasoconstriction of blood vessels and is effective in diminishing bleeding and edema. Ice should not be placed directly onto the skin. **Compression** by an elastic bandage is generally determined by the type of injury and the preference of the physician. Some experts disagree on the use of elastic bandages. When used, the bandage should be 3 to 4 inches wide and applied firmly, and toes or fingers should be periodically checked for blue or white discoloration, indicating that the bandage is too tight. **Elevation** is used to reduce swelling. The injured part should be elevated on two or three pillows.
flaccid (flăk′ sĭd)	Lacking muscle tone; *weak, soft,* and *flabby*
heat (hēt)	**Thermotherapy.** The treatment using scientific application of heat may be used 48 to 72 hours after the injury. Types: heating pad, hot water bottle, hot packs, infrared light, and immersion of body part in warm water. Extreme care should be followed when using or applying heat.
hydrotherapy (hī-drō-thĕr′ ă-pē)	Treatment using scientific application of water; types: hot tub, cold bath, whirlpool, and vapor bath
intrinsic (ĭn-trĭn′ sĭk)	Pertaining to internal origin; a muscle or muscles that have their origin and insertion within a structure
involuntary (ĭn-vŏl′ ŭn-tăr″ ē)	Pertaining to action independent of the will

continued

Vocabulary - continued

WORD	DEFINITION
manipulation (măh-nĭp″ŭ-lā′ shŭn)	The process of using the hands to handle or manipulate as in massage of the body
massage (măh-sähzh)	To knead, apply pressure and friction to external body tissues
muscular dystrophy (mŭs′ kū-lār dĭs′ trō-fē)	A chronic, progressive wasting and weakening of muscles. It is a familial disease and onset is usually at an early age
myositis (mī-ō-sī′ tĭs)	Inflammation of muscle tissue
origin (ŏr′ ĭ-jĭn)	The beginning of anything; the more fixed attachment of a skeletal muscle
position (pō-zĭsh′ ŭn)	Bodily posture or attitude; the manner in which a patient's body may be arranged for examination Types of positions and their descriptions: **Anatomic.** Body is erect, head facing forward, arms by the sides with palms to the front; used as the position of reference in designating the site or direction of a body structure **Dorsal Recumbent.** Patient is on back with lower extremities flexed and rotated outward; used in application of obstetric forceps, vaginal and rectal examination, and bimanual palpation **Fowler's.** The head of the bed or examining table is raised about 18 inches or 46 cm, and the patient sits up with knees also elevated **Knee–Chest.** Patient on knees, thighs upright, head and upper part of chest resting on bed or examining table, arms crossed and above head; used in sigmoidoscopy, displacement of prolapsed uterus, rectal exams, and flushing of intestinal canal **Lithotomy.** Patient is on back with lower extremities flexed and feet placed in stirrups; used in vaginal examination, Pap smear, vaginal operations, and diagnosis and treatment of diseases of the urethra and bladder **Orthopneic.** Patient sits upright or erect; used for patients with dyspnea **Prone.** Patient lying face downward; used in examination of the back, injections, and massage **Sims'.** Patient is lying on left side, right knee and thigh flexed well up above left leg that is slightly flexed, left arm behind the body, and right arm forward, flexed at elbow; used in examination of rectum, sigmoidoscopy, enema, and intrauterine irrigation after labor **Supine.** Patient lying flat on back with face upward and arms at the sides; used in examining the head, neck, chest, abdomen, and extremities and in assessing vital signs

Vocabulary - continued

WORD	DEFINITION
	Trendelenburg. Patient's body is supine on a bed or examining table that is tilted at about 45° angle with the head lower than the feet; used to displace abdominal organs during surgery and in treating cardiovascular shock; also called the "shock position"
prosthesis (prŏs′ thē-sĭs)	An artificial device, organ, or part such as a hand, arm, leg, or tooth
rheumatism (roo′ mă-tĭzm)	A general term used to describe conditions characterized by inflammation, soreness and stiffness of muscles, and pain in joints
rigor mortis (rĭg′ ur mór tĭs)	Stiffness of skeletal muscles seen in death
rotator cuff (rō-tā′ tor kŭf)	A term used to describe the muscles immediately surrounding the shoulder joint. They stabilize the shoulder joint while the entire arm is moved.
strain (strān)	Excessive, forcible stretching of a muscle or the musculotendinous unit
synovectomy (sĭn″ ō-věk′ tō-mē)	Surgical excision of a synovial membrane
tendon (těn′ dŭn)	A band of fibrous connective tissue serving for the attachment of muscles to bones; a giant cell tumor of a tendon sheath is a benign, small, yellow, tumor-like nodule. See Figure 1–8.
torsion (tór′ shŭn)	The process of being twisted

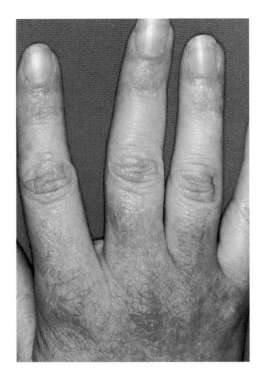

FIGURE 1–6

Dermatomyositis. *(Courtesy of Jason L. Smith, MD.)*

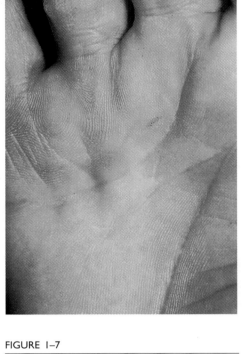

FIGURE 1–7

Dupuytren's contracture. *(Courtesy of Jason L. Smith, MD.)*

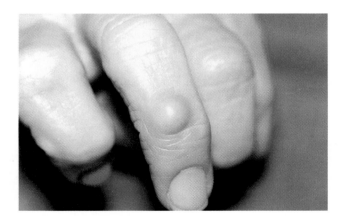

FIGURE 1–8

Giant cell tumor of tendon sheath. *(Courtesy of Jason L. Smith, MD.)*

ABBREVIATIONS

ADP	adenosine diphosphate	LOM	limitation or loss of motion
AE	above elbow	MS	musculoskeletal
AK	above knee	NSAIDs	nonsteroidal anti-inflammatory drugs
ALD	aldolase		
AST	aspartate transaminase	PM	physical medicine
ATP	adenosine triphosphate	PMR	physical medicine and rehabilitation
BE	below elbow		
BK	below knee	ROM	range of motion
Ca	calcium	SGOT	serum glutamic oxaloacetic transaminase
CPK	creatine phosphokinase		
CPM	continuous passive motion	SGPT	serum glutamic pyruvic transaminase
DTRs	deep tendon reflexes		
EMG	electromyography	sh	shoulder
FROM	full range of motion	TBW	total body weight
Ht	height	TJ	triceps jerk
IM	intramuscular	Wt	weight
LDH	lactic dehydrogenase		

DRUG HIGHLIGHTS

Drugs that are generally used for muscular system diseases and disorders include skeletal muscle relaxants and stimulants, neuromuscular blocking agents, anti-inflammatory agents, and analgesics. See Module F, Chapter 3, The Skeletal System, Drug Highlights for a description of anti-inflammatory agents and analgesics.

Skeletal Muscle Relaxants

Used to treat painful muscle spasms that may result from strains, sprains, and musculoskeletal trauma or disease. Centrally acting muscle relaxants act by depressing the central nervous system (CNS) and can be administered either orally or by injection. The patient must be informed of the sedative effect produced by these drugs. Drowsiness, dizziness, and blurred vision may diminish the patient's ability to drive a vehicle, operate equipment, or climb stairs.
Examples: Paraflex (chlorzoxazone), Flexeril (cyclobenzaprine HCl), and Robaxin (methocarbamol).

Skeletal Muscle Stimulants

Used in the treatment of myasthenia gravis. This disease is characterized by progressive weakness of skeletal muscles and their rapid fatiguing. Skeletal muscle stimulants act by inhibiting the action of acetylcholinesterase, the enzyme that halts the action of acetylcholine at the neuromuscular junction. By slowing the destruction of acetylcholine, these drugs foster accumulation of higher concentrations of this neurotransmitter and increase the number of interactions between acetylcholine and the available receptors on muscle fibers.
Examples: Mytelase (ambenonium chloride), Tensilon (edrophonium chloride), and Prostigmin Bromide (neostigmine bromide).

Neuromuscular Blocking Agents   Used to provide muscle relaxation. These agents are used in patients undergoing surgery and/or electroconvulsive therapy, endotracheal intubation, and to relieve laryngospasm.
Examples: Tracrium (atracurium besylate), Flaxedil (gallamine triethiodide), and Norcuron (vecuronium).

DIAGNOSTIC AND LABORATORY TESTS

Test	Description
aldolase (ALD) blood test (ăl′ dō-lāz blod test)	A test performed on serum that measures ALD enzyme present in skeletal and heart muscle. It is helpful in the diagnosis of Duchenne's muscular dystrophy before symptoms appear.
calcium blood test (kăl′ sē-ŭm blod test)	A test performed on serum to determine levels of calcium. Calcium is essential for muscular contraction, nerve transmission, and blood clotting.
creatine phosphokinase (CPK) (krē′ ă-tĭn fŏs″ fō-kīn′ āz)	A blood test to determine the level of CPK. It is increased in necrosis or atrophy of skeletal muscle, traumatic muscle injury, strenuous exercise, and progressive muscular dystrophy.
electromyography (EMG) (ē-lĕk″ trō-mī-ŏg′ ră-fē)	A test to measure electrical activity across muscle membranes by means of electrodes that are attached to a needle that is inserted into the muscle. Electrical activity can be heard over a loudspeaker, viewed on an oscilloscope, or printed on a graph (electromyogram). Abnormal results may indicate myasthenia gravis, amyotrophic lateral sclerosis, muscular dystrophy, peripheral neuropathy, and anterior poliomyelitis.
lactic dehydrogenase (LDH) (lăk′ tĭk dē-hī-drŏj′ ĕ-nāz)	A blood test to determine the level of LDH enzyme. It is increased in muscular dystrophy, damage to skeletal muscles, after a pulmonary embolism, and during skeletal muscle malignancy.
muscle biopsy (mŭs′ ĕl bī′ ŏp-sē)	An operative procedure in which a small piece of muscle tissue is excised and then stained for microscopic examination. Lower motor neuron disease, degeneration, inflammatory reactions, or involvement of specific muscle fibers may indicate myopathic disease.
serum glutamic-oxaloacetic transaminase (SGOT) (sē′ rŭm gloo-tăm′ ĭk ŏks″ ăl-ō-ă-sē′ tĭk trăns ăm′ ĭn-āz)	A blood test to determine the level of SGOT enzyme. It is increased in skeletal muscle damage and muscular dystrophy. This test is also called aspartate transaminase (AST).

Test	Description
serum glutamic pyruvic transaminase (SGPT) (sē′ rŭm gloo-tăm′ ĭk pī-roo′ vĭk trăns-ăm′ ĭn-āz)	A blood test to determine the level of SGPT enzyme. It is increased in skeletal muscle damage. This test is also called alanine aminotransferase (ALT).

COMMUNICATION ENRICHMENT

This segment is provided for those who wish to enhance their ability to communicate in either English or Spanish.

▶ Related Terms

English	Spanish	English	Spanish
muscle	músculo (*mūs*-kū-lō)	shoulder	hombro (*ōm*-brō)
muscle spasm	espasmo muscular (ĕs-*păs*-mō *mŭs*-kū-lăr)	stiffness	tiesura (tĭ-ĕ-*sŭ*-ră)
		contraction	contracción (cōn-trăk-sĭ-*ō n*)
raise your:	levante su: (lĕ-*uăn*-tĕ sū)	twitch	crispamiento (*krĭs*-pă-mĭ-ĕn-tō)
arm	brazo (*bră*-zō)	tighten	estrechar (ĕs-trĕ-chăr)
leg	pierna (pĭ-ĕr-nă)	walk	caminar (*kă*-mĭ-năr)
muscle biopsy	biopsia muscular (bĭ-*ōp*-sĭ-ă *mŭs*-kū-lăr)	limitation of movement	limitación de movimiento (lĭ-mĭ-tă-sĭ-*ōn* dĕ *mō*-vĭ-mĭ-ĕn-tō)
weight	peso (*pĕ*-sō)	tendon	tendón (*tĕn*-dōn)
height	altura (ăl-*tū*-ră)	neck	cuello (*kwā*-yō)
malaise	malestar (*mă*-lĕs-tăr)	finger, toe	dedo (*dĕ*-dō)
painful	doloroso (dō-lō-*rō*-sō)		

English	Spanish	English	Spanish
fiber	fibra (*fĭ*-bră)	amputate	amputar (ăm-pū-*tăr*)
bend	vuelta (*vū*-ĕl-tă)	sport	deporte (dĕ-*pōr*-tĕ)
motion	moción (*mō*-sĭ-ōn)	heat	calor (kă-*lōr*)
weakness	debilidad (dĕ-bĭ-lĭ-*dăd*)	massage	masaje (mă-*să*-hĕ)
fatigue	fatiga (*fă*-tĭ-gă)	harden	endurecer (ĕn-*dū*-rĕ-sĕr)
tone	tono (*tō*-nō)	tense	tenso (*tĕn*-sō)
flaccid	flacido (*flă*-sĭ-dō)	nourishment	nutrimento (nū-trĭ-mĭ-*ĕn*-tō)
position	posición (pō-sĭ-sĭ-*ōn*)	two	dos (dōs)
development	desarrollo (dĕ-să-*rō*-jō)	slow	lento (*lĕn*-tō)
exercise	ejercicio (ĕ-hĕr-*sĭ*-sĭ-ō)		

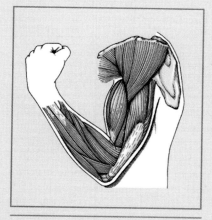

2

ANATOMY AND PHYSIOLOGY OF THE MUSCULAR SYSTEM

OBJECTIVES

On completion of this chapter, you should be able to:

- Describe the properties and functions of muscle tissue.

- Describe the organization of skeletal muscle.

- Describe the structure of a sarcomere.

- Describe the sliding-filament model of muscle contraction.

- Describe the relationship between muscle contractions and motor units.

- Contrast isotonic and isometric muscle contractions.

- Distinguish between aerobic and anaerobic exercise.

- Identify the major axial muscles of the body.

- Identify the major appendicular muscles of the body.

- Describe the effects of exercise and aging on muscle tissue.

It is hard to imagine what our lives would be like without muscle tissue. We would be unable to sit, stand, walk, speak, or grasp objects. Blood would not circulate, because there would be no heartbeat to propel it through blood vessels. The lungs could not rhythmically empty and fill, nor could food move through the digestive tract.

Three different types of muscle tissue move the body and the materials within it. *Skeletal muscle tissue* moves the body by pulling on the bones of the skeleton. *Cardiac muscle tissue* contracts the chambers of the heart, pushing blood through the vessels of the circulatory system. *Smooth muscle tissue* pushes and squeezes fluids and solids along the digestive tract and performs a variety of other functions. All three muscle tissues share the following properties: **excitability**, the ability to respond to stimulation; **contractility**, the ability to shorten; and **elasticity**, the ability of a muscle to rebound toward its original length after a contraction.

This chapter focuses on skeletal muscle tissue. It begins by examining the microscopic structure of skeletal muscle tissue and ends with an overview of the major muscle groups of the body.

▶ SYSTEM BRIEF

The muscular system is made up of some 700 skeletal muscles. Together, they make up about 45 percent of the body weight of a male and 35 percent of the weight of a female. These muscles perform the following important functions:

1. **Produce movement**: Contracting muscles attached to the bones of the skeleton produce movement.
2. **Maintain posture and body position**: Constant muscular contractions permit us to sit upright without collapsing and stand without toppling over.
3. **Maintain body temperature**: Contracting muscles generate heat that keeps our body temperature in the normal range.

▶ THE STRUCTURE OF SKELETAL MUSCLE

Skeletal muscles are the organs of the muscular system and, like any organ, contain a variety of tissues. Each skeletal muscle contains connective and neural tissues as well as skeletal muscle tissue. A typical skeletal muscle appears in Figure 2-1.

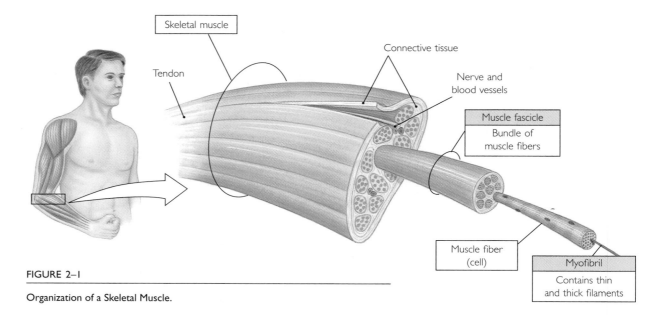

FIGURE 2–1

Organization of a Skeletal Muscle.

Connective tissue is an important part of each muscle. Three layers (outer, middle, and inner) are found in all skeletal muscles. The outer layer surrounds the entire muscle, separating it from surrounding tissues and organs. The connective tissue of the middle layer divides the skeletal muscle into a series of compartments, each containing a group of muscle cells. Each group is called a **fascicle** (FA-si-kul), from the Latin word *fasciculus*, meaning "a bundle." The middle connective tissue layer also contains blood vessels and nerves that supply the surrounding fascicles. Within a fascicle, an inner layer of connective tissue surrounds each skeletal muscle cell and ties adjacent muscle cells together.

At each end of the muscle, the connective tissue layers usually converge to form cordlike **tendons.** Tendons attach skeletal muscles to bones. Any contraction of the muscle will pull on the tendon and, in turn, on the attached bone. Sometimes muscles attach to bones or other muscles through broad sheets of connective tissue rather than through cordlike tendons. Such a sheet is called an **aponeurosis** (ap-ō-noo-RŌ-sis).

STRUCTURE OF A MUSCLE FIBER

Skeletal muscle tissue consists of elongated cells called *muscle fibers*. Muscle fibers, shown in Figure 2-1, are quite different from the "typical" cells. One obvious difference is their enormous size. For example, a skeletal muscle fiber from a thigh muscle could have a diameter of 100 μm (0.1 mm) and a length equal to that of the entire muscle (30 to 40 cm). In addition, each skeletal muscle fiber is *multinucleate*, containing hundreds of nuclei just beneath the cell membrane.

Like a package of spaghetti noodles, each muscle fiber contains hundreds of long, cylindrical structures called **myofibrils**. (*Myo* is Latin for "muscle.") Each myofibril (one of the "noodles")

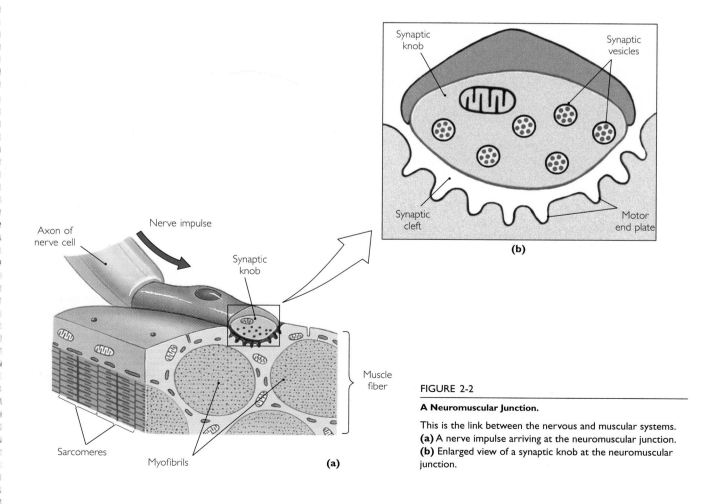

FIGURE 2-2

A Neuromuscular Junction.

This is the link between the nervous and muscular systems. **(a)** A nerve impulse arriving at the neuromuscular junction. **(b)** Enlarged view of a synaptic knob at the neuromuscular junction.

contains bundles of threadlike proteins, or *filaments*, responsible for the contraction of the muscle fiber. There are two types of filaments: **thin filaments,** consisting primarily of the protein *actin*, and **thick filaments,** composed primarily of the protein *myosin*. The filaments in each myofibril are organized in repeating units called *sarcomeres*.

THE NERVE CELL–MUSCLE CELL LINK

Skeletal muscles normally contract in response to a signal from the nervous system. Skeletal muscles are controlled by nerve cells called *motor neurons*. The link between a motor neuron and a skeletal muscle fiber occurs at a specialized connection called a **neuromuscular junction.** As Figure 2-2 shows, the neuromuscular junction contains a *synaptic knob*, the expanded tip of a process from the motor neuron. The synaptic knob contains membranous sacs (*synaptic vesicles*), each filled with **neurotransmitter** molecules. Binding of a neurotransmitter to receptors at the muscle fiber will trigger an electrical impulse in the cell membrane of the muscle fiber. A thin space, the *synaptic cleft*, separates the synaptic knob from the *motor end plate* of the muscle fiber. Folds in the muscle cell membrane in this region increase the surface area of the muscle fiber exposed to neurotransmitter released by the synaptic knob. When neurotransmitter molecules trigger the formation of an electrical impulse in the muscle fiber membrane, that impulse stimulates the release of calcium ions stored within the endoplasmic reticulum of the muscle fiber. These calcium ions then trigger the contraction of the muscle fiber.

▶ HOW A MUSCLE FIBER CONTRACTS

sarco-, muscle + *meros*, part

sarcomere: the smallest contracting unit in a muscle fiber; each myofibril consists of a chain of sarcomeres

Sarcomeres (SAR-kō-mērs) are the working units of a skeletal muscle fiber. Each myofibril contains thousands of sarcomeres. The regular arrangement of thick and thin filaments within each sarcomere produces the striped appearance of a myofibril. All the myofibrils are arranged parallel to the long axis of the cell, with their sarcomeres lying side by side. As a result, the entire muscle fiber has a banded, or *striated*, appearance that corresponds to the bands of the individual sarcomeres.

SARCOMERE STRUCTURE

The structure of the sarcomere provides a key to understanding how a muscle fiber contracts. Figure 2-3a shows a diagrammatic view of an individual sarcomere at rest. The thick filaments lie

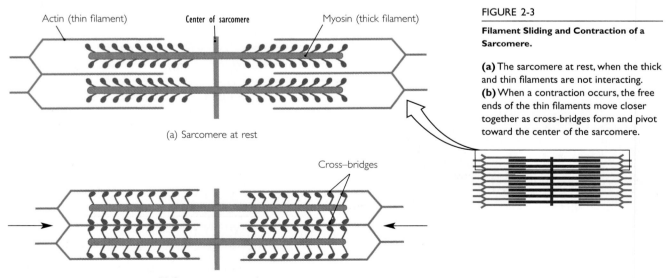

Actin (thin filament)   Center of sarcomere   Myosin (thick filament)

(a) Sarcomere at rest

Cross–bridges

(b) Sarcomere contracting

FIGURE 2-3

Filament Sliding and Contraction of a Sarcomere.

(a) The sarcomere at rest, when the thick and thin filaments are not interacting. **(b)** When a contraction occurs, the free ends of the thin filaments move closer together as cross-bridges form and pivot toward the center of the sarcomere.

in the center of the sarcomere. Thin filaments are attached to either end of the sarcomere and extend toward the center of the sarco-mere, passing among the thick filaments. Sliding of the thin filaments toward the center of the sarcomere causes the unit to shorten, or contract (Figure 2-3). This explanation of muscle contraction is called, not surprisingly, the *sliding filament model.*

SARCOMERE FUNCTION

What causes filament sliding? Sliding occurs after the **cross-bridges**, or "heads," of the thick filaments attach to the thin filaments. Each cross-bridge then pivots at its base, pulling the thin filament toward the center of the sarcomere. This pivoting, called a *power stroke*, shortens the sarcomere (Figure 2-3b). The sliding of thin filaments continues as each cross-bridge detaches, pivots, and reattaches, much like an individual pulling in a rope grabs, pulls, releases and then grabs again, hand over hand. A molecule of ATP must bind to the myosin head before it can detach from the thin filament; the energy provided by the ATP will be used in the next power stroke.

What triggers a contraction? Cross-bridge formation can occur only in the presence of calcium ions. Calcium ions are normally stored within the endoplasmic reticulum of the muscle fiber. The calcium ions are released into the cytoplasm around the myofibrils when one or more electrical impulses travel across the surface of the muscle fiber, in response to the arrival of neurotransmitter at the motor end plate. As soon as the impulse, or impulses, have passed, the calcium ions are pumped back into the endoplasmic reticulum. This is an active transport process that requires ATP. The muscle contraction ends when calcium ion concentrations in the cytoplasm return to their normal low levels. Under these circumstances, cross-bridge formation can no longer occur.

Each time ATP is broken down, some of the energy is released as heat. Muscle contractions release large amounts of heat, and skeletal muscle activity is largely responsible for maintaining body temperature. That is why we shiver when we get cold—the muscle contractions generate heat that can elevate (or at least stabilize) body temperature.

Concept Questions

✔ Why does skeletal muscle appear striated when viewed with a microscope?

✔ Where would you expect to find the greatest concentration of calcium ions in resting skeletal muscle?

 Clinical Note

What Is Rigor Mortis?

When death occurs, circulation stops, and the skeletal muscles are deprived of nutrients and oxygen. Within a few hours, the skeletal muscle fibers have run out of ATP, and the endoplasmic reticulum becomes unable to remove calcium ions from the cytoplasm. Calcium ions diffusing into the cell from the extracellular fluid or leaking out of their storage area (the endoplasmic reticulum) then trigger a sustained contraction. Without ATP, the myosin cannot detach from the cross-bridges, and the muscle locks in the contracted position. All the body's skeletal muscles are involved, and the individual becomes "stiff as a board." This physical state, called **rigor mortis**, lasts until the muscle fibers begin to decompose 15–25 hours later.

► THE WORK OF MUSCLE

Skeletal muscles perform work by pulling on the bones of the skeleton. The bones serve as levers, with the pull of the muscles providing the force to lift a weight or move the body. The nerve supply to muscles allows us to control when and how we move.

HOW NERVES AND MUSCLES WORK TOGETHER

During normal movements, whenever a muscle fiber contracts, it contracts fully, and it always produces the same amount of pull, or *tension*. There is no mechanism to control the amount of tension produced by the contraction of a single muscle fiber: The muscle fiber is either ON (contracting completely) or OFF (relaxing). This is known as the **all-or-none principle**.

Our skeletal muscles would not be very useful to us, however, if the entire muscle could contract only completely or not at all. Fortunately, the all-or-none principle applies only to individual muscle fibers—not to an entire muscle. The amount of tension produced in a skeletal muscle *as a whole* is determined by how many of its muscle fibers are stimulated at one time.

A typical skeletal muscle contains tens of thousands of muscle fibers. Each muscle fiber receives instructions from a motor neuron at a single neuromuscular junction. Although some motor neurons control only a few muscle fibers, most motor neurons contro l hundreds of muscle fibers. All the muscle fibers controlled by a single motor neuron form a **motor unit**.

When we decide to perform a particular movement, specific groups of motor neurons are stimulated. The amount of tension in a muscle depends on how many motor units are then "recruited"; the greater the number called into action, the stronger the muscle's contraction. The size of the motor units within a muscle determines the degree of control available over the tension produced. In the muscles of the eye, where precise control is quite important, each motor neuron may control as few as two or three muscle fibers. On the other hand, we have less precise control over the force exerted by our leg muscles, where one motor neuron may control as many as 2000 muscle fibers.

Some of the motor units within any particular muscle are always active, even when the entire muscle is not contracting. The contractions of these motor units do not produce enough tension to cause movement, but they do tense and firm the muscle. This background tension in a resting skeletal muscle is called **muscle tone**. A muscle with little muscle tone appears limp and soft, whereas one with moderate muscle tone is quite firm and solid.

HOW MUSCLES AND BONES WORK TOGETHER

Bones and muscles are closely interconnected. The physical relationships among bones and muscles, especially the location of muscle attachments relative to the joints involved, determine the power, speed, and direction of body movements. These principles can best be understood in mechanical terms. A **lever** is a rigid structure—such as a crowbar—that moves on a fixed point, called the **fulcrum,** in response to an applied force. In the body each bone is a lever, each joint is a fulcrum, and our muscles apply the forces that produce movement. A force that resists or opposes movement is called a **resistance**. Body weight or an external weight (like a brick in the hand) are examples of resistances that can oppose movement.

Three classes of levers are found in the body. They differ in the placement of the fulcrum (the joint) in relation to the applied force (the muscle attachment) and the position of the resistance (the weight to be moved). An everyday example of the use of a lever is shown in Figure 2-4a. The most common levers in the body are *third-class levers* (Figure 2-4b). In this type of lever, the applied force lies between the fulcrum and the resistance. The point of force application and the resistance move in the same direction, but the resistance moves farther. Thus third-class levers increase the speed and range (distance traveled) of body movements. Figure 2-4c shows how this type of lever action is used to raise the forearm and hand.

Origins, Insertions, and Actions

Consider a muscle that extends between two articulating bones. Typically, when that muscle contracts, one bone will move while the other remains fixed in position. The end of the muscle attached to the stationary bone is called the **origin**, and the end attached to the bone that moves is called the **insertion.** The **action** is the specific movement produced when the muscle contracts. We usually indicate the action in terms of the joint involved. Figure 2-4c shows that for the *biceps brachii* muscle, there are two points of origin on the scapula and a single insertion on the radius of the forearm. We thus say that the biceps brachii originates on the scapula and inserts on the radius. The primary movement produced when the biceps brachii contracts is flexion of the elbow. (The various types of body movements are discussed in Module F.)

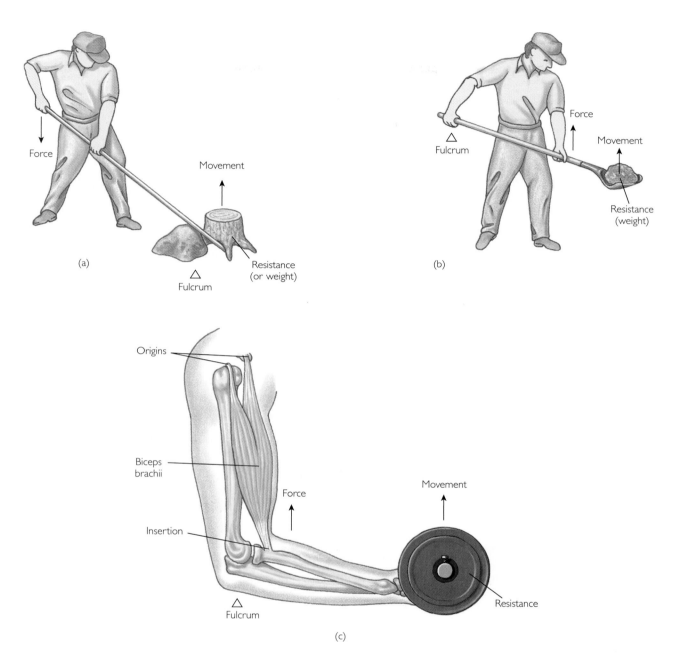

FIGURE 2-4

Levers and Muscle Action.

(a) First-class lever action results in an increase in force (or strength) on the resistance (the stump). **(b)** Third-class lever action results in increased speed and range of movement. **(c)** Third-class lever action at the elbow joint results in the upward movement (flexion) of the forearm and the barbell.

Skeletal muscles do not work in isolation. Generally, individual muscles or groups of muscles work in pairs; as one contracts, the other relaxes. Muscles can be grouped and described according to their primary actions. A muscle whose contraction is chiefly responsible for producing a particular movement is a **prime mover**. The *biceps brachii,* which produces flexion of the elbow, is an example of a prime mover. **Antagonists** are prime movers whose actions oppose that of the muscle under consideration. For example, the *triceps brachii* is a prime mover that extends the elbow and is an antagonist of the biceps brachii.

iso, same + tonos, tension

isotonic contraction: a muscle contraction where tension rises until movement begins, and then remains at that level throughout the contraction

Concept Questions

✔ A motor unit from a skeletal muscle contains 1500 muscle fibers. Would this muscle be involved in fine, delicate movements or powerful, gross movements? Explain.

✔ Is it possible for a muscle to contract without shortening? Explain.

✔ How would you distinguish between the origin and insertion of a particular muscle?

hyper, over + trophē, nourishment

hypertrophy: an enlargement of skeletal muscles in response to repeated stimulation

aero, air + bios, life

aerobic metabolism: chemical reactions that require oxygen for the generation of ATP; the oxygen is obtained from the air at the lungs and distributed by the cardiovascular system

Isotonic and Isometric Contractions

Muscle contractions may be classified as *isotonic* or *isometric* based on the pattern of tension produced in the muscle and its overall change in length. In an **isotonic** contraction, enough tension is generated to produce movement, and tension remains at that same level until the movement stops, and relaxation occurs. During isotonic contractions, the muscle shortens and the bone at the insertion is pulled toward the origin. Lifting an object off a desk, walking, running, and so forth involve isotonic contractions.

Contracting muscles do not always produce movement, however. Have you ever strained to lift something so heavy you were unable to move it, no matter how hard you tried? Although your muscles were contracting, no movement was produced. Contractions in which the muscle tension increases but the muscle length stays the same are called **isometric**, from the Greek for "same measure." Familiar examples of isometric contractions include pushing against a wall or trying to pick up a car. Although these are rather unusual movements, less obvious isometric contractions are actually quite common. For example, the muscle contractions that keep our bodies upright when standing or sitting involve the isometric contractions of muscles that oppose gravity.

Normal daily activities involve a combination of isotonic and isometric muscular contractions. As you sit reading this text, isometric contractions stabilize your vertebrae and maintain your upright position. When you next turn a page, the movements of your arm, forearm, hand, and fingers are produced by isotonic contractions.

MUSCLES AND EXERCISE

Muscle performance improves with exercise. Athletes use different training methods depending upon whether their sport is primarily supported by **aerobic** (oxygen-requiring) or **anaerobic** (without oxygen) energy production.

Aerobic sports involve sustained activities such as jogging and distance swimming. Aerobic exercises are designed to extend the length of time over which a muscle can continue to contract. Aerobic training exercises stimulate an increase in the number of mitochondria and the amount of *myoglobin,* an oxygen-binding pigment, within muscle fibers. The presence of additional mitochondria improves the ability of the muscle fibers to generate the ATP needed to support contractions. **Myoglobin** (MĪ-ō-glō-bin) binds oxygen molecules inside a muscle fiber, just as a related pigment, *hemoglobin*, binds oxygen in the blood. Myoglobin provides an oxygen reserve that can be used during a contraction.

Anaerobic sports include such activities as a 50-yard dash or swim, a pole vault, or a weight-lifting competition. The frequent, brief, and intensive training workouts used by athletes engaged in such sports stimulate an increase in the number of myofibrils and sarcomeres within their muscle fibers. The result is an enlargement, or **hypertrophy**, of the stimulated muscles. The effects are dramatic—for example, champion weight lifters and bodybuilders have hypertrophied muscles. We are born with almost all the muscle fibers we will ever have, and hypertrophy results from the enlargement of existing muscle fibers, rather than from the formation of new muscle fibers.

Muscle Fatigue

Skeletal muscle is considered *fatigued* when it can no longer contract, despite continued stimulation. Muscle fatigue may be caused either by a lack of ATP or by the buildup of *lactic acid*.

What causes a lack of ATP? Skeletal muscle fibers, like most cells in the body, generate ATP through oxygen-requiring chemical reactions in their mitochondria. Because these reactions use oxygen, this process of energy production is called **aerobic metabolism**. If a muscle's contractions require no more ATP than the amount generated by its mitochondria, and oxygen supplies remain adequate, the muscle fiber can function aerobically for long periods. Under these conditions, sufficient ATP is available, and fatigue occurs only after relatively long periods. For example, the muscles of long-distance athletes may become fatigued only after several hours of moderate exertion, when the muscle fibers run out of organic compounds suitable for mitochondria.

An athlete sprinting the 100-yard dash, however, may suffer from the muscle fatigue associated with lactic acid buildup. A muscle working at *peak* levels of exertion consumes ATP much faster than its mitochondria can produce it. The additional ATP is produced through **anaerobic** (non-oxygen–requiring) **metabolism**, in a process called *glycolysis* (glī-KOL-i-sis). In glycolysis, glucose molecules are split in half to form pyruvic acid molecules and a small amount of ATP. This reaction occurs in the cytoplasm, not in the mitochondria. Although glycolysis can supply straining muscles with ATP, problems develop as the excess pyruvic acid is converted to **lactic acid**. Lactic acid releases hydrogen ions that cause a dangerous decline in pH in and around the muscle fiber. After a relatively short time (seconds to minutes), the pH change inactivates key enzymes, and the muscle can no longer function normally.

a-, without + *aeros*, air + *bios*, life

anaerobic metabolism: chemical reactions that can generate ATP in the absence of oxygen

Muscle Recovery

After exertion, conditions inside the muscle gradually return to normal levels during the *recovery period*. During this period, lactic acid is removed and the muscle fibers rebuild their energy reserves (especially glycogen). In addition, the body as a whole must lose the heat generated during intense muscular contraction; that's why you continue to perspire after an exercise period ends.

During the recovery period, the body's oxygen demand goes up considerably. The extra oxygen is used by mitochondria (1) in liver cells, where ATP is required for the conversion of lactic acid to glucose, and (2) in muscle fibers, where ATP is needed to restore the cell's reserves of ATP and glycogen to pre-exertion levels. The additional oxygen required during the recovery period is often called the **oxygen debt**. While repaying an oxygen debt the body's breathing rate and depth of breathing must increase. This is why you continue to breathe heavily for some time after you stop exercising.

Muscle Atrophy

a-, without + *trophē*, nourishment

atrophy: the degeneration of unstimulated muscle fibers

A common fitness slogan is "use it or lose it." Skeletal muscles that are not "used," or stimulated, on a regular basis will become smaller and weaker. This process is called **atrophy.** Individuals whose muscles are paralyzed by spinal injuries first lose muscle tone and then undergo gradual muscle atrophy. Even a temporary reduction in muscle use can lead to muscular atrophy. This can easily be seen by comparing limb muscles before and after a cast has been worn. Muscle atrophy is reversible in its early stages, but once muscle fibers die, they are replaced by fibrous tissues, and the atrophy is permanent. That is why physical therapy is crucial to individuals temporarily unable to move normally.

▶ MAJOR MUSCLES OF THE BODY

Concept Questions

✔ Why would a sprinter experience muscle fatigue before a marathon runner would?

✔ Which activity would be more likely to create an oxygen debt, swimming laps or lifting weights?

The muscular system includes all the nearly 700 skeletal muscles that can be controlled voluntarily. Figure 2-5 shows some of the major superficial muscles of the human body.

In the last chapter we described the skeletal system by dividing it into axial and appendicular divisions. We will use the same divisions in our discussion of the muscular system.

- The **axial muscles** are associated with the axial skeleton only. They position the head and spinal column and also move the rib cage, assisting in the movements that make breathing possible. Roughly 60 percent of the skeletal muscles in the body are axial muscles.
- The **appendicular muscles** stabilize or move the bones of the appendicular skeleton.

Understanding the meaning of the muscle names will thus help you remember and identify them. The name of a muscle may refer to (1) its location (for example, the *temporalis* attaches to the temporal bone); (2) its action (for example, the *flexor digitorum* flexes the fingers); or (3) its shape (for example, the *deltoid* muscle has the shape of the Greek letter *delta* [Δ]). Examples are given in Table 2-1.

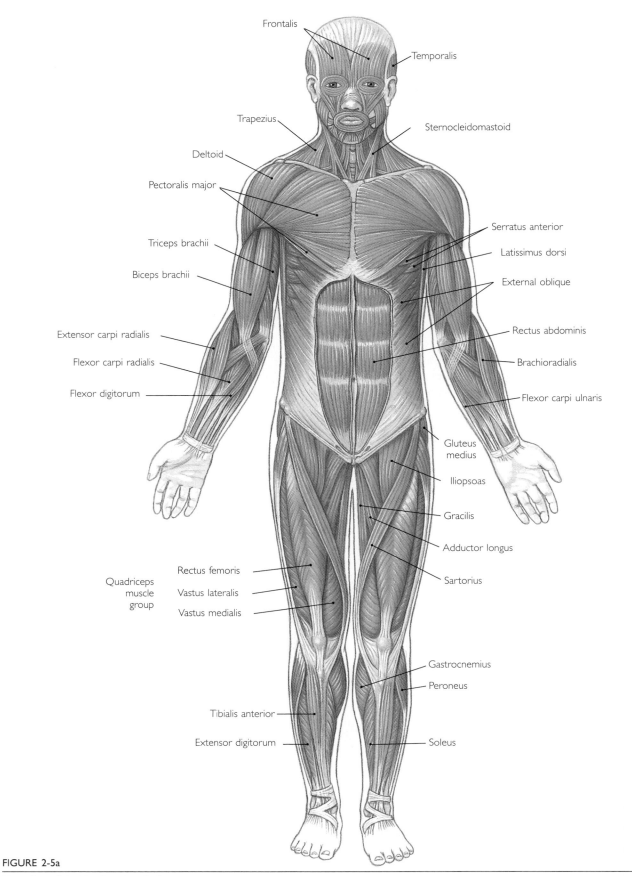

Frontalis

Temporalis

Trapezius

Sternocleidomastoid

Deltoid

Pectoralis major

Serratus anterior

Latissimus dorsi

Triceps brachii

External oblique

Biceps brachii

Rectus abdominis

Extensor carpi radialis

Brachioradialis

Flexor carpi radialis

Flexor digitorum

Flexor carpi ulnaris

Gluteus
medius

Iliopsoas

Gracilis

Adductor longus

Quadriceps
muscle
group

Rectus femoris

Vastus lateralis

Sartorius

Vastus medialis

Gastrocnemius

Peroneus

Tibialis anterior

Extensor digitorum

Soleus

FIGURE 2-5a

Major Superficial Muscles of the Body.
Anterior view.

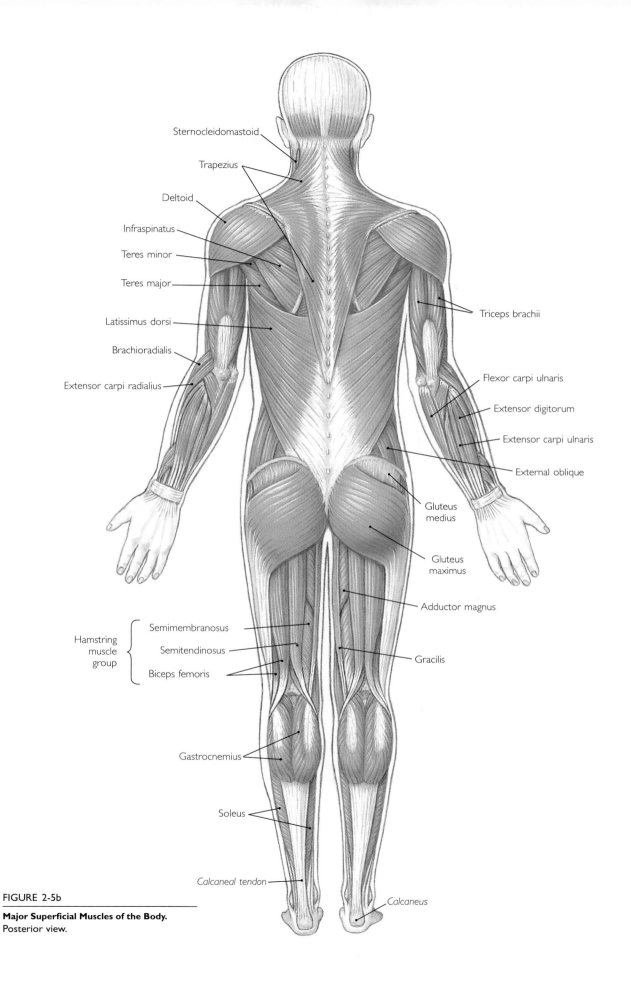

Sternocleidomastoid

Trapezius

Deltoid

Infraspinatus

Teres minor

Teres major

Latissimus dorsi

Brachioradialis

Extensor carpi radialius

Triceps brachii

Flexor carpi ulnaris

Extensor digitorum

Extensor carpi ulnaris

External oblique

Gluteus medius

Gluteus maximus

Adductor magnus

Hamstring muscle group {
Semimembranosus

Semitendinosus

Biceps femoris

Gracilis

Gastrocnemius

Soleus

Calcaneal tendon

Calcaneus

FIGURE 2-5b

Major Superficial Muscles of the Body.
Posterior view.

Table 2-1	Muscle Terminology		
Terms Indicating Direction Relative to Axes of the Body	**Terms Indicating Specific Regions of the Body**	**Terms Indicating Structural Characteristics of the Muscle**	**Terms Indicating Actions**
Anterior (front)	Abdominis (abdomen)	**Origin**	**General**
Externus (superficial)	Carpi (wrist)	Biceps (two heads)	Abductor
Inferioris (inferior)	Cleido/clavius (clavicle)	Triceps (three heads)	Adductor
Lateralis (lateral)	Costalis (ribs)	Quadriceps (four heads)	Depressor
Medialis/medius (medial, middle)	Femoris (femur)	**Shape**	Extensor
	Ilio- (ilium)	Deltoid (triangle)	Flexor
Obliquus (oblique)	Lumborum (lumbar region)	Orbicularis (circle)	Levator
Posterior (back)	Oculo- (eye)	Serratus (serrated)	Pronator
Rectus (straight, parallel)	Oris (mouth)	Teres (long and round)	Rotator
Superficialis (superficial)	Psoas (loin)	Trapezius (trapezoid)	Supinator
Superioris (superior)	Radialis (radius)	**Other Striking Features**	**Specific**
Transversus (transverse)	Temporalis (temples)	Gracilis (slender)	Buccinator (trumpeter)
	Thoracis (thoracic region)	Latissimus (widest)	Sartorius (like a tailor)
	Tibialis (tibia)	Longissimus (longest)	
	Ulnaris (ulna)	Longus (long)	
		Magnus (large)	
		Major (larger)	
		Maximus (largest)	
		Minor (smaller)	
		-tendinosus (tendinous)	
		Vastus (great)	

THE AXIAL MUSCLES

The major axial muscles can be placed into three groups. The first group, the *muscles of the head and neck*, includes muscles responsible for facial expressions, chewing, and swallowing. The second group, the *muscles of the spine*, includes flexors and extensors of the spinal column. The third group, the *muscles of the trunk*, form the muscular walls of the thoracic and abdominopelvic cavities, and the floor of the pelvic cavity. Table 2-2 summarizes the location and actions, or movements, of the major axial muscles.

Muscles of the Head and Neck

The muscles of the head and neck are shown in Figure 2-6 and listed in Table 2-2. The muscles of the face originate on the surface of the skull and insert into the dermis of the skin. When they contract, the skin moves, changing our facial expression. The largest group of facial muscles is associated with the mouth. The **orbicularis oris** (or-bik-ū-LA-ris ŌR-is) constricts the opening, and other muscles move the lips or the corners of the mouth. The **buccinator** (BUK-si-nā-tor), another

Table 2-2	Axial Muscles		
Region/Muscle		**Location**	**Action**
Muscles of the Head and Neck			
Frontalis		Forehead	Raises eyebrows, wrinkles forehead
Orbicularis oculi		Encircles eyelids	Closes eye
Buccinator		Lines the cheek	Pushes food into teeth, blowing, sucking
Orbicularis oris		Encircles lips	Purses lips; "kissing" muscle
Zygomaticus		Upper cheek	Raises corner of mouth; "smiling" muscle
Depressor anguli oris		Side of chin	Pulls corner of mouth down
Temporalis		Side of head above ear	Raises jaw
Masseter		Rear of cheek	Raises jaw
Sternocleidomastoid		Side of neck	Together, both flex the neck; alone, turns head to one side
Muscles of the Spine			
Erector spinae		Along back from head to sacrum	Extend spinal column
Quadratus lumborum		Hip to lower vertebrae and adjacent surface of ribs	Flexes spinal column
Muscles of the Trunk			
Intercostals		Between each rib and adjacent ribs	Externals raise ribs; internals lower ribs
Diaphragm		Separates thoracic and abdominal cavities	Expands and reduces size of lung cavities
Obliques (external and internal) and transversus abdominis		Make up three layers of the abdominal wall	Compress abdomen
Rectus abdominis		Anterior surface of abdominal wall, from ribs to pelvis	Flexes spinal column; the "sit-up" muscle
Muscles of the Pelvic Floor			
Urethral sphincter		Encircles urethra	Closes urethra; provides voluntary control of urination
Anal sphincter		Encircles anus	Closes anal opening; provides voluntary control of defecation
Levator ani		Forms much of the pelvic floor	Supports internal organs

Concept Questions

✔ If you were contracting and relaxing your masseter muscle, what would you probably be doing?

✔ Which muscle would best be described as the "kissing" muscle?

muscle associated with the mouth, compresses the cheeks, as when pursing the lips and blowing forcefully. During chewing, contraction and relaxation of the buccinator moves food back across the teeth from the space inside the cheeks. The chewing motions are primarily produced by contractions of the **masseter** (MAS-se-tur), with assistance from the **temporalis** (tem-pō-RA-lis).

Smaller groups of muscles control movements of the eyebrows and eyelids, the scalp, the nose, and the external ear. Other muscles of the neck control the position of the larynx, lower the mandible, tense the floor of the mouth, and provide a stable foundation for muscles of the tongue and pharynx. One of these, the **sternocleidomastoid** (ster-nō-klī-dō-MAS-toyd) extends from the clavicles and the sternum to the mastoid region of the skull. It can rotate the head or flex the neck.

Muscles of the Spine

The muscles of the spine are covered by more superficial back muscles, such as the trapezius and latissimus dorsi (see Figure 2-5b). Spinal extensor muscles include the **erector spinae** (the *sacrospinalis,*

FIGURE 2-6

Muscles of the Head and Neck.

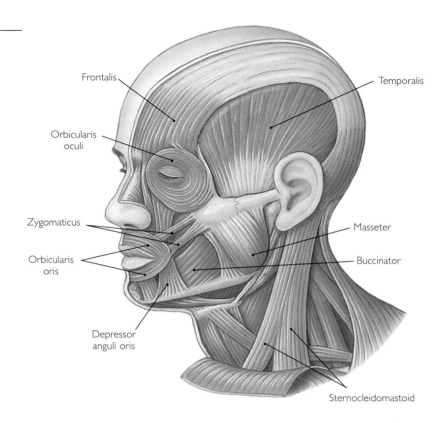

Frontalis

Temporalis

Orbicularis
oculi

Zygomaticus

Masseter

Orbicularis
oris

Buccinator

Depressor
anguli oris

Sternocleidomastoid

iliocostalis, *longissimus*, and *spinalis*), which keep the spine and head erect (Figure 2-7 and Table 2-2). When contracting together, these muscles extend the spinal column. When only the muscles on one side contract, the spine is bent laterally. The erector spinae are opposed by the *quadratus lumborum* and the various abdominal muscles that flex the spinal column.

Muscles of the Trunk

The muscles of the trunk include (1) the **external** and **internal intercostals** and **obliques**, (2) the **transversus abdominis,** (3) the **rectus abdominis,** (4) the muscular **diaphragm** that separates the thoracic and abdominopelvic cavities, and (5) the muscles that form the floor of the pelvic cavity.

The dome-shaped diaphragm is important in breathing. Because of its shape and its position inferior to the lungs, contraction of the diaphragm increases the size of the pleural cavities and expands the lungs. This action pulls air into the respiratory system. When it relaxes, the diaphragm moves upward, compressing the lungs and pushing air out of the respiratory system. The intercostal muscles, located between the ribs, are also involved in breathing. The external intercostals raise the rib cage and expand the lungs, and the internal intercostals lower the rib cage and compress the lungs.

The floor of the pelvic cavity is called the **perineum** (pe-ri-NĒ-um). It is formed by a broad sheet of muscles that extend from the sacrum and coccyx to the ischium and pubis. Prominent muscles in this region include the **levator ani**, which supports most of the organs within the pelvic cavity, and the **urethral** and **anal sphincter muscles**, which provide voluntary control of urination

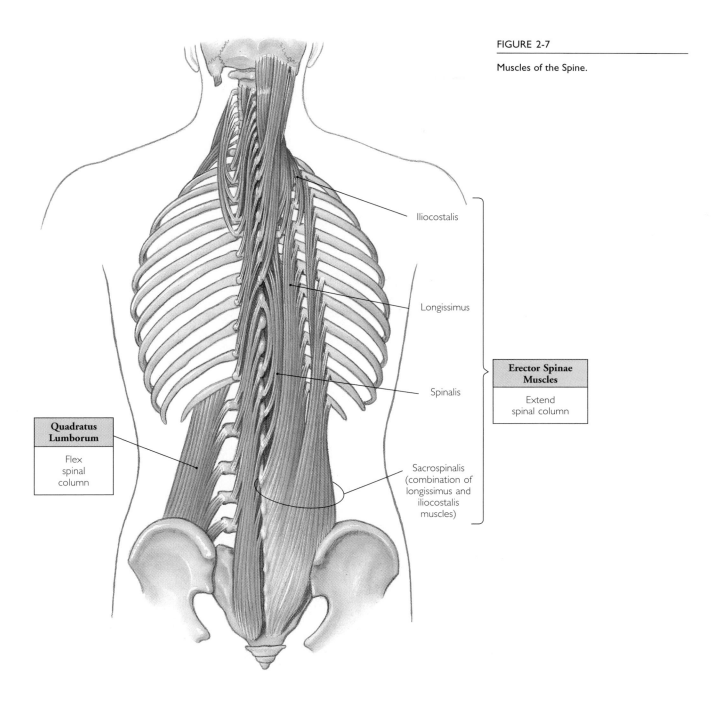

FIGURE 2-7

Muscles of the Spine.

Iliocostalis

Longissimus

Spinalis

Erector Spinae Muscles

Extend spinal column

Quadratus Lumborum

Flex spinal column

Sacrospinalis (combination of longissimus and iliocostalis muscles)

Concept Questions

✔ Which muscles of the spine and trunk would you use while doing sit-ups?

✔ The perineum forms the floor of what body cavity?

and defecation. Both superficial and deep muscles of the perineum are shown in Figure 2-8. Note that there are no differences between the deep muscles in males and females.

The oblique muscles are broad muscular sheets that form the walls of the abdomen (Figure 2-9 and Table 2-2). Contraction of the oblique muscles can compress organs in the abdominopelvic cavity or rotate the spinal column, depending on whether one side or both sides are contracting. The *rectus abdominis* is an important flexor of the spinal column.

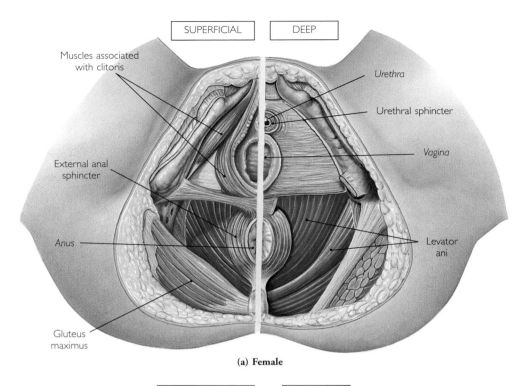

SUPERFICIAL   DEEP

Muscles associated
with clitoris

Urethra

Urethral sphincter

External anal
sphincter

Vagina

Anus

Levator
ani

Gluteus
maximus

(a) Female

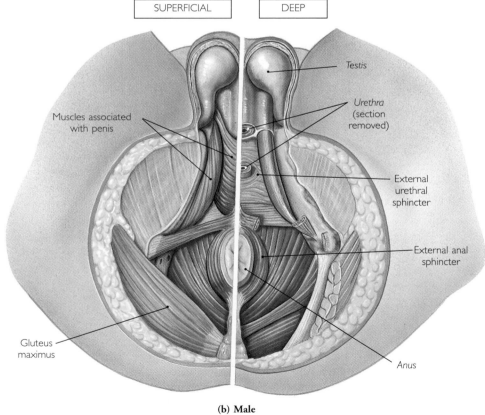

SUPERFICIAL   DEEP

Testis

Muscles associated
with penis

Urethra
(section
removed)

External
urethral
sphincter

External anal
sphincter

Gluteus
maximus

Anus

(b) Male

FIGURE 2-8

Muscles of the Male and Female Pelvic Floor.
There are no differences in the deep muscles between male and female.

FIGURE 2-9

Muscles of the Trunk.

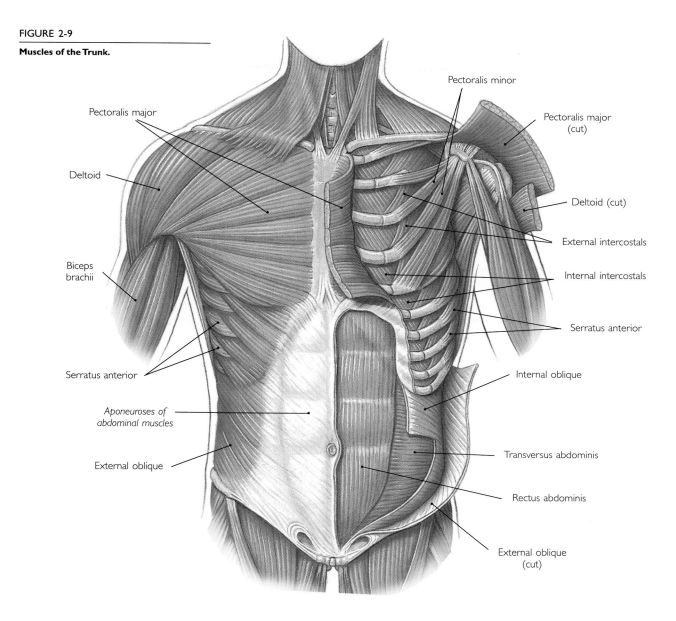

THE APPENDICULAR MUSCLES

The appendicular muscles include (1) the muscles of the shoulders and upper limbs and (2) the muscles of the pelvic girdle and lower limbs. There are few similarities between the two groups because the functions and required ranges of motion are very different.

Muscles of the Shoulder and Upper Limb

The large, superficial **trapezius** (tra-PĒ-zē-us) muscle covers the back and portions of the neck, reaching to the base of the skull (see Figures 2-5a and b). This muscle forms a broad diamond. Its actions are quite varied because specific regions can be made to contract independently.

On the chest, the **serratus** (ser-RA-tus) **anterior** originates along the anterior surfaces of several ribs and inserts along the vertebral border of the scapula. When the serratus anterior contracts, it pulls the shoulder forward.

The primary muscles of the arm are shown in Figure 2-5. They include (1) the superficial muscle of the shoulder, the **deltoid** (DEL-toyd) (Figure 2-5a), which is the major abductor of the arm;

(2) the **infraspinatus** (in-fra-spī-NĀ-tus), **teres** (TER-ēz) **major**, and **teres minor** (Figure 2-5b), which rotate the arm and are often called the muscles of the *rotator cuff*; and (3) the **pectoralis** (pek-tō-RA-lis) **major** (Figure 2-5a) and the **latissimus dorsi** (la-TIS-i-mus DOR-sē) (Figure 2-5b). The pectoralis major flexes the shoulder, and the latissimus dorsi extends it. These two muscles also work together to adduct and rotate the arm. All these muscles provide substantial support for the loosely built shoulder joint. The muscles of the rotator cuff are a frequent site of sports injuries. Powerful, repetitive arm movements, such as pitching a fastball at 95 mph for nine innings, can place intolerable stresses on the muscles of the rotator cuff, leading to muscle strains (a tear or break in the muscle), bursitis (inflammation of bursae), and other painful injuries.

Although most of the muscles that insert on the forearm and wrist originate on the humerus, there are two noteworthy exceptions. The **biceps brachii** and the **triceps brachii** insert on the forearm and originate on the scapula. Their primary actions are on the elbow. For example, the triceps brachii extends the elbow during push-ups, while the biceps brachii makes a prominent bulge as it both flexes the elbow and supinates the forearm.

Other important muscles of the upper limb include the following:

- The **brachioradialis** flexes the elbow, opposed by the triceps brachii.
- The **flexor carpi ulnaris** and the **flexor carpi radialis** work together to produce flexion of the wrist. Note that the flexor muscles are on the anterior and medial surfaces of the forearm.
- The **extensor carpi radialis** and the **extensor carpi ulnaris** produce extension of the wrist. Note that the extensor muscles are on the posterior and lateral surfaces of the forearm.
- The **flexor digitorum** and **extensor digitorum** muscles perform flexion and extension of the fingers.

The muscles of the forearm provide strength and crude control of the palm and fingers. Fine control of the hand involves small muscles that originate on the carpal and metacarpal bones. No muscles originate on the phalanges, and only tendons extend across the distal joints of the fingers.

Table 2-3 summarizes the major muscles of the shoulder and upper limb.

Muscles of the Hip and Lower Limb

The muscles of the lower limb can be divided into three groups: (1) muscles that move the thigh, (2) muscles that move the leg, and (3) muscles that affect the ankles and feet.

The following muscles that move the thigh may be located in Figure 2-5, pp. 46-47:

- **Gluteal muscles** cover the lateral surface of the ilia. The **gluteus maximus** is the largest and most posterior of the gluteal muscles, which extend the hip and rotate and abduct the thigh.
- The adductors of the thigh include the **adductor magnus**, the **adductor longus**, and the **gracilis** (GRAS-i-lis). When an athlete suffers a *pulled groin*, the problem is a strain in one of these adductor muscles.
- The largest flexor of the hip is the **iliopsoas** (il-ē-ō-SŌ-us) muscle. It inserts at the greater trochanter of the femur.

The general pattern of muscle distribution in the lower limb is that extensors are found along the anterior and lateral surfaces of the limb, and flexors lie along the posterior and medial surfaces.

- The flexors of the knee include three muscles collectively known as the *hamstrings* (the **biceps femoris**, the **semimembranosus** (sem-ē-mem-bra-NŌ-sus), and the **semitendinosus** (sem-ē-ten-di-NŌ-sus) and the **sartorius** (sar-TŌR-ē-us).
- Collectively the extensors of the knee are known as the **quadriceps femoris**. The three **vastus** muscles (only two are shown in Figure 2-5) and the **rectus femoris** insert on the patella, which is attached to the tibia by the *patellar ligament*.

Most of the muscles that move the ankle produce the plantar flexion involved with walking and running.

- The large **gastrocnemius** (gas-trok-NĒ-mē-us) of the calf is assisted by the underlying **soleus** (SŌ-lē-us) muscle. These muscles share a common tendon, the **calcaneal tendon**, or *Achilles tendon*.

Concept Questions

✔ What muscles are you using when you pull your shoulders forward?

✔ Baseball pitchers sometimes suffer from rotator cuff injuries. What muscles are involved in this type of injury?

✔ Injury to the flexor carpi ulnaris would impair what two movements?

Table 2-3	Muscles of the Shoulder and Upper Limb	
Region/Muscle	**Location**	**Action**
Shoulder		
Trapezius	Upper back, back of head and neck, to clavicle and scapula	Varied movements of scapula; elevates clavicle; extends head and neck
Serratus anterior	Between ribs and scapula	Pulls shoulder forward (protraction)
Muscles That Move the Arm		
Deltoid	Tip of shoulder to humerus	Raises (abducts) arm
Latissimus dorsi	Middle of back to humerus	Lowers (adducts) arm and extends shoulder
Pectoralis major	Upper chest to humerus	Flexes shoulder and adducts arm
Infraspinatus	Shoulder blade of scapula to humerus	Lateral rotation of humerus
Teres minor	Posterior, inferior edge of scapula to humerus	Lateral rotation of humerus
Teres major	Posterior, inferior edge of scapula to humerus	Medial rotation of humerus
Muscles That Move the Forearm		
Biceps brachii	Anterior surface of arm	Flexes the elbow
Brachioradialis	Extends from lower humerus and adjacent forearm to lateral tip of radius	Flexes the elbow
Triceps brachii	Posterior surface of arm	Extends elbow; opposes biceps brachii
Muscles That Move the Hand and Fingers		
Flexor carpi muscles	Anterior side of forearm	Flex wrist
Extensor carpi muscles	Posterior side of forearm	Extend wrist
Flexor and extensor digitorum muscles	Anterior and posterior sides of the forearm tendons extending to bones of the fingers	Flex and extend the fingers at the interphalangeal joints

Concept Questions

✔ You often hear of athletes suffering a "pulled hamstring." To what does this phrase refer?

✔ How would you expect a torn calcaneal tendon to affect movement of the foot?

- The **peroneus** (per-Ō-nē-us) muscle produces eversion as well as plantar flexion, as when you twist the sole of your foot outward or point your toes.
- The large **tibialis** (tib-ē-A-lis) **anterior** opposes the gastrocnemius and soleus, and dorsiflexes the foot, as when you "dig in your heels" and pull on a rope while playing tug-of-war.

Important muscles that move the toes originate on the surface of the tibia, the fibula, or both. Table 2-4 notes four muscles that move the toes, although only the relatively superficial **extensor digitorum** is shown in Figure 2-5a. The other digital muscles lie deep within the leg. Several smaller muscles involved with fine movement of the toes originate on the tarsal and metatarsal bones.

▶ AGING AND THE MUSCULAR SYSTEM

As the body ages, there is a general reduction in the size and power of all muscle tissues. The effects on the muscular system can be summarized as follows:

1. *Skeletal muscle fibers become smaller in diameter.* The overall effect is a reduction in muscle strength and endurance, and a tendency to fatigue more rapidly.

Table 2-4	Muscles of the Lower Limb	
Group/Muscle	**Location**	**Action**
Muscles That Move the Thigh		
Gluteus maximus	Large buttock muscle	Extends hip
Gluteus medius	Under the gluteus maximus between hip and upper femur	Abducts thigh
Adductors	Medial (inner) region of thigh	Adduct thigh and flex hip
Gracilis	Medial (inner) region of thigh	Adducts thigh and flexes knee
Iliopsoas	Anterior, superior thigh	Flexes hip
Muscles That Move the Leg		
Hamstring Muscles Biceps femoris Semimembranosus Semitendinosus	Posterior surface of thigh; extends from lower pelvis to tibia and fibula	Flexors of the knee
Sartorius	Crosses anterior thigh; extends from pelvis to tibia	Flexes hip and knee
Quadriceps Muscles Rectus femoris Vastus lateralis Vastus medialis	Anterior surface of thigh; extends from lower pelvis to tibia and fibula	Extensors of the knee
Muscles That Move the Foot		
Tibialis anterior	Anterior and lateral side of tibia; extends to foot	Dorsiflexion of foot ("digging in the heels")
Gastrocnemius	Posterior leg ("calf") between femur and heel	Flexes knee, plantar flexes foot ("on tiptoe")
Peroneus	Posterior leg; extends from fibula and tibia to foot	Plantar flexes and everts foot (turns sole outward)
Soleus	Posterior leg; extends from fibula and tibia to heel	Plantar flexes and inverts foot (turns sole inward)
Flexor and extensor digitorum muscles (several)	Anterior and posterior leg; extends to bones of toes	Flex and extend toes at interphalangeal joints

2. *Skeletal muscles become smaller and less elastic.* Aging skeletal muscles develop increasing amounts of fibrous connective tissue, a process called *fibrosis*. Fibrosis makes the muscle less flexible, and the collagen fibers can restrict movement and circulation.

3. *The tolerance for exercise decreases.* A lower tolerance for exercise results in part from the tendency for rapid fatigue and in part from a decreased ability to control body temperature, which leads to overheating.

4. *The ability to recover from muscular injuries decreases.* When an injury occurs, repair capabilities are limited, and scar tissue formation is the usual result.

The rate of decline in muscular performance is the same in all individuals, regardless of their exercise patterns or lifestyle. Therefore to be in good shape late in life, one must be in *very* good shape early in life. Regular exercise helps control body weight, strengthens bones, and generally improves the quality of life at all ages. Extremely demanding exercise is not as important as regular exercise. In fact, extreme exercise in the elderly may lead to problems with tendons, bones, and joints. Although it has obvious effects on the quality of life, there is no clear evidence that exercise prolongs life expectancy.

CHAPTER REVIEW SECTION

KEY WORDS

aerobic:	Requiring the presence of oxygen.
anaerobic:	Without oxygen.
aponeurosis:	A broad sheet of connective tissue that may serve as the origin or insertion of a skeletal muscle.
atrophy:	Wasting away of muscle tissue from lack of use.
fascicle:	A small bundle of muscle fibers
glycolysis (glī-KOL-i-sis):	An anaerobic process that breaks down glucose to form pyruvic acid and small amounts of ATP; occurs in the cytoplasm, not in the mitochondria.
insertion:	In a muscle, the point of attachment to the bone that is more movable.
isometric contraction:	A muscular contraction characterized by increasing tension but no change in length.
isotonic contraction:	A muscular contraction during which tension increases and then remains stable as the muscle shortens.
lactic acid:	Acid produced during anaerobic glycolysis; the amount of lactic acid can build up in muscle tissue and cause fatigue.
motor unit:	All the muscle fibers controlled by a single motor neuron.
myofibrils:	Collections of thin and thick filaments that lie within skeletal muscle fibers and cardiac muscle cells.
neuromuscular junction:	A functional connection between a motor neuron and a skeletal muscle fiber.
origin:	In a muscle, the point of attachment to the bone that is less movable.
prime mover:	In a muscle group, the muscle primarily responsible for performing a specific action.
sarcomere:	The smallest contractile unit of a skeletal muscle cell; lie end to end within myofibrils.
sphincter:	Muscular ring that contracts to close the entrance or exit of an internal passageway.

STUDY OUTLINE

INTRODUCTION

1. There are three types of muscle tissue: skeletal muscle, cardiac muscle, and smooth muscle. All muscle tissues share the properties of **excitability**, **contractility**, and **elasticity**. The muscular system includes all the skeletal muscle tissue that can be controlled voluntarily.

SYSTEM BRIEF

1. **Skeletal muscles** attach to bones directly or indirectly and perform these functions: (1) produce skeletal movement, (2) maintain posture and body position, and (3) maintain body temperature.

THE STRUCTURE OF SKELETAL MUSCLE

1. Layers of connective tissue surround and interconnect each muscle fiber, each bundle of muscle fibers, and the entire muscle. **Tendons** at the ends of muscles attach them to bones.

STRUCTURE OF A MUSCLE FIBER

2. A muscle cell contains numerous **myofibrils** that run the length of the cell. The myofibrils contain **thin filaments** (*actin*) and **thick filaments** (*myosin*) that aid in contraction.
3. The filaments in each myofibril are organized into short, repeating units called **sarcomeres.**

THE NERVE CELL–MUSCLE CELL LINK

4. Muscles contract in response to signals from the nervous system.
5. Each skeletal muscle fiber is controlled by a neuron at a **neuromuscular junction**.
6. **Neurotransmitter** molecules released at the neuromuscular junction cause an electrical impulse to develop in the muscle fiber that leads to the release of calcium ions.

HOW A MUSCLE FIBER CONTRACTS

1. Sarcomeres are the functional, contracting units of muscle fibers.

SARCOMERE STRUCTURE

2. The relationship between the thick and thin filaments changes as the muscle contracts and shortens. The ends of the sarcomeres move closer together as the thin filaments slide past the thick filaments.

SARCOMERE FUNCTION

3. The contraction process involves temporary binding between myosin on the thick filament and actin on the thin filaments. The presence of calcium ions permits the myosin **cross-bridges** to attach to the thin filaments.
4. Muscle contraction requires calcium ions and large amounts of ATP.

THE WORK OF MUSCLE

1. During normal muscular activity, the number of activated muscle fibers determines the tension developed by an entire skeletal muscle.

Section Two

CLINICAL LABORATORY
PROCEDURES

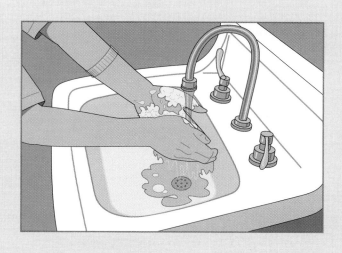

Medical Assistant Role Delineation Chart

Highlight indicates material covered in this chapter

ADMINISTRATIVE

ADMINISTRATIVE PROCEDURES

- Perform basic clerical functions
- Schedule, coordinate, and monitor appointments
- Schedule inpatient/ outpatient admissions and procedures
- Understand and apply third party guidelines
- Obtain reimbursement through accurate claims submission
- Monitor third-party reimbursement
- Perform medical transcription
- Understand and adhere to managed care policies and procedures
- *Negotiate managed care contracts (adv)*

PRACTICE FINANCES

- Perform procedural and diagnostic coding
- Apply bookkeeping principles
- Document and maintain accounting and banking records
- Manage accounts receivable
- Manage accounts payable
- Process payroll
- *Develop and maintain fee schedules (adv)*
- *Manage renewals of business and professional insurance policies (adv)*
- *Manage personal benefits and maintain records (adv)*

CLINICAL

FUNDAMENTAL PRINCIPLES

- Apply principles of aseptic technique and infection control
- Comply with quality assurance practices
- Screen and follow up patient test results

DIAGNOSTIC ORDERS

- Collect and process specimens
- Perform diagnostic tests

PATIENT CARE

- Adhere to established triage procedures
- Obtain patient history and vital signs
- Prepare and maintain examination and treatment areas

- Prepare patient for examinations, procedures, and treatments
- Assist with examinations, procedures, and treatments
- Prepare and administer medications and immunizations
- Maintain medication and immunization records
- Recognize and respond to emergencies
- Coordinate patient care information with other health care providers

GENERAL (TRANSDISCIPLINARY)

PROFESSIONALISM

- Project a professional manner and image
- Adhere to ethical principles
- Demonstrate initiative and responsibility
- Work as a team member
- Manage time efficiently
- Prioritize and perform multiple tasks
- Adapt to change
- Promote the CMA credential
- Enhance skills through continuing education

COMMUNICATION SKILLS

- Treat all patients with compassion and empathy
- Recognize and respect cultural diversity
- Adapt communications to individual's ability to understand
- Use professional telephone technique
- Use effective and correct verbal and written communications
- Recognize and respond to verbal and non-verbal communications
- Use medical terminology appropriately
- Receive, organize, prioritize, and transmit information
- Serve as liaison
  Promote the practice through positive public relations

LEGAL CONCEPTS

- Maintain confidentiality
- Practice within the scope of education, training, and personal capabilities
- Prepare and maintain medical records
- Document accurately
- Use appropriate guidelines when releasing information
- Follow employer's established policies dealing with the health care contract
- Follow federal, state, and local legal guidelines
- Maintain awareness of federal and state health care legislation and regulations
- Maintain and dispose of regulated substances in compliance with government guidelines
- Comply with established risk management and safety procedures
- Recognize professional credentialing criteria
- Participate in the development and maintenance of personnel, policy, and procedure manuals
- *Develop and maintain personnel, policy, and procedure manuals (adv)*

INSTRUCTION

- Instruct individuals according to their needs
- Explain office policies and procedures
- Teach methods of health promotion and disease prevention
- Locate community resources and disseminate information
- *Orient and train personnel (adv)*
- *Develop educational materials (adv)*
- *Conduct continuing education activities (adv)*

OPERATIONAL FUNCTIONS

- Maintain supply inventory
- Evaluate and recommend equipment and supplies
- Apply computer techniques to support office operations
- *Supervise personnel (adv)*
- *Interview and recommend job applicants (adv)*
- *Negotiate leases and prices for equipment and supply contracts (adv)*

SOURCE: Reprinted by permission of the American Association of Medical Assistants from the AAMA Role Delineation Study: Occupational Analysis of the Medical Assisting Profession.

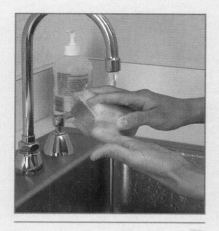

INFECTION CONTROL: ASEPSIS

3

OBJECTIVES

After completing this chapter, you should:

- Define and spell the glossary terms for this chapter.
- Describe the conditions required for the infection process to occur.
- Discuss the body's defenses against infection.
- Explain the immune system.
- Discuss the steps to follow in the infection control systems listed below.
  a. Standard Precautions
  b. OSHA
- Define medical asepsis.
- Explain the correct procedure for handwashing.
- Define surgical asepsis.
- Explain the difference between sanitization, disinfection, and sterilization.
- Discuss the five types of hepatitis and their level of contagion.
- Describe the means of transmission for HIV.

CLINICAL PERFORMANCE COMPETENCIES

After completing this chapter, you should perform the following tasks:

- Demonstrate the proper handwashing technique for medical asepsis.
- Demonstrate the procedure for wrapping materials for the autoclave.
- Demonstrate the correct procedure for disposing of sharps.
- Disinfect, sanitize, and sterilize materials.
- Demonstrate procedure for applying nonsterile gloves.
- Demonstrate procedure for applying and removing isolation gown.

Glossary

aerobic   Microorganism which is able to live only in the presence of oxygen.

anaerobic   Microorganism which thrives best or lives without oxygen.

aseptic   Germ free.

bactericidal   Ability to destroy disease-causing bacteria.

bloodborne pathogens   Disease producing organisms transmitted by means of blood and body fluids containing blood.

carrier(s)   Individual who is unaware he or she has a disease but is capable of transmitting it to someone else (for example "Typhoid Mary" who, legend has it, spread the disease typhoid).

incubation   Period of time during which a disease develops after the person is exposed.

immunity   Resistance to disease.

medical asepsis   Killing organisms after they leave the body.

nosocomial infection   Infection that is acquired after a person has entered the hospital. It is caused by the spread of an infection from one patient or person to another.

opportunistic infections   Infections, such as pneumonia, that occur in a body with a reduced immune system (for example, as seen in AIDS).

pathogens   Disease producing microorganisms.

permeable   Material that allows something to penetrate or pass through.

phagocytosis   Process of engulfing, digesting, and destroying pathogens.

reservoir   Source of the infectious pathogen.

sterile   All microorganisms and spores are killed.

surgical asepsis   A technique practiced to maintain a sterile environment.

syndrome   A set of symptoms or disorders which occur together and indicate the presence of a disease.

WARNING!

**For all patient contact, adhere to Standard Precautions.
Wear protective equipment as indicated.**

Pathogenic, or disease producing organisms, are everywhere. The healthy individual has some resistance to pathogens. However pathogens are especially important to control in the medical office setting since patients who may be already suffering from a disease are more susceptible to infection. The medical assistant must be aware of how easily pathogens can be spread from one person to another or from an inanimate object to a person since lack of knowledge can cause infections to occur.

▶ HISTORY OF ASEPSIS

Methods for controlling the spread of infection were used before early man understood the infection process. Religions, such as the Jewish faith, emphasize the careful preparation and cleanliness associated with foods. About 500 years ago, microorganisms known as germs were suspected to be the cause of some diseases. But, it was not until 100 years ago that Semmelweiss, Lister, and Pasteur (discussed in Chapter 2) contributed discoveries to our understanding of germ theory.

Louis Pasteur discovered that many diseases are caused by bacteria and that bacteria can be killed by excess heat. The heat method for killing germs in milk is called pasteurization in his honor. Joseph Lister discovered that germs could be killed using carbolic acid. He was the first to insist on cleaning surgical wounds by spraying the surrounding tissue with carbolic acid. This introduced the principles of **aseptic,** or germ free, technique in surgery. Lister introduced the concept of clean techniques in hospitals which greatly reduced the death rate from amputations from 45 to 15 percent. Semmelweiss taught his medical students to wash their hands before delivering babies. This simple precaution had an immediate effect on reducing the death rate from puerperal sepsis (childbed fever) in new mothers.

Today, we have a better understanding of germs and bacteria thanks to high powered microscopes. Sophisticated equipment can disinfect and sterilize equipment and materials. However, sterilization is meaningless if good aseptic technique is not practiced. With the advent of communicable diseases such as hepatitis, acquired immune deficiency syndrome (AIDS), and tuberculosis (TB) the need for adherence to aseptic technique has become critical.

MICROORGANISMS

Microorganisms are small, living organisms capable of causing disease, which can only be seen with the aid of a microscope. Microorganisms are normally found on the skin, in the urinary and gastrointestinal tract, and in the respiratory tract.

Microorganisms, also called microbes, are bacteria, fungi, protozoa, and viruses. The sizes of microorganisms can be expressed in micrometers. A micrometer is one millionth part of a meter or one thousandth of a millimeter. These microorganisms are listed with descriptions and examples of each in Table 3-1.

See Figure 3-1 for an illustration of pathogens (cocci, bacilli, virus). The study of each of these microorganisms represents a separate science:

- Bacteriology—the study of bacteria.
- Mycology—the study of fungi.
- Protozoonology—the study of protozoa.
- Virology—the study of viruses.

TABLE 3-1   Microorganisms

Microorganism	Description	Example
Bacteria	Most numerous of all microorganisms	(See cocci, bacilli, and spirilla below.)
	Unicellular	
	Many are pathogenic to humans	
	Identified by shape and appearance	
• **Cocci**	3 types of spherical bacteria	
1. Staphlococci	Form grape-like clusters of pus producing organisms	Boils, pimples, acne, osteomyelitis
2. Streptococci	Form chains of cells	Rheumatic heart disease, scarlet fever, strep throat
3. Diplococci	Form pairs of cells	Pneumonia, gonorrhea, and meningitis
• **Bacilli**	Rod shaped bacteria	Gram positive bacilli: tuberculosis, tetanus, diphtheria, gas gangrene
		Gram negative bacilli: *Escherichia coli* (urinary tract infection), *Bordetella pertussis* (whooping cough)
• **Spirilla**	Spiral shaped organisms	Syphilis and cholera
		(Continued on next page)

TABLE 3-1   *(Continued)*

Microorganism	Description	Example
Fungi	Parasitic and some non-parasitic plants and molds Depend on other life forms for their nutrition, such as dead or decaying organic material Reproduction method is budding Yeast is a typical fungus Fungus means "mushroom" in Latin Feed on antibiotics and flourish on antibiotic therapy	*Histoplasma capsulatum* (histoplasmosis), tinea pedis (athlete's foot), candidiasis (yeast infection), and ringworm
Protozoa	One-celled organisms Both parasite and non-parasite Can move with cilia or false-feet Typically 2 to 200 mm in size	Amebic dysentery, malaria, and trichomonas vaginitis
Rickettsia	Visible under a standard microscope Susceptible to antibiotics Transmitted by insects (ticks, fleas)	Rocky Mountain Spotted Fever
Virus	Smallest of microorganisms Can only be seen with electron microscope Can only multiply within a living cell (host) Difficult to kill with chemotherapy since they become resistant to the drug Can be destroyed by heat (autoclave sterilization) but generally not by chemical disinfection More viruses than any other category of microbial agents Feed on antibiotics and flourish on antibiotic therapy	Herpes virus, HIV, ARC, AIDS, common cold, influenza virus, smallpox, hepatitis A, hepatitis B, rabies, mumps, shingles

How Microorganisms Grow

Microorganisms occur everywhere in nature and have several requirements to grow: food, moisture, darkness, and a suitable temperature. In addition, some bacteria require oxygen (**aerobic**) or the absence of oxygen (**anaerobic**) to live. Table 3-2 presents the four conditions necessary for the growth of bacteria.

Some microorganisms, such as certain types of fungi and bacteria, are necessary for normal body function. For example, normal flora within the digestive system breaks down food and converts

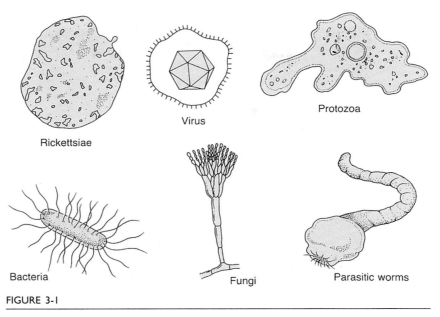

FIGURE 3-1

Pathogens.

TABLE 3-2   Conditions Required for Bacterial Growth

Condition	Explanation
Moisture	Bacteria grow best in moist areas: skin, mucous membranes, wet dressings, wounds, dirty instruments.
Temperature	Thrive at body temperature (98.6°F).
	Low temperatures (32°F and below) retard, but do not kill, bacterial growth.
	Temperatures of 107°F and above will kill most bacteria.
Oxygen	Aerobic bacteria require oxygen supply to live.
	Anaerobic bacteria can survive without oxygen.
Light	Darkness favors the growth of bacteria.
	Bacteria will die if exposed to direct sunlight or light.

unused food into waste products. In some cases the normal flora will invade areas of the body where they do not belong, and thus, convert to **pathogens**, which are disease producing microorganisms. For example, *Escherichia coli* (E. coli) is a normal bacteria within the colon where it aids in food digestion. When E. coli moves into the bladder or bloodstream, through improper hygiene habits, such as improper handwashing, it can cause urinary and blood infections.

Those microorganisms which are capable of producing disease (pathogens) grow best at body temperature (98.6°F) destroy and use human tissue as food, and give off waste toxins that are absorbed and poison the body. Table 3-3 lists several disease-causing pathogens as they relate to areas within the human body.

TABLE 3-3   Disease-Producing Microorganisms

Body Location	Disease
Respiratory system (Nose and throat)	Strep throat (streptococcus)
	Diphtheria
	Scarlet fever
	Influenza (*Haemophilius influenzae* Type b)
	Upper Respiratory Tract Infection (URI)
Cerebrospinal system	Meningitis
Lungs	Pneumonia
	Tuberculosis
Heart and blood	Endocarditis
	Rheumatic fever
Liver	Hepatitis B (Serum hepatitis)
Immune system	AIDS
Intestines	Dysentery
	Typhoid
	Pinworms
	Hepatitis A (Acute infective hepatitis)
Organs of reproduction	Gonorrhea
	Syphilis
Skin	Boils (staphylococcus)
	Impetigo
	Scabies
	Head lice
Tissues	Gas gangrene
	Rheumatic fever (heart tissue)
	Tetanus

▶ TRANSMISSION

Scientists have determined that certain germs can multiply every twelve minutes. If not controlled, germs may spread infection and diseases rapidly from one person to another. The principles of asepsis are applied in the hospital setting to prevent the spread of **nosocomial** (hospital-acquired) **infection**. The same emphasis on halting the spread of infection takes place in the medical office setting.

The presence of a pathogenic organism, or microorganism, is not enough to cause an infection to occur. Several factors must be in place for infection to occur. These are

1. The pathogen needs to be present.
2. A reservoir, or source, of disease including individuals who are ill with a disease and human carriers of disease who are unaware they have the disease but can still spread it.
3. A portal of exit, or means of escape, from the reservoir, for example through respiratory tract secretions, intestinal waste products, reproductive tract secretions, blood and blood products, and across the placenta barrier.
4. A means of transmission for the pathogen to pass directly from the reservoir to the new host. That is transmission of the pathogen directly from one person to another or indirect transmission as in the case when an inanimate object, such as milk or water, harbors the pathogen until it is transmitted to a human.
5. A portal of entry, or means of entry, such as the respiratory tract, skin and mucus membranes, reproductive and urinary tracts, blood, and across the placenta, for the pathogen into the new host.
6. A susceptible host which cannot fight off the pathogen.

Microorganisms normally found on the skin may enter the body through a portal of entry and then become pathogens. A portal of entry occurs where the body's defense, such as the skin, has broken down and allows direct access into the body. This can occur when the skin is cut as in a surgical incision, an injury causing a skin break, or in any invasive procedure such as the insertion of a needle in venipuncture. Figure 3-2 illustrates a chain of infection. The stages of the infection process are described in Table 3-4.

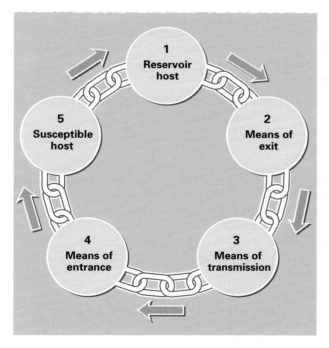

FIGURE 3-2

Chain of infection.

TABLE 3-4   Stages of the Infection Process

Stage	Description
Invasion	Pathogen enters the body through the portal of entry: respiratory, digestive, reproductive, urinary tracts, and skin.
Multiplication	Reproduction of pathogens.
Incubation period	May vary from several days to months or years during which time the disease is developing but no symptoms appear.
Prodromal period	First mild signs and symptoms appear. A highly contagious period.
Acute period	Signs and symptoms are evident and most severe.
Recovery period	Signs and symptoms begin to subside.

▶ THE INFECTION CONTROL SYSTEM

The body has several natural defense mechanisms to prevent the spread of infection. These include:

- Dietary intake of sufficient nutrients to promote health
- Age of the person—the young and aged are more susceptible to diseases of the immune system due to immaturity of the immune system in the young and decrease in effectiveness of the system in the aged
- Adequate amount of rest
     Mechanisms which promote the spread of infection include:
- Presence of other disease processes in the body—diseases such as diabetes and pneumonia can weaken the system
- Genetic inheritance such as diabetes, anemia, cystic fibrosis

The spread of microorganisms can be prevented in two ways: by preventing their spread and by destroying the microorganisms themselves.

PREVENTION

The human body has several natural barriers to infection. These include the skin, mucous membranes, gastrointestinal tract, lymphoid and blood system. The largest natural barrier to infection is the intact skin. The acid pH of the skin inhibits bacterial action. Mucous membranes lining the body's orifices, respiratory, digestive, reproductive, and urinary tracts also assist in repelling microorganisms. The gastrointestinal tract, containing hydrochloric acid (HCl), causes a **bactericidal** action which destroys disease-producing bacteria.

Lymphoid and Blood System

The lymphoid and blood systems produce antibodies that protect the body from disease. Leukocytes (white blood cells) actively fight pathogenic microorganisms with the process of **phagocytosis.** The process of phagocytosis is shown in Figure 3-3. During the process of inflammation, phagocytes engulf, digest, and destroy pathogens. Lymphocytes produce antibodies during the antigen-antibody reaction.

The Antigen-Antibody Reaction

Antibodies, which are protein substances produced by lymphocytes in the spleen, lymph nodes and tissue, and the bone marrow, react in response to antigens (foreign substances). Antibodies have the

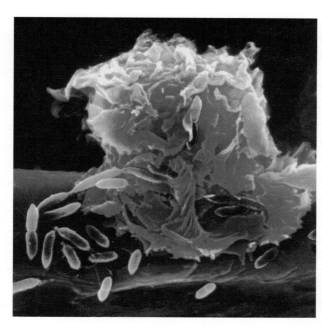

FIGURE 3-3

Phagocytosis.

ability to neutralize antigens or make them more susceptible to phagocytosis. The antibody-antigen reaction occurs in reaction to an invasion of antigens. **Immunity**, a resistance to disease, is said to have occurred when enough antibodies have been produced to provide protection for weeks, months, or years. The body has a natural protective mechanism called immunity.

Immunity can either be genetic or acquired. Genetic immunity does not involve antibodies. Species immunity protects humans from certain animal diseases such as chicken cholera. It also protects animals from certain human diseases such as measles and influenza.

Acquired immunity, on the other hand, does involve the development of antibodies. This type of immunity may be either natural or artificial and may be acquired either through an active or passive means. Active immunity occurs when antigens are produced by the body. There are two types of active immunity: natural (person is born with this immunity) and acquired (from an immunization or having had the disease such as with measles). Passive immunity develops when antibodies are artificially introduced into the body.

Active and passive immunity can be produced by both natural and acquired methods. Natural acquired immunity results from having recovered from a disease, such as measles, or being exposed to disease and becoming a carrier, such as in tuberculosis.

Artificial active immunity is the result of receiving vaccinations with inactivated (dead) or attenuated (weakened) organisms. For example, inactivated vaccines include influenza, whooping cough, typhoid, and the polio vaccine (Salk). Examples of attenuated vaccines are measles, polio (Sabin), smallpox, German measles (rubella), and mumps. Artificial passive immunity is produced by injecting a commercially prepared product to produce antibodies. Gamma globulin, used to prevent viral hepatitis, is an example. Acquired immunity is described in Table 3-5.

The Inflammatory Process

The body may react to the invasion of a foreign substance, such as bacteria or a virus, with an acute inflammatory process. This inflammatory process is the result of a tissue invasion of microorganisms from an injury, infection, or an allergy (antigen-antibody reaction).

The inflammatory process produces dilation of blood vessels due to an increased blood flow, production of watery fluids and materials (exudate), and the invasion of monocytes (white blood

TABLE 3-5   Acquired Immunity

Type of Immunity	Description
Active acquired natural	By having the disease which results in production of antibodies and "memory cells" which respond when the antigen reappears again.
Active acquired artificial	Administration of a vaccine which stimulates production of antibodies and "memory cells" to prevent that disease from occurring.
Passive acquired natural	Acquired from someone else's antibodies such as from the mother to the fetus through the placenta or through breast milk.
Passive acquired artificial	Temporary protection from gamma globulin (examples tetanus immune globulin, rabies antiserum).

cells) and neutrophils into the injured tissues to produce phagocytosis. After phagocytosis occurs, the process of repair begins. The signs and symptoms of the inflammatory process are both local and systemic or traveling throughout the body system. See Table 3-6 for a description of this process.

TABLE 3-6   Acute Inflammatory Process

Local	Systemic
Redness	Leukocytosis
Heat	Fever
Swelling/edema	Increased pulse rate
Pain	Increased respiration rate
Stiffness	

▶ STANDARD PRECAUTIONS

The Centers for Disease Control and Prevention (CDC) in 1994 issued new isolation guidelines that emphasize two tiers of approach to infection control. The first and most important tier, or level, contains precautions designed to care for all patients in a health care setting regardless of their diagnosis or risk of infection. This tier contains precautions designed to decrease the risk of transmission of disease through body fluids. It is referred to as "Standard Precautions" and is used regardless of the patient's diagnosis or whether or not the patient has a known infectious disease. It uses the major features of universal precautions and body substance isolation, which alerts those in the health care field to handle all materials as if they are contaminated.

Standard Precautions apply to 1) blood, 2) all body fluids (except sweat) regardless of whether they contain blood, 3) non-intact skin, and 4) mucus membranes. Body fluids include:

- Blood
- Body fluids containing visible blood
- Tissue specimens
- Semen
- Vaginal secretions
- Amniotic fluid
- Cerebrospinal fluid
- Pleural fluid
- Pericardial fluid
- Peritoneal fluid
- Interstitial fluid

Also included are feces, nasal secretions, sputum, tears, urine, vomitus, saliva, and breast milk which contain visible blood.

Standard Precautions promote handwashing and the use of gloves, masks, eye protection, or gowns when appropriate for patient contact. Masks, protective eyewear, gowns and gloves are referred to as a barrier type of protection. Standard Precautions are discussed in Table 3-7.

TABLE 3-7   Standard Precautions—Equipment and Situations

Precaution	Description
Gloves	Must be worn when in contact with blood, all body fluids, secretions, excretions (except sweat) regardless of whether or not they contain visible blood, mucous membranes, nonintact skin, or contaminated articles.
Gown	Must be worn during procedures (or situations) in which there may be exposure to blood, body fluids, mucous membranes, or draining wounds. Wash hands after removing gown.
Mask/Protective Eyewear (goggles/shield)	Must be worn during procedures that are likely to generate droplets of blood or body fluids (splashes or sprays) as when a patient is coughing excessively.
Handwashing	Hands must be washed both before and after gloves are removed. Hands must be washed immediately if contaminated with blood or body fluids, between patient contact, and when indicated to prevent transfer of microorganisms between other patients and the environment.
Transportation	Precautions must be taken when transporting a patient to minimize the risk of transmitting microorganisms to other patients or environmental surfaces or equipment.
Multiple-use	Common multiple-use equipment, such as blood pressure cuffs or stethoscopes, must be cleaned and disinfected after use or when it becomes soiled with bodily fluids or blood. Single use items are discarded.
Needles and sharp instruments	Must be discarded into a puncture-proof container. Needles should not be recapped.

The second tier of the CDC guidelines is focused on the patients who are either suspected of carrying an infectious disease or are already infected. This second tier, which requires extra precautions in addition to the "Standard Precautions," is known as "Transmission-based Precautions." It includes three types of categories: Airborne Precautions, Droplet Precautions, and Contact Precautions.

- *Airborne Precautions* are designed to reduce the transmission of certain diseases, such as tuberculosis (TB), measles, or chickenpox. In addition to practicing Standard Precautions, use Airborne Precautions for patients who are known to be infected with microorganisms which are transmitted via airborne droplet nuclei (smaller than 5 microns) that can remain suspended in the air and widely dispersed throughout a room by air currents. Airborne precautions include isolation of the patient in a private room if hospitalized, with a mask and protective gown used by the health care worker. Hands must be washed before gloving and after gloves are removed. The transport of the patient should be as limited as possible with the patient wearing a mask during transport. All re-usable patient care equipment should be cleaned and disinfected before use on another patient.

- *Droplet Precautions* are used for patients known or suspected to be infected with microorganisms transmitted by droplets generated by a patient during coughing, sneezing, talking or performance of procedures that induce coughing. Examples of these illnesses include: invasive *Haemophilus influenzae* Type b disease (meningitis, pneumonia), invasive Neisseria meningitis disease (meningitis, pneumonia, and sepsis), diptheria, pertussis, streptococcal pneumonia, scarlet fever, mumps, and rubella. Precautions include isolation of the patient in a private room if hospitalized. Hands must be washed before and after gloves are worn. Gloves and gowns must be worn if coming into contact with bodily fluids or blood of the patient. A mask should be worn if the medical assistant is within three feet of the patient and transport of the patient should be limited. All re-usable equipment should be cleaned and disinfected.

- *Contact Precautions* are used for patients known to be infected with a microorganism that is not easily treated with antibiotics and which can be transmitted easily between the patient

TABLE 3-8   Summary of Standard Precautions

1. Wear protective barrier equipment (for example, face mask, eye shield, or goggles), when there is any risk of splashing, splattering or aerosolization (becoming airborne in small particles) of potentially infectious body fluids.

2. Wear gloves when there is any potential for exposure to blood or body fluids, secretions, excretions, and contaminated items. This includes performing routine clinical work, touching mucous membranes and the nonintact skin of patients, handling tissue and clinical specimens (Figure 3-4).

3. Wear gloves when drawing blood, including finger and heel sticks on infants, and during preparation of blood smears.

4. Change gloves after each patient. Wash hands before putting on gloves and after removing them.

5. Change gloves if they become contaminated with blood or other body fluids and dispose of properly in bio-hazardous container.

6. Wash hands or other skin surfaces if they become contaminated with potentially infectious blood or body fluids.

7. Care for linens and equipment that are contaminated with blood, blood products, body fluids, excretions, and secretions in a manner that avoids contact with your skin and mucous membranes or cross-contamination to another person.

8. Wear a gown or other protective clothing when there is a risk of splashing, splattering or other means of exposure to the patient's body fluids.

9. Wear a mask if a patient has an air-borne disease. A special mask is recommended if a patient has an active case of tuberculosis (TB).

10. Use care with needles, scalpels and other sharp instruments to avoid unintentional injury.

11. Dispose of needles and other sharp items in a rigid, puncture-resistance sharps container.

12. Do not recap or handle used needles.

13. Store reusable sharp instruments and needles in a puncture-resistant container.

14. Avoid mouth-to-mouth breathing in all but life threatening situations. Use a mechanical device or mask barrier instead.

15. Use a solution of household bleach (1:10 dilution) to disinfect environmental surfaces and reusable equipment.

16. Use hazardous waste containers for contaminated materials.

Adapted from "Guidelines for Isolation Precaution in Hospitals" developed by the Centers for Disease Control (CDC) and the Hospital Infection Control Practices Advisory Committee (HICPAC), January 1996.

and health care worker or from patient to patient. Examples of these illnesses include: enteric (intestinal) infections, gastrointestinal, respiratory, skin, or wound infections, diphtheria, herpes simplex virus, impetigo, Hepatitis A, scabies, pediculosis, and zoster. Precautions include isolation of the patient in a private room if hospitalized. Gloves and gowns must be worn if coming into contact with the patient. A mask and eyewear should be worn if there is potential for exposure to infectious body materials and fluids. When possible do not use patient care equipment on other patients.

Standard Precautions are summarized in Table 3-8.

▶ OSHA

The CDC precautions are required and enforced by OSHA. On December 2, 1991, The Occupational Safety and Health Administration (OSHA) issued its final standard on Occupational

Bloodborne Pathogens which resulted from a concern that healthcare workers face a significant health risk in the occupational exposure to **bloodborne pathogens**, or disease producing organisms transmitted via the blood. All health care agencies were required to comply with this law by July 6, 1992.

This OSHA directive is aimed at minimizing exposure of health care workers to Hepatitis B virus (HBV) and Human Immunodeficiency Virus (HIV). The OSHA federal standard is now a law which states that Universal Precautions against transmission of bloodborne pathogens cannot just be recommended. They are law and must be observed by employers of health care personnel.

The OSHA guidelines apply to facilities in which the employees could be "reasonably anticipated" to come into contact with potentially infectious materials: body fluids, saliva, and tissues.

> **Med Tip:** The CDC's "Standard Precautions" are similar to "Universal Precautions" since both are directed at body fluids that are blood, blood-related, or fluids that contain blood. However, "Standard Precautions" are broader since they include precautions for any moist body substance.

▶ PHYSICAL AND CHEMICAL BARRIERS

Effective physical and chemical barriers are used to maintain infection control. The development of a nosocomial infection, or hospital/medical facility acquired infection, is prevented when careful medical and surgical asepsis is maintained.

▶ MEDICAL ASEPSIS

Medical asepsis refers to the destruction of organisms after they leave the body. Techniques, such as handwashing, using disposable equipment, and wearing gloves, can help reduce the number and transfer of pathogens. Aseptic technique is a means of reducing the transfer of pathogens in the medical office.

Ordinary hygiene habits of everyday life are a form of medical asepsis. These include handwashing when handling food or after using the bathroom and covering one's mouth during a cough or sneeze. One of the most effective means of reducing pathogenic transmission is through handwashing. This is considered the first stage of infection control since the hands are a primary method for infection to transfer from the host to the receiver. In order to keep the skin free of harmful organisms, there must be frequent handwashing using a disinfectant soap, friction, and warm running water. Jewelry, such as rings, allows germs to hide and grow. See Figure 3-5 for an illustration of hands with jewelry that is likely to catch pathogens.

Medical asepsis is used during "clean" procedures which involve body parts which normally are not **sterile**. Something is sterile when all microorganisms and spores are dead. Situations involving medical asepsis would include taking oral, aural, and rectal

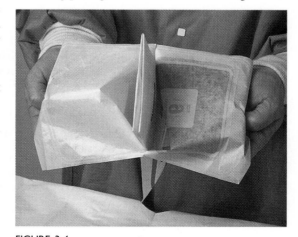

FIGURE 3-4

Sterile glove packet used for surgery.

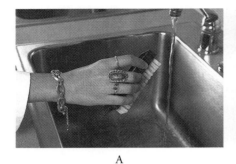
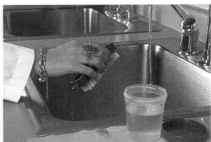
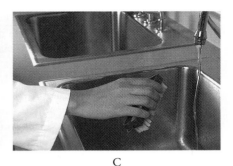

A   B   C

FIGURE 3-5 A-C

Jewelry provides places for pathogens to hide and grow.

temperatures; obtaining throat or vaginal cultures or smears; obtaining urine, stool, or sputum specimens; administering medications; and cleaning treatment rooms.

Aseptic techniques which can cause a break in the chain of infection include

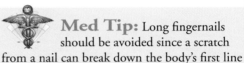

Med Tip: Long fingernails should be avoided since a scratch from a nail can break down the body's first line of defense—the skin. In addition, long nails can puncture gloves allowing pathogens to enter.

- Washing hands before and after any contact with patients or equipment.
- Handling all specimens and materials as though they contain pathogens.
- Using gloves to protect yourself when handling contaminated articles or materials, such as specimens.
- Not wearing jewelry which can attract bacteria.
- Using disposable equipment whenever possible. Dispose of all equipment properly after use.
- Cleaning all nondisposable equipment as soon as possible after patient use.
- Using only clean or sterile supplies for each patient.
- Using a protective covering over your clothes if there is any danger of contaminated materials or supplies coming into contact with your uniform.
- Discarding items that fall on the floor if they cannot be cleaned. All floors are considered contaminated. If in doubt, throw it out!
- Placing all wet or damp dressings and bandages in a waterproof bag to protect persons handling the garbage.

HANDWASHING

Handwashing provides the first defense against the spread of disease and should be done often. See Figure 3-6 for a demonstration of proper handwashing technique.

PROTECTIVE CLOTHING AND EQUIPMENT

Protective clothing, such as gowns, gloves, and masks, are worn for two reasons. They are

1. To protect the patient from any microorganisms that might be present on the health care worker's street clothing.
2. To protect the health care worker from carrying microorganisms away from the patient.

In addition, protective devices, such as gloves and masks, assist in protecting the health care worker from contamination with bloodborne pathogens. Nonsterile gowning technique is used for procedures, such as drawing blood, specimen collection, infant handling, and when in contact with a patient who is in isolation. Figure 3-7 A-D illustrates nonsterile gown technique.

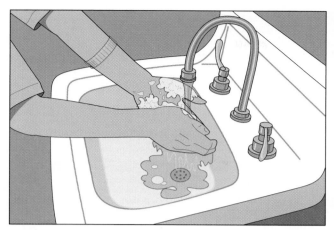

A Hold hands lower than elbows.

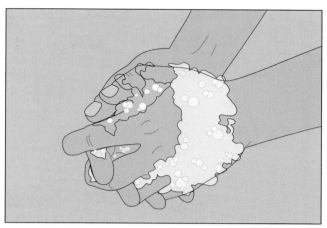

B Interlace fingers and thumbs.

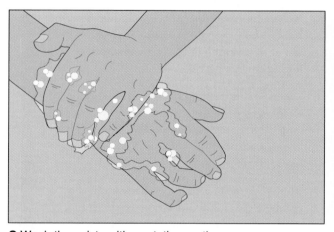

C Wash the wrists with a rotating motion.

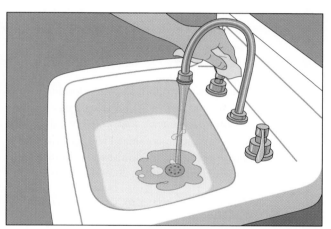

D Turn the water off with a dry paper towel.

FIGURE 3-6

Handwashing.

Figure 3-8 shows proper technique for putting on an isolation gown and Figure 3-9A-I illustrates how to remove an isolation gown. Proper step-by-step technique for removing gloves is shown in Figure 3-10 A-E.

▶ SURGICAL ASEPSIS

Surgical asepsis refers to the techniques practiced to maintain a sterile environment. It is the destruction of organisms before they enter the body.

There are three important steps to take to reach sterility, which is the absence of microorganisms. These methods for preventing the spread of disease in the medical office are sanitization, disinfection, and sterilization. Sanitization inhibits or inactivates pathogens by means of scrubbing and washing items. Disinfection destroys most or all pathogens on inanimate objects with the use of chemicals such as iodine, chlorine, alcohol and phenol. Sterilization is the destruction of all living organisms and spores with the use of pressurized steam, extreme temperatures, or radiation.

PROCEDURE: Handwashing

Terminal Performance
Competency: Student will perform handwashing procedure without error.

Equipment and Supplies
    Soap in liquid soap dispenser
    Nail brush or orange cuticle stick
    Hot running water
    Paper towels
    Waste container

Procedural Steps

1. Remove jewelry (includes rings with the exception of wedding band, watch, bracelets). ***Rationale:*** Jewelry has crevices and grooves which can harbor bacteria and dirt.

2. Stand at sink without allowing clothing to touch sink. Turn water on using paper towel. Discard paper towel. ***Rationale:*** Avoid direct contact with contaminated faucets. Sinks are also considered contaminated. Paper towel is contaminated after touching the faucet(s).

3. Adjust running water to correct lukewarm temperature. Discard paper towel. ***Rationale:*** Hot water may burn skin and cold water will not allow soap lather to form. Improper water temperature can cause chapping and cracking of skin which allows pathogens to enter.

4. Wet hands under running water and place liquid soap (size of a nickel or 1 teaspoon) into palm of hand. If using bar soap, keep the bar in hands and use enough soap to form a lather. Work soap into a lather by moving it over palms, sides, and backs—the entire surface—of both hands for 2 minutes. Use a circular motion and friction. Interlace fingers and move soapy water between them.

Rationale: Friction assists in removing organisms and dirt. If soap bar falls into sink or onto floor during the procedure the medical assistant must start procedure over again. Only use bar soap if liquid soap is unavailable. Soap bars allow the growth of bacteria to occur and must be thoroughly rinsed after each use.

5. Keep hands pointed downward with hands and forearms at elbow level or below during the entire handwashing procedure. ***Rationale:*** Water will run off hands and not back up onto arms for further contamination.

6. Use hand brush and/or orange cuticle stick to clean under fingernails. Thoroughly scrub wedding band if present. ***Rationale:*** Running water and soap may not be sufficient to remove dirt particles under nails.

7. Rinse hands under running water with fingers pointed down using care not to touch the sink or faucets. ***Rationale:*** The sink is not sterile (only clean) and may have contaminants present. Running water will wash away dirt and organisms.

8. Reapply soap and wash wrists and forearms for 1 more minute using circular motions.

9. Rinse hands under running water.

10. Dry hands thoroughly with paper towel. Discard paper towel.

11. Using a dry paper towel turn faucet off. ***Rationale:*** Paper towel will protect clean hands from coming into contact with contaminated faucet handles.

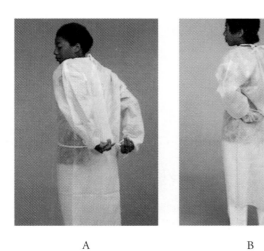
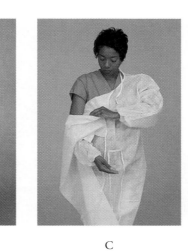
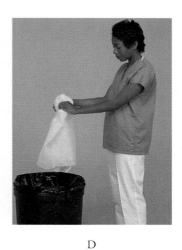

A   B   C   D

FIGURE 3-7 A-D

(A) Tie the neck piece of the gown and over lap the flaps. (B) Tie the gown securely at the waist. If gloves are to be worn, put them on now. (C) To take off a gown, remove and dispose of gloves properly if you are wearing them. Untie neck and waist. Grasp shoulders. Turn gown inside out as you remove it. (D) Fold up the gown and discard. Do not reuse a gown. Wash your hands.

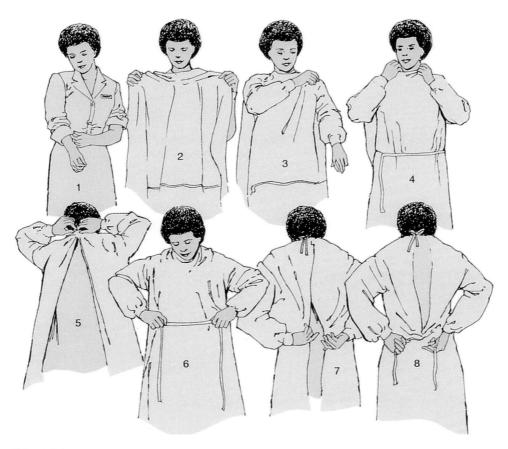

FIGURE 3-8

Putting on an isolation gown.

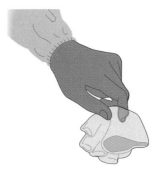

A Remove gloves.

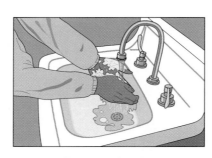

B Wash hands.

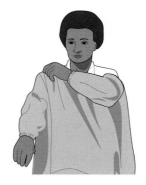

C Grasp each shoulder of gown near neck to remove sleeves.

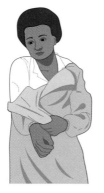

D As you remove sleeves turn them inside out.

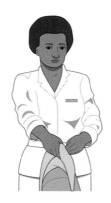

E Fold the gown inside out, holding it away from you.

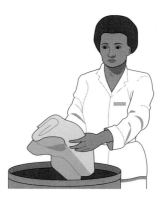

F Roll up the gown and discard it.

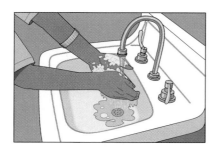

G Wash your hands.

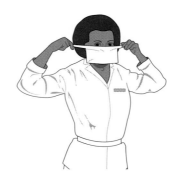

H Remove your mask.

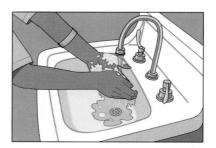

I Wash your hands.

FIGURE 3-9 A-I

Removing an isolation gown.

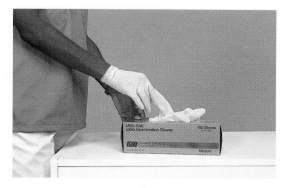

A

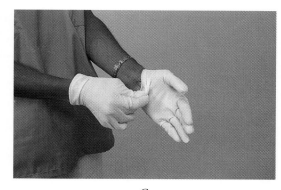

C

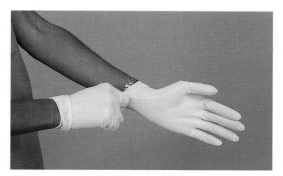

B

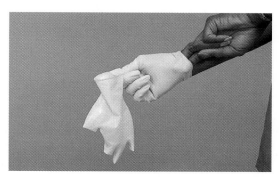

D

FIGURE 3-10 A-E

Removing gloves. (A) Use a clean pair of gloves for each patient contact. (B) Grasp the glove just below the cuff. (C) Pull the glove over your hand while turning the glove inside out. (D) Place the ungloved index finger and middle finger inside cuff of the glove, turning the cuff downward. (E) Pull the cuff and glove inside out as you remove your hand from the glove.

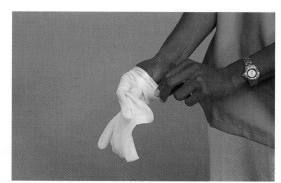

E

SANITIZATION

Sanitization includes the careful scrubbing of equipment and instruments using a brush and detergent with a neutral pH, such as a soapless soap, rinsing in hot water, and air drying. Sanitization cleans items, but microorganisms and bacteria are not destroyed. Supplies and equipment that do not come into direct contact with the patient or touch only the skin surface must be sanitized. If contaminated material cannot be sanitized immediately, then it should be soaked in detergent and water according to the manufacturer's instructions.

Another means of sanitizing equipment is with the use of ultrasound. In this case the instruments and equipment are placed into a bath tank and sound waves vibrate to break up the contamination. The articles are then rinsed thoroughly. Always follow the instructions of your supervisor regarding the proper procedure for sanitizing instruments or use the procedure provided here.

PROCEDURE: Sanitizing Instruments

Terminal Performance
Competency: The student will able to clean and sanitize instruments with no visible contamination remaining.

Equipment and Supplies

Disposable gloves

Rubber (utility) gloves

Plastic Brush

Towel

Sink

Running Water

Container which will hold all the instruments

Low-sudsing (low pH) detergent or germicidal agent

Note: Instruments should be rinsed under warm running water immediately after surgery to remove gross blood, body fluids and tissue. If it is not possible to clean them immediately, instruments should be submerged in water containing a low pH detergent.

Procedural Steps

1. Apply both disposable and rubber gloves. ***Rationale:*** Instruments have sharp edges which can cut through disposable gloves. Instruments are contaminated with blood and other waste materials.

2. Place low-sudsing (low pH) detergent or germicidal agent in large container with water. Rinse all instruments. ***Rationale:*** This will clean off gross blood and waste products.

A low pH detergent prevents staining on stainless steel surfaces.

3. Rinse instruments in clear water in either sink or container. Delicate and sharp instruments should be separated from general instruments.

4. Scrub each instrument individually with brush and detergent under running water. Open instruments to thoroughly scrub all serrated edges and hinge areas. ***Rationale:*** Blood and other debris collect in hinges, cracks and on serrated edges.

5. Rinse instrument thoroughly under hot water. ***Rationale:*** Any detergent left on instrument will prevent the disinfection process.

6. If instruments cannot be cleaned immediately after use then soak them in a solution of water and a blood solvent. When ready to wash instruments begin with step 1. ***Rationale:*** Soaking instruments prevents blood and other organic material to harden. Hardened blood is difficult to remove.

7. After thoroughly rinsing cleaned instruments, roll them in a towel to dry them. ***Rationale:*** Drying instruments prevents rust.

8. Check condition of all instruments for defects or remaining soil.

9. Wrap instrument(s) for sterilization.

DISINFECTION

Disinfection involves a soaking and wiping process. Disinfection destroys or inhibits the activity of disease-causing organisms. Disinfecting agents include chemical germicides, flowing steam, and boiling water. Chemical germicides are used to disinfect heat-perishable objects in the medical office, including some rubber and plastic items, clean floors, and office furniture. Two common disinfectants are zephrin chloride and chlorophenyl.

Contaminated instruments and equipment are completely immersed in a germicidal solution according to the manufacturer's instructions from 1 to 10 hours. They are then rinsed in water. (Instruments are rinsed in distilled water to prevent rust and corrosion.) Instruments must be dried after disinfection and rinsing.

Disinfectants can eliminate many organisms, but are not effective against spores (dormant stage of some bacteria), spore-forming bacteria, and some viruses. Some disinfectants, while effective on objects, may be too strong to use on patients (as for example, formaldehyde). The disinfectants, alcohol, and betadine are used when preparing a patient's skin for surgical procedures or injections since antiseptics prevent the growth of some microorganisms.

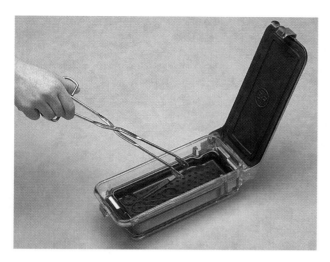

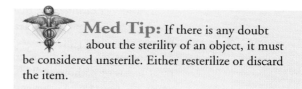

Med Tip: If there is any doubt about the sterility of an object, it must be considered unsterile. Either resterilize or discard the item.

FIGURE 3-11

Cold chemical sterilizer.

Objects that come into contact with mucous membranes, such as vaginal speculums, laryngoscopes or thermometers, should be disinfected or even sterilized, if possible. Instruments that cannot be soaked, such as scopes, computers, and electrical instruments) are wiped thoroughly with a germicidal solution. To be effective the entire instrument or item must be fully submersed. Items are generally left in the solution for 15 to 45 minutes. Germicidal solutions must be changed frequently according to the manufacturer's instructions. The chemical disinfection process is referred to as a "cold" process since no heat is used or generated (Figure 3-11).

Chemical disinfectants used for soaking and wiping include soap, alcohol, phenol, acid, alkalines (such as bleach), and formaldehyde. Some of these are discussed in Table 3-9.

TABLE 3-9   Disinfection Methods

Method	Description and Use
Alcohol (70% isopropyl)	Used for skin surfaces, equipment such as stethoscopes and thermometers, and table surfaces
	Causes damage to rubber products, lens, and plastic
	Flammable
Chlorine (sodium hypochlorite or bleach)	Use in dilution of 1:10 (one part bleach to 10 parts water)
	Used to eliminate a broad spectrum of microorganisms
	Corrosive effect on instruments, rubber, and plastic products
	Can cause skin irritation
	Inexpensive
Formaldehyde	Used to disinfect and sterilize
	Dangerous product which is regulated by OSHA—must have clearly marked labels
Hydrogen peroxide	Effective disinfectant only for use on non-human surfaces and products
	May damage rubber, plastic, and metals
Glutaraldehyde	Effective against viruses, bacteria, fungi and some spores
	Regulated by OSHA—must have clearly marked labels and use in well ventilated area
	Must wear gloves and masks when using

A means of disinfection that is used in operating rooms is ultra violet rays. Equipment that cannot be soaked is placed under the ultraviolet lamps for a specified period of time. This will kill microorganisms.

Another means of disinfection is the use of boiling water. Moist heat of up to 212°F will kill most forms of pathogens. This is not useful for killing viruses, such as the hepatitis virus or spores which are resistant to other methods of disinfection. Sterilization cannot occur at this temperature. Stainless-steel, glassware, and instruments can be boiled without damage. The articles are submerged in a container filled with cold water. The water must completely cover the articles to be disinfected. Distilled water should be used when boiling instruments or stainless steel to prevent sediment or deposits from forming. The water is then brought to the boiling point and continues to boil for 20 to 30 minutes for disinfection. When the boiling time has elapsed, the disinfected materials are allowed to cool. To maintain disinfection they must be touched only with sterile forceps.

STERILIZATION

Sterilization results in killing all microorganisms, both pathogenic and nonpathogenic. The use of heat (steam or dry), chemicals, high-velocity electron bombardment, or ultraviolet light radiation are used for this process. Heat sterilization, produced by an autoclave under steam pressure, is able to kill spores, bacteria, and other microorganisms. Dry heat is used for dense ointments such as petroleum jelly.

All supplies including dressings, needles, and instruments that come into contact with internal body tissue or an open wound must be sterile. Once a sterile article is touched by hands or another unsterile object, it is considered contaminated. Sterile gloves must be used when touching sterilized items.

▶ AUTOCLAVE

The methods used for sterilization include the autoclave and chemical (cold) sterilization. The autoclave process is an effective means of sterilization in the medical office. Types of autoclaving include: steam under pressure, dry heat (320°F for 1 hour), dry gas, or radiation.

Autoclaving is steam under pressure which destroys the organisms by causing them to explode. This method of sterilization requires 15 pounds of pressure and a temperature of 250-270°F depending on manufacturer's recommendations. Distilled water must be used in the steam autoclave. The autoclave consists of an outer chamber (jacket), which creates a build-up of steam that is forced into the inner chamber, and an inner chamber in which the materials to be sterilized are placed (Figure 3-14). Depending on the model type there may be three gauges on the autoclave 1) a jacket pressure gauge to indicate pressure in outer chamber; 2) a chamber pressure gauge to indicate the steam pressure in inner chamber; and 3) a temperature gauge to indicate temperature in inner chamber in which items are placed. Some of the newer models have only one gauge. The temperature used in autoclaving (250°F) must be reached before autoclaving the materials. Figure 3-15 displays an ultraclave automatic autoclave/sterilizer.

The microorganisms are killed in autoclaving by the condensation of steam on each of the items, not by the heat produced. Heat is actually transferred to the items by way of the steam condensation. Steam sterilization is not effective if air pockets are present within the packs. A pump within the autoclave will first remove air from the chamber. The pressure level and temperature levels within the autoclave chamber can be built up only after the air is removed. Therefore the gauges indicating pressure and temperature must be monitored by the medical assistant. Table 3-10 describes autoclave sterilization time requirements.

The autoclave should be thoroughly cleaned (sanitized) and free of any materials or lint before using. If detergent or other cleaner is used for cleaning, it should be completely rinsed before placing objects into the autoclave. The air exhaust valve must be cleaned and free of lint after each use.

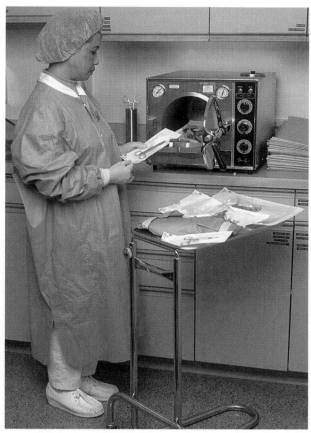

FIGURE 3-14

Autoclave.

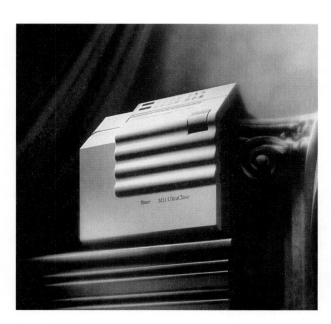

FIGURE 3-15

Ritter M11 Ultra Clave™ Automatic Sterilizer.

The wrapping in which the instruments and materials, such as dressings, to be sterilized are placed must be **permeable**, or allow steam to pass through and be strong enough to hold together during the steam process. Wrapping materials include heavy paper, muslin, plastic, and stainless steel containers. See Figure 3-16 A-D for an illustration of how to wrap instruments for the autoclave. Instruments with hinges should be open, tubing free of any kinks, and syringes unassembled before wrapping.

The wrapping generally consists of two layers of permeable materials. All items must be completely covered with the wrapping material and fastened with tape which states the date of sterilization and identifies the item. Figure 3-17 displays tapes that have changed color during the sterilization process.

Sterilization pouches or bags are often used for individual instruments. Careful inspection must be made to make sure the bag has not ruptured or been punctured during the autoclave process. Small, lightweight instruments are suitable for pouches. The pouches have sterilization indicators both inside and outside the bag.

Instruments which will be used immediately can be placed in perforated trays and autoclaved unwrapped. Instruments can be sterilized in instrument trays. The lid for the tray is placed next

TABLE 3-10   Sterilization Time Requirements

Time	Article
15 minutes	Glassware
	Metal Instruments (open tray or individual wrapping with hinges open)
	Syringes (unassembled)
	Needles
20 minutes	Instruments—partial metal in double-thickness wrapper or covered tray
	Rubber products: gloves, tubing, catheters wrapped or unwrapped
	Solutions in a flask (50-100 mL)
30 minutes	Dressings—small packs in paper or muslin
	Solutions in a flask (500-1000 mL)
	Syringes—unassembled individually wrapped in gauze
	Syringes—unassembled individually wrapped in glass tubes
	Needles—individually packaged in paper or glass tubes
	Sutures—wrapped in paper or muslin
	Instrument and treatment trays—wrapped in paper or muslin
	Gauze—loosely packed
60 minutes	Petroleum jelly—in dry heat

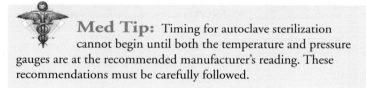

Med Tip: Timing for autoclave sterilization cannot begin until both the temperature and pressure gauges are at the recommended manufacturer's reading. These recommendations must be carefully followed.

to the open tray of instruments. The lid is immediately placed over the instruments after sterilization. A towel is usually placed under the instruments to absorb moisture during autoclaving.

Items should be wrapped in individual packs which can be handled for storage and use by their outer wrapping without contaminating the inner items. When the autoclaved package is opened, the contents are removed without contaminating them. The autoclave chamber must not be overloaded or the steam will not be able to penetrate the wrapping and sterilize the instruments and materials. Items should be placed on their edges to permit the proper penetration with moisture and heat.

Containers and jars of supplies should be placed on their sides for full sterilization to occur. Solutions should be autoclaved separately since they may boil over during autoclaving. The lid of plastic containers and bags will become sealed upon sterilization.

The time or pressure required for autoclaving, according to the manufacturer's recommendations, must never be shortened. If proper timing and pressure is not observed when autoclaving, the items will become warm but not sterile.

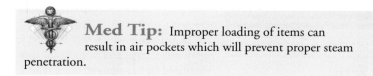

Med Tip: Improper loading of items can result in air pockets which will prevent proper steam penetration.

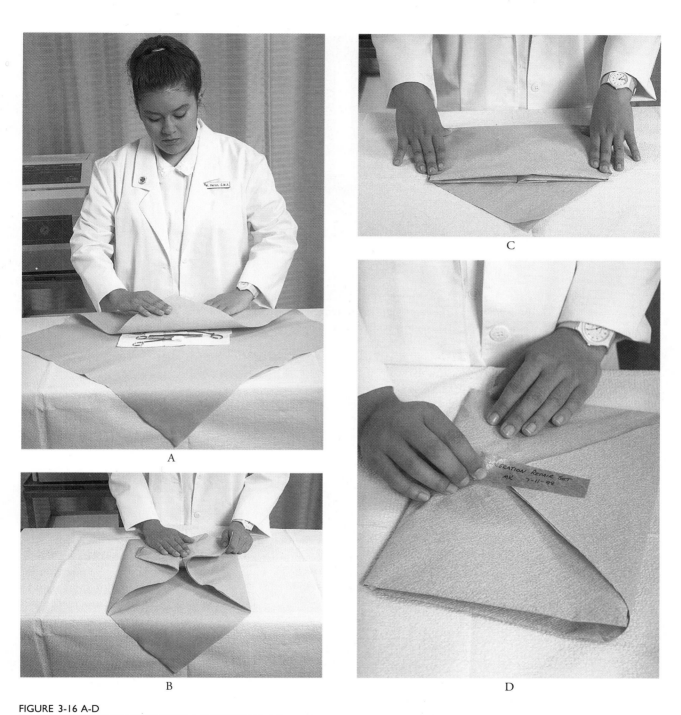

FIGURE 3-16 A-D

Wrapping instruments for the autoclave.

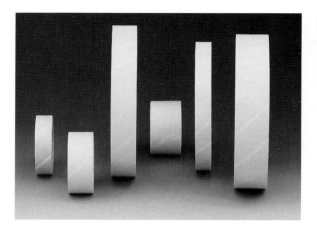

FIGURE 3-17

Autoclave indicator tape.

DRYING AUTOCLAVED GOODS

After the process is complete, the drying process is almost as important as the correct temperature and pressure in autoclaving. Wetness on items ("wet packs") can cause a break in sterility since moisture will allow bacteria to grow and be transmitted into the inside of the package. A towel can be placed in the bottom of the autoclave tray to absorb some moisture. "Wet Packs" can be avoided by allowing for a drying period at the end of autoclaving. To do this open the door of the autoclave 3/4 inch (but no more) just before the drying cycle on the autoclave. Run the dry cycle according to the manufacturer's directions.

 Med Tip: Do not open the autoclave door all the way during the drying cycle since the cold air from the room will enter the autoclave and cause condensation to form on the packs and instruments. The rule to follow is that all autoclaved materials should be completely dry when they are removed and remain dry for 1 hour after removal.

STERILIZATION INDICATORS

Indicators are used to signify sterilization. Note that the change of color or dots appearing in an indicator strip only indicate that steam has entered the chamber and not that the instruments are sterile. OK strips are placed inside the wrapper or in the chamber. Autoclaving tape turns black after autoclaving. Indicators come in a variety of types including strips and tape. The strips are placed in the center of a pack to indicate that the inner contents have been exposed to the conditions for sterility: correct temperature, correct time, and exposure to moisture. Figure 3-18 illustrates sterility checks.

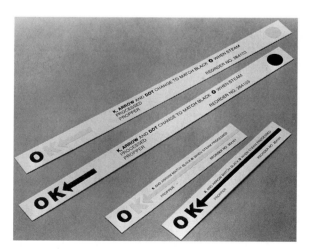

FIGURE 3-18

Sterility checks.

SHELF-LIFE

Autoclaved packages are stored with the date visible and the oldest date in front of the stack so that it is used first. Instruments are considered sterile for 21-30 days (21 days in plastic bags and 30 days in muslin), with a shelf-life of approximately one month. Shelf-life is dependent upon the type of wrapper used. The individual manufacturer's guidelines should be followed concerning when to reclean and resterilize the item. Autoclaved packages cannot be reautoclaved in the same packages without washing, rinsing, drying and rewrapping each item.

▶ HEPATITIS AND AIDS

Two diseases that require special attention during a discussion of infection control are hepatitis and AIDS since both these diseases affect several million people.

HEPATITIS

Hepatitis is a viral disease of the liver resulting in inflammation and infection. Forms of hepatitis are A, B, C, D, and E.

Hepatitis A (Acute Infective Hepatitis)

Hepatitis A is transmitted by fecal waste contamination of food and the water supply. This occurs when food and water become contaminated with fecal waste products of animals or humans. The **incubation** period, or period of time during which the disease develops after exposure into symptoms, is from 14 to 50 days with a very slow onset of symptoms including fever, loss of appetite, jaundice, nausea, vomiting, malaise, dark urine, and whitish stools.

Hepatitis B (Serum Hepatitis)

Hepatitis B, also called HBV, is transmitted through body fluids including blood, semen, saliva, and breast milk which are contaminated with the virus. This potentially fatal disease can be passed from one drug user to another when sharing a contaminated needle. Hepatitis B is on the increase due to its appearance in persons with HIV and AIDS. The incubation period for this liver infection is 60 to 90 days with a rapid onset of symptoms. HBV symptoms include

- Fever
- Chills
- Diarrhea with clay-colored stools
- Nausea and vomiting
- Orange-brown urine

- Headache
- Anorexia
- Enlarged liver
- Jaundice

The diagnosis of HBV is made through a liver biopsy to identify the virus. Treatment for all forms of hepatitis is a high-protein diet and rest. Treatment for HBV may last for several weeks with the possibility of relapse.

There are two types of vaccine available for HBV: one made from human serum and the other a synthetic product. HBV vaccine is administered in three doses; the second dose one month after the first and the third dose six months later.

Pediatricians and health officials are now recommending that infants and adolescents be vaccinated for hepatitis B due to the rising incidence of this disease. The schedule for infants is for the first dose to be given at time of birth.

 Med Tip: Immunization against HBV is required by OSHA for all health care workers. Others who should be counseled to receive this vaccine are intravenous drug users and persons with multiple sexual partners.

Hepatitis C

Hepatitis C, also referred to as non-A and non-B hepatitis, is the most common form of new hepatitis cases every year. The symptoms and treatment are similar to those of hepatitis B.

Hepatitis D

Hepatitis D, also called delta hepatitis, is the most recently identified form of hepatitis. The symptoms of this form of hepatitis can be more severe than with other forms of hepatitis. Hepatitis D is spread through the use of intravenous drugs and intimate contact. There is a rapid growth of this form of hepatitis due to the increased number of HIV and AIDS cases in which it is seen.

Hepatitis E

Hepatitis E is the result of exposure to food contaminated with human feces. It is a major infectious disease in developing countries due to poor sanitary conditions.

HIV/AIDS

Acquired immune deficiency syndrome (AIDS) was first documented in the United States in 1980. This disorder of the immune system was first noted when five homosexual young men were treated for an unusual form of pneumonia, *Pneumocystis carinii,* in Los Angeles. At approximately the same time, doctors were noticing the occurrence of a rare blood vessel malignancy, Kaposi's sarcoma, in homosexual young men in California and New York. The combination of these disorders came to be associated with a **syndrome** caused by a virus, the human immunodeficiency virus (HIV). Figure 3-19 depicts the AIDS virus.

The Centers for Disease Control in Atlanta reports that about 1.5 million Americans have been infected with HIV and over one-quarter million have AIDS. Globally, the World Health Organization (WHO) suspects there are as many as 15 million cases of HIV and 5 millions cases of AIDS. There is not a cure for HIV or AIDS at this time and people with the disease will have it for the rest of their lives.

This infectious virus causes the immune system, which is the body's shield against infection, to break down and eventually become ineffective by invading the body's macrophages and T-cells, which fight disease. When the T-cells are invaded they render the macrophages useless for fighting off pathogenic invasions.

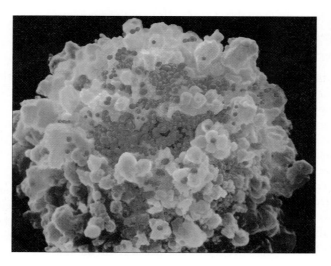

FIGURE 3-19

The AIDS virus.

The various means by which the AIDS virus can enter the body are listed below. They are

- Vaginal, anal, or oral intercourse with a person who has the virus
- Sharing needles or syringes with a person who has the virus
- Receiving transfusions of blood or blood products donated by someone who has the virus
- Receiving organ transplants from a donor who has the virus
- Contaminating open wounds or sores with blood, semen, or vaginal secretions infected with the virus
- Having artificial insemination with the sperm of a man who has the virus

A mother's fetus, or unborn child, may become infected if she contracts the virus before or during her pregnancy. An infant could become infected by being breast fed by a woman with the virus.

The virus can survive well in body fluids such as blood, semen, and vaginal secretions. The virus can stay in cells for months, and even years. During this time the cells will replicate, or reproduce, themselves. The body's defensive T-cells are eventually destroyed by the new viral cells.

Some HIV victims will develop AIDS-related complex (ARC) which has less serious symptoms than AIDS. ARC symptoms include loss of appetite and weight loss, diarrhea, skin rash, fatigue, night sweating, swollen lymph glands, and poor resistance to infection.

Not all HIV patients develop AIDS or any other HIV-related condition. Estimates, according to the CDC, range from 50 percent to 90 percent of patients developing full-blown AIDS. It may take eight to ten years for symptoms of HIV infection to develop and 12 years or more for symptoms of AIDS to develop. The stages of HIV infection are listed below:

- After becoming infected with HIV, it may take a person six weeks to three years to develop antibodies (which means they will not test positive for HIV). Before developing these antibodies, some people with HIV have symptoms that are usually brief but not severe. These might include slight fever, headaches, fatigue, and swollen glands for a few weeks.
- After antibodies develop, the person will test positive for HIV. However, another period with no symptoms may occur. This "incubation period" can last several years. However, even though there are no symptoms, the immune system becomes increasingly damaged during this time.
- Next, a person with HIV may experience a long period of swelling of the lymph glands in the throat, armpits, and groin. This condition is called "persistent generalized lymphadenopathy" and may last a number of years.
- When HIV has seriously damaged the immune system, a condition called AIDS-related complex (ARC) may occur. These symptoms can include a white coating of the mouth and throat (thrush), similar infections of the skin and mucous membranes of the anus and genital area, and severe viral infections such as herpes.

AIDS, the final stage of an HIV infection, includes a variety of viral, fungal, bacterial, parasitic infections, nervous disorders, and cancers. These infections are often present in the healthy body and can be overcome by the immune system. However, in the AIDS patient, the immune

Med Tip: It is not possible to tell if a person has HIV just by looking at the person. Many people do not know they have HIV because they have no symptoms. In order to be protected, you must use standard precautions as if everyone you come into contact with has HIV or AIDS.

system is no longer effective and, hence, the infections become life-threatening. These infections, called **opportunistic infections**, include:

- *Pneumocystis carinii* pneumonia (PCP)
- Kaposi's sarcoma—a type of skin cancer
- Toxoplasmosis—infestation of parasites that infect the brain and central nervous system

> **Med Tip:** Note that testing positive for HIV antibodies does not necessarily mean that a person has, or will develop, AIDS. Positive test results, if leaked to an employer or insurance company, can lead to loss of job, on-the-job harassment, or other serious consequences, even though such actions may be illegal.

Tuberculosis (TB) is seen with increasing frequency among persons infected with HIV. HIV infection is one of the strongest known risk factors for the progression of TB from infection to disease. However, of the diseases associated with HIV infection, TB is one of the few that is transmissible, treatable, and preventable. An estimated 5% of all AIDS patients have TB according to the CDC.

AIDS is diagnosed based on several factors: functioning ability of the immune system based on tests such as T-cell counts, the presence of one or more opportunistic infections, and the presence of HIV antibodies. The HIV or AIDS Antibody test, known as ELISA (Enzyme-Linked Immuno-Sorbent Assay), is used as a screening test. With a positive ELISA, a patient is said to be HIV positive or HIV antibody positive. The Western Blot test is used to confirm results of the ELISA.

HIV does not survive well outside the human body, and it is not transmitted through air, food, water, pets, or bugs. The virus has been found in tears, saliva, urine, and breast milk. HIV is destroyed by a 1:10 household bleach solution or an application of heat treatment at 132°F (56° C) for 10 minutes. Standard Precautions which include the use of aseptic technique, gloving, careful handling of needles and syringes to avoid puncture wounds, can prevent contracting the virus by health care workers.

HIV and AIDS are no longer considered to be diseases of the homosexual population since they have become increasingly prevalent in women and children.

The symptoms of AIDS are described below:

- T-cell count less than 200 (normal range for T-cells is 500 cells per cubic millimeter of blood).
- Unexplained weight loss of 10-15 pounds in less than 2 months that is not associated with diet or exercise.
- Long-lasting occurrences of diarrhea.
- Unexplained fever, chills, and drenching night sweats for more than 2 weeks.
- Unexplained extreme fatigue.
- Swelling or hardening of lymph glands located in the throat, groin, or armpit.
- Periods of continued, deep, dry coughing that are not due to other illnesses or smoking.
- Increased shortness of breath.
- Appearance of discolored or purplish growths on the skin or inside the mouth.
- Unexplained bleeding from growths on the skin, mucous membranes, or from any opening on the body.
- Severe numbness or pain in the hands and feet, loss of motor control and reflex, paralysis or loss of muscular strength.
- Altered state of consciousness, personality change, or mental deterioration.

There is presently no cure for AIDS. The drugs AZT (zidovudine) and ddC (zalcitabie) have been found effective in boosting the immune system and prolong-

> **Med Tip:** HIV cannot be obtained from donating blood. The disease is not transmitted through casual contact such as touching.

ing life. A combination of these two drugs has resulted in an increase of T-cell counts in some individuals. Supportive measures to improve the quality of life for the AIDS patient include delivery of home meals, nutritional supplements, and hospice care.

The medical assistant may be asked to provide information to a caregiver. Recommendations for caring for someone with AIDS are presented in Table 3-11.

TABLE 3-11   Caring for Someone with AIDS

To protect themselves from infection, caregivers should be reminded to do the following:

- Handle all needles with care. Never replace caps back on needles or remove needles from syringes. Dispose of all needles in puncture-proof containers out of the reach of children.

- Wear latex or rubber gloves if they have any contact with blood, blood-tinged body fluids, urine, feces, or vomit.

- Wash hands after removing gloves.

- Any cut, open sore, or breaks on exposed skin of either the patient or caregiver should be covered with a bandage.

- Flush all liquid waste containing blood down the toilet using care to avoid splashing during pouring. Non-flushable items such as paper towels, sanitary pads and tampons, wound dressings, or items soiled with blood, semen, or vaginal fluid should be enclosed in a plastic bag and tightly sealed. Check with your local health department or physician to determine trash disposal regulations for your area.

- Use a disinfection solution of one part bleach to 10 parts water to disinfect such items as floors, showers, tubs, sinks. Discard solution in toilet after using.

To protect the person with AIDS from infection:

- If the caregiver has a cold or flu, and there is no one else available to care for the AIDS patient, a surgical-type mask should be worn.

- Wash your hands before touching the AIDS patient.

- Any one with boils, fever blisters (herpes simplex), or shingles (zoster) should avoid close contact with the patient.

- Gloves should be worn if the caregiver has a rash or sores on their hands.

- Persons living with or caring for an AIDS patient should have received all the recommended childhood immunizations and booster shots, including the hepatitis vaccine.

- The AIDS patient should not be in the same room with a person who has, or is recovering from, chickenpox.

The caregiver should:

- Call the local AIDS service organization for support.

- Seek the help of clergy, counselors, and other health care professionals to help cope with feelings of frustration and stress.

- Not be afraid to touch the person with AIDS.

- Encourage the patient to become involved in their own care. Assist them in being active as long as possible.

- Not be afraid to discuss the disease with the patient.

When patients come in for HIV or AIDS testing, they should receive counseling from the physician before and after the test. The counseling should include information on methods for safe sex.

For more information on HIV or AIDS, write to the CDC National AIDS Clearinghouse, P.O. Box 6003, Rockville, MD 20849-6003 or call 1-800-458-5231. The Spanish hotline is 1-800-344-7432. The deaf access hotline is 1-900-AIDS-TTY.

LEGAL AND ETHICAL ISSUES

There is a grave responsibility for the medical assistant to maintain aseptic technique. An ethical concern is that every break in aseptic technique must be reported and corrected immediately. Even when one cannot see a needle puncture in a glove, the wearer of the glove may know there has been a puncture resulting in a break in the barrier to infection. The medical assistant must readily admit if a barrier has been broken so that corrective action can be taken.

The identity of an employee or patient who is HIV positive or has AIDS or hepatitis is confidential and must be respected.

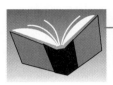

PATIENT EDUCATION

Handwashing must be stressed for all patients. Special emphasis should be placed on washing hands before and after eating, using the toilet, handling contaminated items such as door knobs, or coming into contact with any bodily fluids. Personal hygiene such as daily bathing, oral hygiene, and clean clothes has to be stressed.

Patients truly believe they are carrying out good infection control procedures, when, in fact, there are breaks in the barriers against infection, and as a result infection spreads. The medical assistant must carefully instruct patients concerning the importance of thorough handwashing with soap and warm water before performing such procedures as changing dressings, handling wounds, and colostomy care. Diabetic patients need special instructions on procedures to use to prevent infections developing since they are an at risk population.

Remind the patients that they cannot see germs with the naked eye. Commercial disinfectants are encouraged when cleaning bathrooms and kitchens.

Patients of all ages who are sexually active should be instructed on the proper use of condoms for protection against AIDS, other sexually transmitted diseases, and hepatitis B.

Summary

Good aseptic technique is everybody's business. The medical assistant is often the first barrier against infection in the office. The meticulous attention given to sterilization of all reusable materials and equipment is often the full responsibility of the medical assistant. This is a serious responsibility. All who handle waste products must be trained in safety measures such as Standard Precautions. Document waste removal.

When practicing aseptic technique, know the right way to do something and then never deviate from that method. Never take shortcuts with asepsis.

Competency Review

1. Define and spell the glossary terms for this chapter.
2. Describe the disease transmission process.
3. Develop an infection control plan for a medical office.
4. Wrap and label instruments for autoclave sterilization.
5. Correctly load an autoclave.
6. Correctly follow the step-by-step procedure for sterile gowning and gloving.
7. Call the 800 number of the CDC to request educational brochures that can be used to develop patient teaching materials.

PREPARING FOR THE CERTIFICATION EXAM

Test Taking Tip — Do not look for cues to correct answers by studying the pattern of correct responses. Answers occur in a random pattern.

Examination Review Questions

1. A commonly used disinfectant is
   (A) formaldehyde
   (B) Lysol
   (C) 70% alcohol
   (D) soap
   (E) phenol

2. Most sterilization indicators operate on what principle?
   (A) a color change will revert back when item is contaminated
   (B) original color reappears after 6 weeks
   (C) color change indicates the package has been properly sealed
   (D) color change indicates sterilization is complete
   (E) none of the above

3. Dry heat sterilization is used for
   (A) plastic items
   (B) dressings
   (C) gloves
   (D) surgical instruments
   (E) ointments and powders

4. Steam under pressure, dry heat, and chemical-gas mixtures are used in
   (A) disinfection
   (B) sterilization
   (C) sanitization
   (D) cleaning
   (E) fumigation

5. Before removing sterilized items from the autoclave, they should be allowed to
   (A) change color
   (B) cool
   (C) dry
   (D) depressurize
   (E) all of the above

6. Sterile materials which are wrapped in paper or cloth can be stored for
   (A) one year
   (B) only 10 days
   (C) 6 months
   (D) 21-30 days
   (E) two years

7. Instruments which are being disinfected in boiling water should remain immersed for NOT less than
   (A) 90 minutes
   (B) 60 minutes
   (C) 30 minutes
   (D) 45 minutes
   (E) 15 minutes

8. After the autoclave temperature reaches 250°F, the timer for sterilizing wrapped surgical instruments should be set for
   (A) 10 minutes
   (B) 15 minutes
   (C) 30 minutes
   (D) 50 minutes
   (E) 60 minutes

9. Which of the following is NOT a cause of incomplete sterilization when using the autoclave?
   (A) trapping pockets of air in the autoclave
   (B) setting the timer before the correct temperature has been reached
   (C) opening the door completely during the drying cycle
   (D) placing instruments overlapping one another
   (E) placing only one instrument in each packet

10. What conditions are necessary for bacterial growth to occur?
    (A) moisture
    (B) body temperature
    (C) oxygen
    (D) light
    (E) all of the above

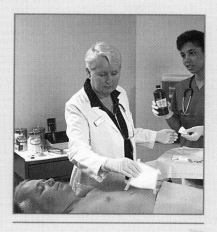

ASSISTING WITH MINOR SURGERY

OBJECTIVES

After completing this chapter, you should:

- Define and spell the glossary terms for this chapter.
- Discuss all 6 guidelines for surgical aseptic technique.
- List and differentiate between the types of ambulatory surgery.
- Describe the differences between medical asepsis (clean technique) and surgical asepsis (sterile technique).
- List and describe instruments for: cutting, dissecting, grasping, clamping, probing and dilating.
- Explain the rules for handling instruments.
- Give 5 examples of suture materials, including gauge ranges, with examples of when they may be used.
- Describe the preparation of the patient for minor surgery.
- List equipment and supplies used for preparing the patient's skin for surgery.
- Define "informed consent." Discuss the medical assistant's role in the process.
- Describe at least 5 surgical procedures that can be performed in the physician's office and indicate the responsibility of the medical assistant for each procedure.

CLINICAL PERFORMANCE COMPETENCIES

After completing this chapter, you should perform the following tasks:

- Demonstrate proper technique for a surgical scrub and sterile gloving.
- Demonstrate proper method for opening surgical packs to assure sterility.
- Demonstrate surgical aseptic technique for preparing the patient's skin for minor surgery.
- Select, assemble, and prepare equipment for a minor surgical procedure.
- Identify by name and use the instruments used in minor surgical procedures.
- Prepare the patient for a minor surgical procedure.
- Assist the physician during a minor surgical procedure.
- Remove sutures as directed by a physician.
- Apply a sterile dressing.

Glossary

ambulatory surgery   A method for performing surgical procedures which allows the patient to walk into and out of the surgical facility on the same day.

anesthesia   Partial or complete loss of sensation.

biopsy   The removal of tissue for purposes of determining the presence of cancerous (malignant) cells.

cryosurgery   Use of freezing temperatures from a probe to destroy abnormal cells.

hyfrecators   Small electrocautery units used to perform minor cautery procedures in the medical office.

incision(s)   Surgical cut into tissue.

invasive   Enters the skin.

Mayo stand   Small portable tray/table used to hold surgical instruments during a procedure.

outpatient surgery   Surgical procedures, which usually require less than 60 minutes, performed in a setting in which the patient is ambulatory and does not stay in the facility overnight.

scrub assistant   A sterile assistant who passes instruments, swabs (sponges) bodily fluids from the operative site, retracts incisions, and cuts sutures.

sterile field   Work area in surgery in which the area is prepared using sterile drapes (cloths) to cover nonsterile areas.

surgical asepsis   A technique practiced to maintain a sterile environment.

WARNING!

For all patient contact, adhere to Standard Precautions.
Wear protective equipment as indicated.

This chapter discusses surgical aseptic technique, or sterile technique. Procedures requiring sterile technique, such as minor surgical procedures, suture insertion and removal, breast biopsy, incision and drainage, removal of growths, and wound treatment are included. Strict adherence to aseptic technique is necessary when assisting with these procedures. It is important to always remember that an item is either sterile or nonsterile. If there is any doubt about sterility, assume it is nonsterile.

▶ AMBULATORY SURGERY

Ambulatory surgery is a method for performing surgical procedures in which the patient is able to walk into and out of the surgical facility on the day of surgery. This includes outpatient surgery, surgicenter surgery, and office surgery. Since ambulatory surgery is on the increase, the medical assistant is spending more time assisting the physician with surgical procedures.

Outpatient surgery, with its emphasis on surgical procedures performed outside the hospital setting, has resulted in a cost savings to the consumer and to the insurer. Hospitalization is not required unless there is an unexpected complication. The patient is able to return home after a brief recovery time in the outpatient facility or medical office. The disadvantage to this type of surgery is the short time the health care team has to spend assessing the patient's post-operative condition. It is important for each outpatient facility to develop a consistent follow-up procedure to track the patient's condition after leaving.

Outpatient surgery is generally limited to procedures requiring less than 60 minutes to perform. Terminology relating to surgery are

- *Elective:*   Surgery that is considered medically necessary, but can be performed when the patient wishes (for example, removal of benign growths).
- *Emergency:*   Surgery that is required immediately to save a life (for example, hemorrhage) or prevent further injury or infection.
- *Optional:*   Surgery that may not be medically necessary, but the patient wishes to have performed (for example, cosmetic surgery, vasectomy).

- *Outpatient:*   Surgical procedure performed which does not require an overnight stay in a hospital.
- *Surgicenter:*   A medical facility that performs ambulatory surgery.
- *Urgent:*   Surgery that needs to be performed as soon as possible, but is not an immediate or acute emergency (for example, cancer surgery).

▶ PRINCIPLE OF SURGICAL ASEPSIS

Surgical asepsis, or sterile technique, is used when sterility of supplies and the immediate environment is required, as in surgical procedures. Sterile technique results in the killing of all living microorganisms and is necessary during any **invasive** procedure in which the body is entered such as when administering an injection, making a surgical incision, or working with an open wound.

Med Tip: Remember "clean for clean" and "sterile for sterile". Use clean technique when handling nonsterile items (for example, clean hands when applying a dressing to intact skin). Use sterile procedure when handling sterile materials (for example, must use sterile gloves when touching sterile instruments).

Open tissues provide an excellent reservoir (host) for infection. Infections can delay the healing process and result in additional medical costs. Sterile technique prevents infection from microorganisms being introduced into the body, thereby decreasing the risk of infection.

Medical asepsis and surgical asepsis are similar in their overall purpose of decreasing the risk of infection. Medical asepsis results in a "clean" approach in which materials can be handled with clean hands or nonsterile gloves. Surgical asepsis requires a sterile hand washing scrub, sterile gloves, and sterile technique when handling materials. See Table 4-1 for a comparison of medical and surgical asepsis.

GUIDELINES FOR SURGICAL ASEPSIS

When practicing surgical asepsis, follow the guidelines presented here or those used in your office as directed by your supervisor.

STERILE SCRUB AND GLOVING

Figure 4-1 A-G demonstrates handwashing for surgical asepsis and Figure 4–2 A-H gloving following sterile scrub.

Med Tip: All personnel should change to street clothes before leaving the medical facility. Nonsterile surgical "scrub suits" should not be worn home. Their purpose is to protect the patient and the health care worker from exposure to pathogenic organisms.

TABLE 4-1   Surgical Asepsis Versus Medical Asepsis

Surgical Asepsis	Medical Asepsis
"Sterile" technique used	"Clean" technique used
Absence of microorganisms	Controls microorganisms
Surgical scrub performed	Basic handwashing procedure used
Sterile equipment and supplies required	Clean equipment and supplies
Sterile field	Clean field

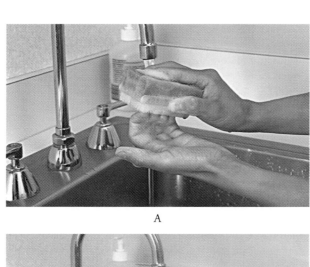

A

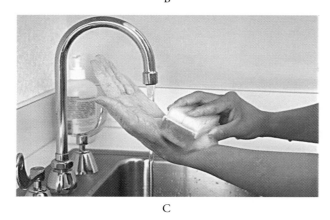

B

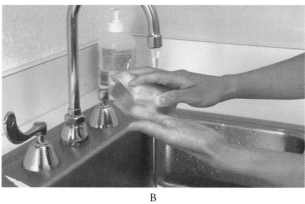

C

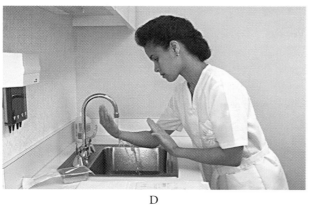

D

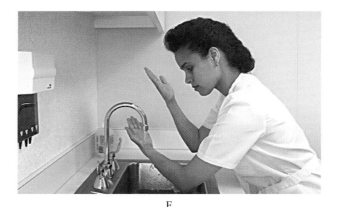

E

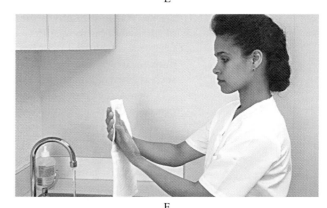

F

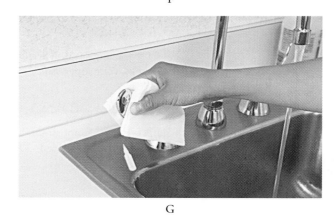

G

FIGURE 4-1 A-G

Sterile scrub handwashing.

PROCEDURE: Surgical Handwashing/Sterile Scrub

Terminal Performance
Competency: Perform surgical scrub on hands and arms using correct procedure for the appropriate length of time.

Equipment and Supplies
Germicidal Dispenser Soap (not bar soap)
Sterile scrub brush
Sterile towel pack (with 2–3 sterile paper or cloth towels)
Paper towels
Sterile gloves (prepackaged)
Running water (foot pedal preferable)
Nail file

Procedural Steps
1. Remove all jewelry. With nail file remove any gross dirt from beneath fingernails before scrubbing. *Rationale:* microorganisms can accumulate in crevices of rings or watch and under fingernails.
2. Assemble equipment.
3. Stand at sink without allowing body to touch it. *Rationale:* Sink is considered contaminated with microorganisms.
4. Remove lab coat. Roll sleeves above elbows. Keep hands and arms above waist level at all times. *Rationale:* All areas below the waist are considered contaminated.
5. Regulate running water temperature to warm, not hot. *Rationale:* Hot water can cause hands to chap and crack which can provide a source of cross-infection.
6. Place hands under running water with hands pointed upward. Allow water to run from fingertips to elbows. *Rationale:* If water is running downward from the unscrubbed arm to the hands it would contaminate the scrubbed hands.
7. Apply circle of soap from dispenser and lather well.
8. Vigorously scrub hands and wrists with scrub brush. Wash thoroughly between fingers. Scrub under fingernails. Scrub toward the elbows using 5 minutes on each hand.
9. Raise the hands, bending at the elbow, and place under running water to rinse soap. Allow water to flow from fingertips to elbows.
10. Perform a second lather and scrub if that is the policy in your facility. In this case, use 3 minutes for each scrub.
11. Using a sterile towel (if possible), pat hands dry moving from fingertips to wrists, and then to elbows. The hands should still be held above the elbows.
12. Turn off faucet with fresh towel (if foot lever not available). *Rationale:* The faucet and handles are considered unclean. A towel protects the clean hands from contamination.
13. Glove immediately. Keep hands above the waist and folded together until procedure begins.

STERILE PACKAGING

Sterile packages (packs) are prepared for use in surgery with either individual pieces of equipment or instruments or several items packed together. These packs are then autoclaved with sterilization indicators and dated. These packs are used for various procedures. For example, all the instruments needed for a procedure, such as a biopsy, are packaged together in a tray and autoclaved. See the procedure for opening a sterile packet. Figure 4-4 A-F demonstrates opening a sterile packet.

When assisting the physician/surgeon with the procedure, the medical assistant will "set up" the specific tray or instruments before the procedure begins. The packets are set up on a **Mayo stand,** which is a small portable table with enough room to hold an instrument tray. For some procedures more than one Mayo stand is used.

Figure 4-5 illustrates dropping a sterile packet onto a sterile field.

Sterile Transfer
Figure 4-6 illustrates how to handle the transfer of sterile equipment from a sterile packet using forceps.

Guidelines: Surgical Asepsis

1. When in doubt about sterility, consider the item nonsterile.
2. All supplies and materials used for sterile procedures must be sterilized at the time of use or prior to use. Check the expiration dates.
3. The human body cannot be sterilized. The patient's skin can be prepared using an antiseptic wash, but will not be sterile. Skin is always considered contaminated (nonsterile).
4. When using sterile gloves:

   • Do not touch the outside of the gloves with bare hands.
   • When wearing sterile gloves, touch only sterile articles.
   • If a sterile glove is punctured by a needle or instrument, remove the instrument from the sterile field, remove and dispose of the damaged glove(s), wash hands, and reglove as soon as possible.

5. Sterile pack (packages):

   • Outer wrappings are considered nonsterile and must not be touched by sterile gloves. Bare hands can only touch the outside wrapper of a pack.
   • Always open sterile packs away from you to avoid touching your clothing, which is considered contaminated.
   • Use sterile packs immediately after opening. Never rewrap them for later use. They must be processed and resterilized.

6. **Sterile field:**   A work area which is prepared using sterile drapes (cloth) which hold the sterile supplies during the surgical procedure

   • Never reach or lean across the sterile field. The air above the sterile field is considered part of the field. Contaminated air droplets can fall into the field and cause infection if transferred to the patient.
   • Never talk, sneeze, or cough over the sterile field.
   • Avoid unnecessary movement around the sterile field.
   • Avoid spills on the sterile field. Moisture or wet areas are considered contaminated and must be covered with a sterile drape or towel.
   • Keep all items and gloved hands above waist level or at the level of the sterile field.
   • The sterile field should not be near windows, fans, drafts, or air conditioners since pathogenic microorganisms can be carried through the air currents.
   • A 1-inch perimeter around the outside of the sterile field is considered contaminated since it is in contact with the nonsterile work surface. Therefore place all sterile items in the center of the sterile field.
   • Do not pass anything over a sterile field.
   • Always face the sterile field. If you must turn away or turn your back to the field, cover the sterile field with a sterile towel.

7. All surgical team members (physicians, nurses, medical assistants) wearing sterile clothing must not leave the surgical area unless they rescrub and replace sterile clothing upon reentry.

▶ HANDLING SURGICAL INSTRUMENTS

Surgical instruments have been developed over the past centuries to meet a specific need during an operation such as cutting, suturing, and grasping. In some cases, an instrument developed by a surgeon bears the name of the surgeon, for example Kelly forceps, Halstead mosquito clamp, and the Bozeman uterine forceps.

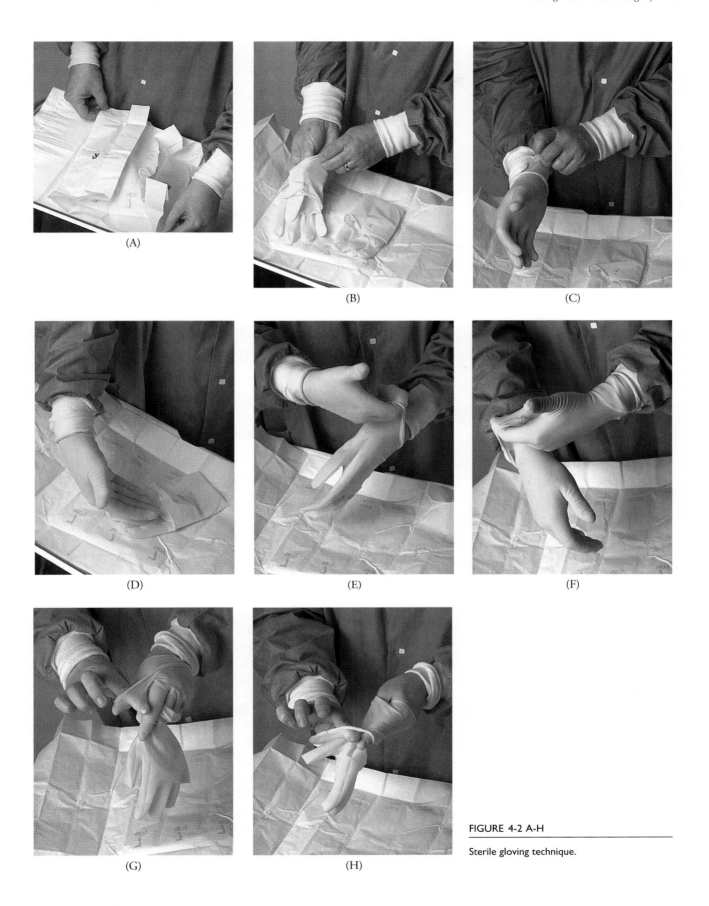

FIGURE 4-2 A-H

Sterile gloving technique.

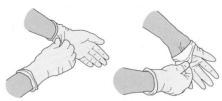
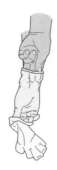
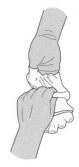

A Grasping the glove just below the cuff with the gloved fingers of the other hand, pull the glove over your hand, while turning it inside out.

B Place the ungloved index and middle fingers inside the cuff of the glove, turning the cuff downward, pulling it inside out, as you remove it from your hand.

FIGURE 4-2 A-B

Guidelines for removing gloves.

FIGURE 4-3

Gloving following sterile scrub.

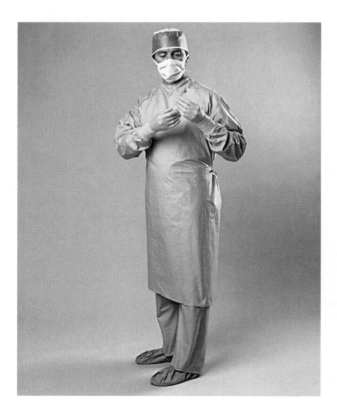

Med Tip: The medical assistant should be able to identify the various types of instruments. It is not necessary to remember the full name, for example Pederson vaginal speculum. However, you should be able to recognize that the instrument is a vaginal speculum. You may wish to develop flash cards of instruments to assist you in memorizing their names and function. *Note:* Some physicians will request an instrument by its full name.

PROCEDURE: Surgical Gloving

**Terminal Performance
Competency:** Apply sterile gloves without a break in sterile technique.

Equipment and Supplies
Double-wrapped sterile glove pack

Note: This procedure follows a surgical hand scrub.

Procedural Steps

1. Assemble equipment and check tape/seal for date and condition of pack.

2. Place the pack on a flat surface at waist height with the cuffed end of the gloves toward you.

3. Open the outside wrapper by touching only the outside of the pack. Leave the opened wrapper in place to provide a sterile work field.

4. Open the inner wrapper without reaching over the pack or touching the inside of the wrapper. Pull inner wrapper edges to each side without touching the inside of the pack. ***Rationale:*** Nonsterile persons or items contaminate a sterile field by reaching across it.

5. Using the thumb and fingers of your left hand (if you are right-handed) pick up the glove on the right side of the pack by grasping the folded inside edge of the cuff. The glove can be "dangled" slightly off the sterile packing material for easier insertion. ***Rationale:*** The folded inside edge of the glove will be placed against the skin and thus will be contaminated. The outer portion of the glove must not be touched by an ungloved hand since it must remain sterile.

6. Pull the glove onto the right hand using only the thumb and fingers of left hand. Do not allow fingers to touch the rest of the glove.

7. Place the fingers of the right gloved hand under the cuff of the left glove and pull onto the left hand and up over the left wrist. *Note:* Thumb of right gloved hand should not touch cuff.

8. With gloved left hand, place fingers under the cuff of the right glove and pull up over the right wrist. Thumb should not touch cuff. ***Rationale:*** The areas under the cuff are considered sterile. Only gloved fingers can touch this area.

9. After the gloves are in place, the fingers can be adjusted, if necessary by using the gloved hands.

10. Removing gloves: Remove the first glove by grasping the edge of that glove (with fingers of the other gloved hand) and pull the first glove over the hand inside out. Discard the first glove into the proper biohazardous waste container. Remove the other glove by grasping edge of the cuff with fingers (of the ungloved hand) and pull the second glove down over hand, inside out. Discard appropriately. ***Rationale:*** Turning the glove inside out seals in blood and body fluids.

INSTRUMENTS USED IN MINOR OFFICE SURGERY

The general classification of instruments is based on their use: cutting, dissecting, grasping, clamping, dilating, probing, visualization and suturing. There are special instruments related to individual specialties such as gynecology, urology, orthopedics, ear, nose, and throat, proctology, obstetrics, and neurology.

A minor surgical setup will include a standard group of instruments such as scalpel, blades, scissors, hemostat, and suture materials. Instruments are usually made of steel and treated to be rust and heat resistant, stain proof and durable.

PROCEDURE: Opening Sterile Packet

Terminal Performance
Competency: Open sterile packet (pack) and use it to set up a sterile field without a break in sterile technique.

Equipment and Supplies
Sterile packet
Mayo stand
Waste container
Sterile forceps

Procedural Steps
1. Wash hands.
2. Assemble equipment. Adjust Mayo stand to correct height.
3. Place packet on Mayo stand so that the folded edge is on top. Place on stand in position so that top flap will fold away from you.
   Rationale: You will not have to reach over sterile field to open last flap.
4. Remove tape or fastener and check sterilization indicator and date. Discard in waste container.
5. Pull the corner of pack that is tucked under and lay this flap away from you. It will hang down over the edge of the Mayo stand.
6. With both hands, pull the next two flaps to each side. The packet will still be covered with the last layer of the outer wrapper.
7. Grasp the corner of the last flap, without reaching over the sterile field, and open toward your body without touching.
8. The inside of this outer wrapper is now your sterile field. If you need to arrange items within this field, use sterile forceps. If an inner packet needs to be opened with an instrument setup, then someone wearing sterile gloves must open it.

CUTTING INSTRUMENTS

Scalpels or knives are used to make **incisions,** which are surgical cuts into tissue. They are small curved instruments which are made to fit easily into the surgeon's hand. A scalpel blade must be inserted into the scalpel handle. Blades come in various sizes depending on the type of incision and tissue: Number 10 and 12 are curved; Number 11 is used for I & D (incisions and drainage); Number 10 is straight; and Number 10 and 15 are used for foreign body removal. Figure 4-7 illustrates a variety of scalpels and blades.

DISSECTING INSTRUMENTS

The most common tool for dissecting or cutting tissue is the scissors. Scissors are also used to cut sutures (thread). Scissors have two blades with sharp edges which come together. The tips of scissors vary greatly since a variety of functions can be performed with the tips. Some scissors have blunt tips which can slide under bandages and dressings to cut without damaging the skin.

Operating scissors or suture scissors are used to cut suture material during surgery. They have a hook on one edge that fits under the suture for ease in suture removal. Dissecting scissors are also called straight or Mayo scissors. Metzenbaum scissors are short curved scissors which are used on delicate tissue. The tips of these scissors are blunt to prevent piercing tissue.

Operating scissors are straight or curved with a combination of blades such as sharp/sharp (s/s), blunt/blunt (b/b), and sharp/blunt (s/b); bandage scissors have a blunt tip and a blunt flat edge to allow it to fit easily under a bandage for cutting. Figure 4-8 illustrates a variety of types of scissors.

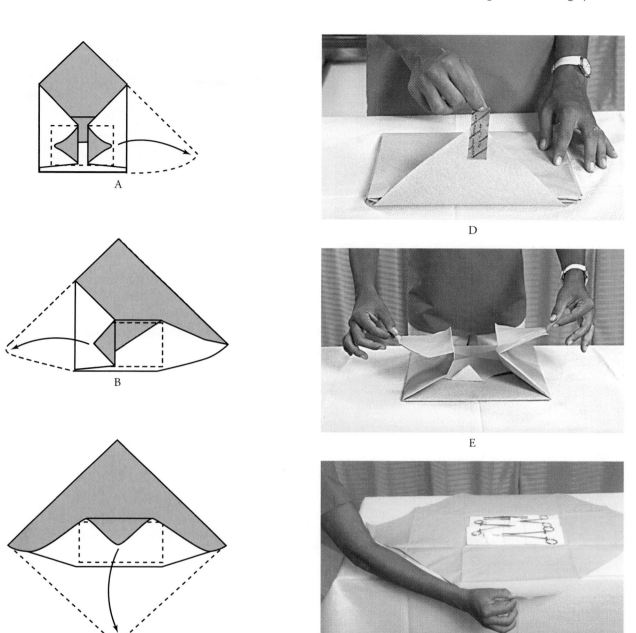

FIGURE 4-4 A-F

Opening a sterile packet.

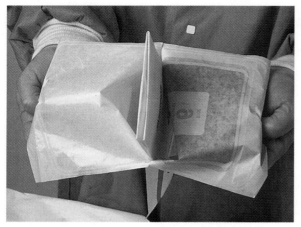

FIGURE 4-5

Dropping a sterile packet onto a sterile field.

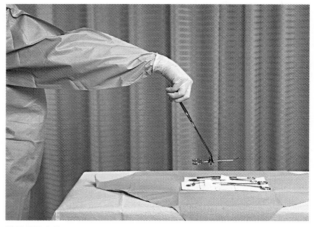

FIGURE 4-6

Proper way to handle a sterile equipment transfer.

PROCEDURE: Dropping Sterile Packet onto Sterile Field

Terminal Performance
Competency: Place (drop) sterile item onto a sterile field or into a gloved hand without contaminating the packet or the field.

Equipment and Supplies
  Sterile pack (containing for example: prepackaged items such as specimen container or needle and syringe in pull-apart packet)

Procedural Steps
  1. Assemble equipment, check date and sealed condition of packet.
  2. Locate the edge on the prepackaged item and pull apart by using thumb and forefinger of each hand. Do not let fingers touch the inside of the packet. **_Rationale:_** The inside of the packet is sterile and the outside is considered contaminated.

  3. Pull the packet apart by securely placing remaining three fingers of each hand against the outside of the packet on each side. The wrapper edges will be pulled back and away from the sterile item.
  4. Holding the item securely 8-10 inches from the sterile field, gently drop the contents inside the field. Instead of having you drop the item, the physician may wish to remove the item from the packet by grasping it firmly with his or her gloved hand. **_Rationale:_** Do not place your unsterile hands and arms over the sterile field.
  5. Discard the paper wrapper in waste container.

GRASPING AND CLAMPING INSTRUMENTS

Forceps are used to grasp tissue or objects (Figure 4-9). One type of forceps is a two-pronged instrument which has a spring-type handle that clamps together tightly to prevent slipping. Another type of closure mechanism is called a ratchet closure or clasp. The ratchet clasp allows the forceps to close with differing degrees of tightness. Forceps often have serration, or teeth-like, edges that prevent tissue slipping out of the forceps.

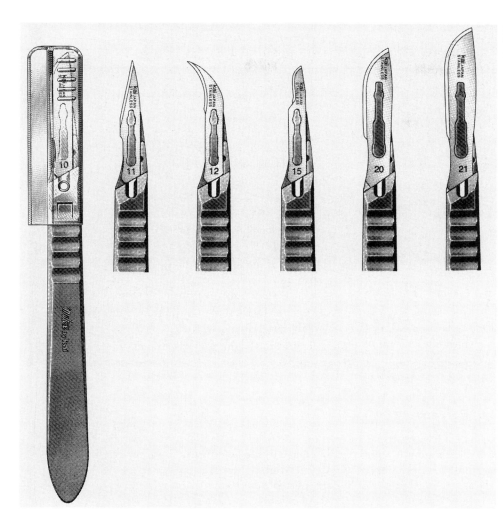

FIGURE 4-7

A variety of scalpels and blades.

PROCEDURE: Transferring Sterile Objects Using Transfer Forceps

Terminal Performance
Competency: Move sterile objects, such as instruments and supplies, within or onto a sterile field or into a gloved hand.

Equipment and Supplies
   Sterile transfer forceps in forceps container with sterilant solution such as Cidex

   Mayo stand with sterile field setup

   Sterile 4 × 4 gauze package, opened

Procedural Steps
   1. Grasp forceps handles firmly without separating the tips and remove vertically from the container. *Rationale:* Open forceps tips could touch the sides of the container which are considered contaminated. Remove vertically to avoid dripping solution onto exposed contaminated portion of forceps.
   2. Holding forceps vertically with tips down, gently tap tips together to drop excess solution onto a dry sterile 4 × 4 gauze or touch the 4 × 4 gauze to dry the tips.
   3. Pick up sterile item to be transferred by holding transfer forceps vertically with tips down. Do not touch the sterile field. Grasp the article to be transferred firmly at its midsection.
   4. Place sterile item within the sterile field. *Rationale:* Remember that the outer 1 inch of the sterile field is considered contaminated.
   5. Place forceps back into container without touching sides of container.
   6. Clean and sterilize the forceps and container in the autoclave once a week. Change solution weekly.

PROCEDURE: Transferring Sterile Solutions onto Sterile Field

**Terminal Performance
Competency:** Pour sterile fluid into a sterile basin on a sterile field without spilling solution or contaminating the field.

Equipment and Supplies
- Sterile saline or other solution as ordered
- Sterile basin
- Mayo stand or side tray
- Waste container

Procedural Steps
1. Wash hands
2. Assemble all equipment. Check expiration dates on solution and sterile basin pack.
3. Set up sterile basin on Mayo tray using inside of wrapper to create a sterile field.
4. Remove cap of solution and place it on a clean surface with outer edge down (inside facing up).

Avoid touching the inner surface of cap. *Rationale:* Inside of cap is considered sterile.

5. Check the label on bottle before pouring the solution.
6. Pour a small amount of the liquid into a waste container for discard. *Rationale:* This will dislodge any bacteria that may have collected on the edge of the bottle after opening.
7. Pour the bottle with the label held against the palm. *Rationale:* Protect the label from drips which can destroy the name of solution.
8. Hold the bottle about 6 inches above the basin and pour slowly to avoid splashing.
9. Replace the lid immediately after using.

Types of Forceps

- Tissue forceps have teeth and are used to grasp tissue.
- Thumb forceps are two-pronged with serrated tips to hold tissue.
- Sponge forceps are used for holding sponges during surgery.
- Towel clamps are used to hold the edges of sterile drapes together.
- Splinter forceps are used to grasp foreign bodies.
- Needle holder forceps are used to grasp needles during suturing.
- Hemostats are applied to blood vessels to hold vessels until they can be sutured.

Figure 4-9 depicts a variety of types of forceps and Figure 4-10 illustrates hemostats.

Guidelines: Handling Instruments

1. Instruments should be rinsed, cleaned, and scrubbed with a brush as soon as possible to prevent a hardening of blood and tissue materials.
2. Handle carefully. Do not throw instruments into the basin for cleaning.
3. Avoid allowing large amounts of instruments to become tangled. They are difficult to separate and could result in damaging your protective gloves.
4. Sharp instruments should remain separate from the rest.
5. Delicate instruments, such as those with lenses, should be handled separately.
6. Instruments with ratchets, should be stored open to prolong their life.
7. Check all instruments for defects before sterilizing them. All tips on instruments should close tightly, scissors should cut evenly, and cutting edges should be smooth.

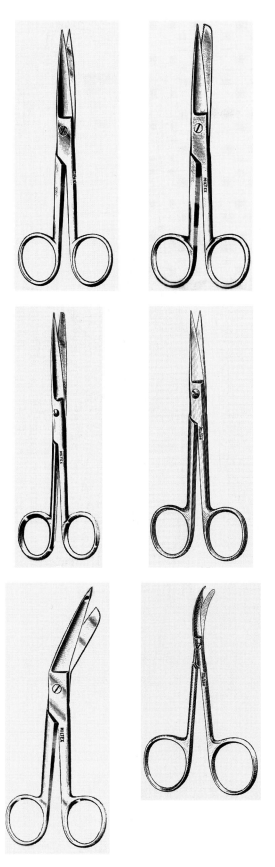

FIGURE 4-8

A variety of types of scissors.

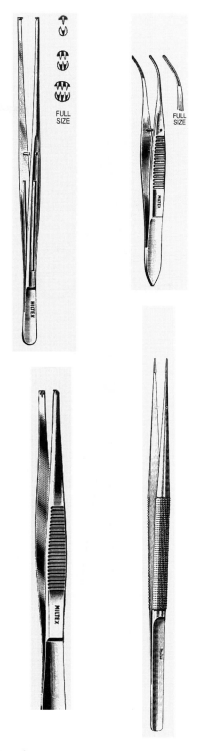

FIGURE 4-9

Types of forceps.

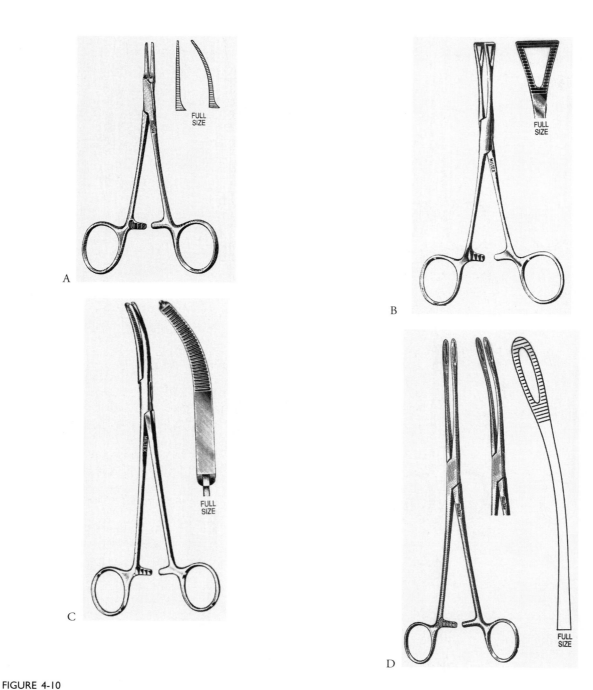

FIGURE 4-10

Hemostats: a) mosquito forceps; b) Pennington Hemostatic forceps; c) curved forceps; and d) sponge forceps.

PROBING AND DILATING INSTRUMENTS

Instruments used to enter body cavities for probing or dilating purposes include:

- *Scope:* An instrument, usually lighted, which is inserted into a body cavity or vessel to visualize the internal structures (Figure 4-11). An obturator is placed inside the scope to guide it into a cavity or canal then removed during visualization of the surgical site. Some obturators have a point which is used to puncture tissue.

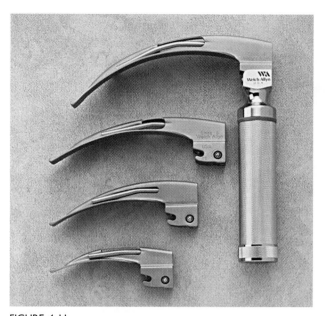

FIGURE 4-11

Laryngoscope.

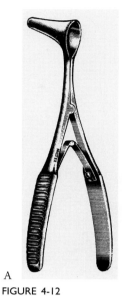
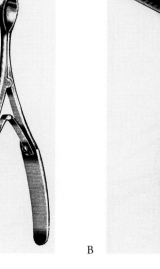
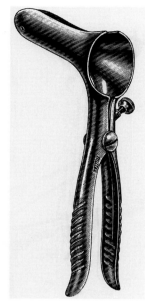

A   B

FIGURE 4-12

Speculum: a) nasal, and b) rectal.

- *Speculum:*   An unlighted instrument with movable parts which when inserted into a cavity such as the vagina, can be spread apart for ease of visualization and tissue sample removal (Figure 4-12).
- *Probe:*   An instrument used to explore wounds and cavities usually with a curved, blunt point to facilitate insertion (Figure 4-13).
- *Trocar:*   An instrument used to withdraw fluids from cavities. It consists of a cannula (outer tube) and a sharp stylette which is withdrawn after the trocar is inserted. Guide tubing or a wire (Figure 4-14).
- *Punch:*   An instrument used to remove tissue for examination and **biopsy** to detect cancerous cells.

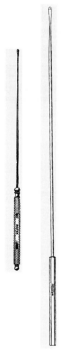

FIGURE 4-13

Probe.

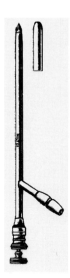

FIGURE 4-14

Trocar.

Specialized instruments are used for disciplines, such as gynecology and obstetrics (Figure 4-15 and 4-16), urology (Figure 4-17), and orthopedics (Figure 4-18).

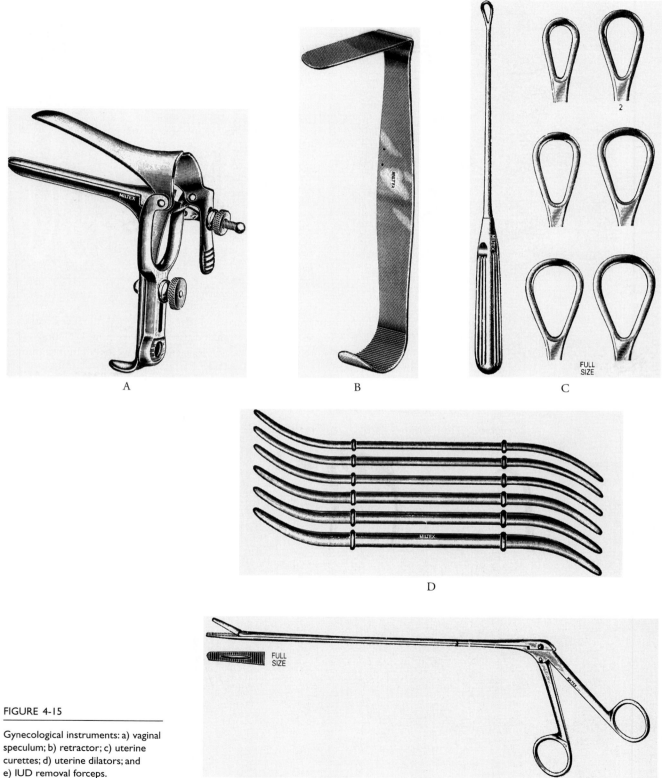

FIGURE 4-15

Gynecological instruments: a) vaginal speculum; b) retractor; c) uterine curettes; d) uterine dilators; and e) IUD removal forceps.
(Continued on next page)

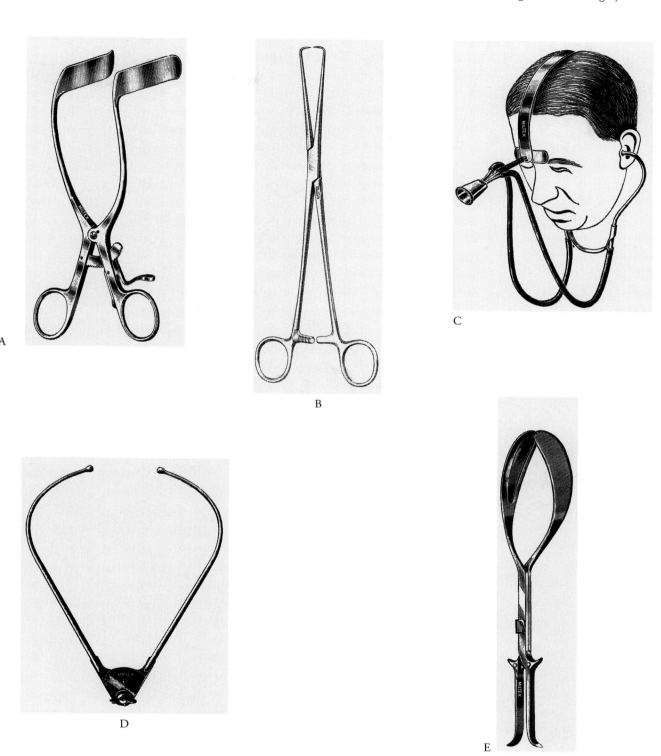

FIGURE 4-16

Gynecological instruments: a) vaginal retractor; b) uterine tenaculum forceps; c) obstetrical stethoscope; d) pelvimeter; and e) OB forceps. *(Continued)*

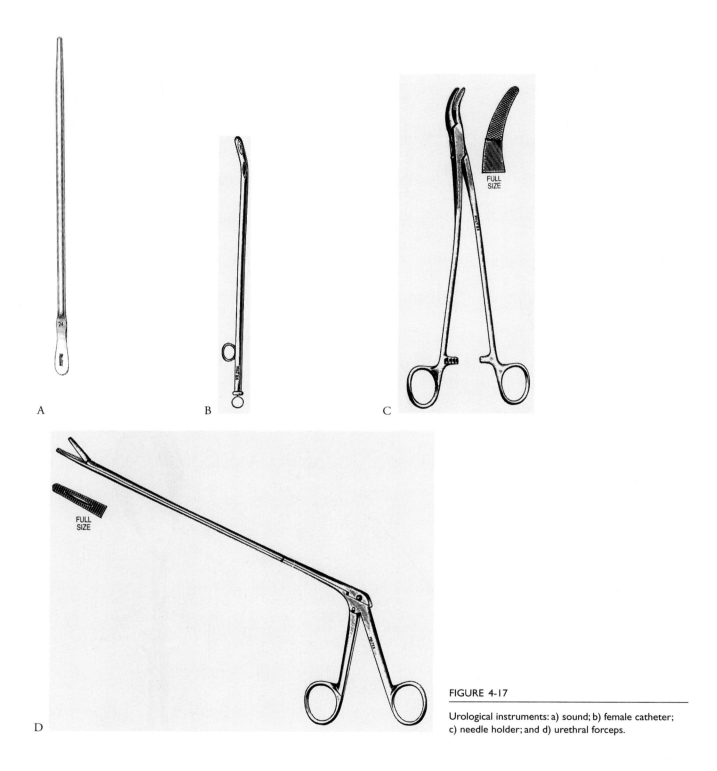

A

B

C

D

FULL
SIZE

FULL
SIZE

FIGURE 4-17

Urological instruments: a) sound; b) female catheter;
c) needle holder; and d) urethral forceps.

Guidelines for Handling Instruments

Surgical instruments are expensive and may be delicate. They require special care and attention. In some instances, there might not be a duplicate of an instrument. Even slight damage to an instrument can result in malfunction at a critical time during surgery.

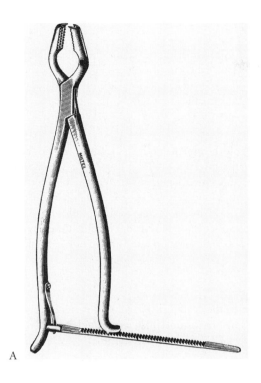

A

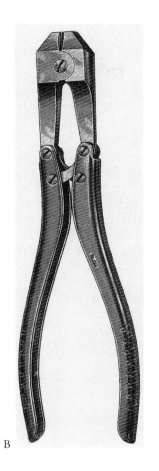

B

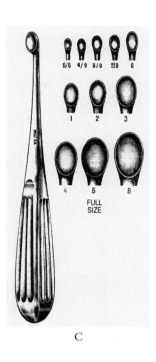

C

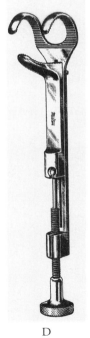

D

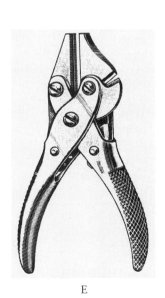

E

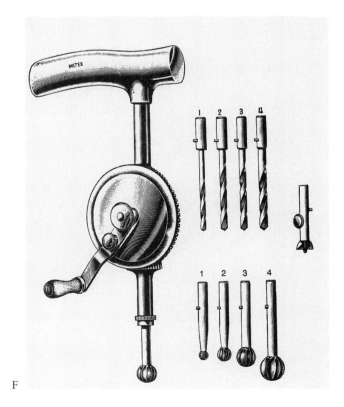

F

FIGURE 4-18

Orthopedic instruments: a) bone holding forceps; b) pin cutter;
c) bone curettes; d) bone clamp; e) wire cutters; and f) drill set.

SUTURE MATERIALS AND NEEDLES

Suture (thread) materials are used to bring together a surgical incision or wound until healing takes place. Suture materials are added to the surgical tray setup when they are needed for a procedure. Sutures come either with or without an attached needle. The package label will indicate type, size, and length of the suture material. Suture types include absorbable and non-absorbable.

Absorbable Sutures

Absorbable sutures are digested by tissue enzymes and absorbed by the body tissues. They do not have to be removed. Absorption usually occurs 5 to 20 days after insertion. This type of suture, such as surgical catgut (made from sheep's intestinal lining), is used for internal organs such as the bladder and intestines, subcutaneous tissue, and ligating, or tying off, blood vessels. They include plain cat gut, surgical cat gut, and chromic cat gut. Plain cat gut is used in areas where there is rapid healing such as highly vascular areas of the lips and tongue. Surgical cat gut is used on tissues in which there is fast healing such as the vaginal area. Chromic cat gut has a slower absorption rate and can be used to hold tissue together longer, such as for muscle repair.

Nonabsorbable Sutures

Nonabsorbable sutures are used on skin surfaces in which they can easily be removed after incisional healing takes place. This type of suture material, such as nylon, cotton, silk, dacron, and stainless steel, is not absorbed by the body. Black silk, which can easily be seen, is the most commonly used nonabsorbable suture.

Suture Material

Suture material varies and is selected based on the circumstances in which it is used.

- *Silk suture,* while the most expensive, is also considered the most dependable. It is widely used, easy to tie, and used as an all-purpose suture.
- *Nylon suture* has an elasticity and strength that makes it ideal for use in joints and skin closure. The disadvantage is the difficulty in forming a tight knot.
- *Polyester suture* is considered the strongest of all the standard suture material, with the exception of steel. Polyester is used in ophthalmic, cardiovascular, and facial surgery which all require a strong unbreakable suture since a broken suture could result in permanent damage to the patient.
- *Steel,* such as used in staples, is the most widely used suture material in major surgery. It is the strongest of all staple material.
- *Cotton suture,* with less strength than other suture materials, is no longer widely used.

The size, which is the gauge or diameter of suture material, is stated in terms of 0s, decreasing in size with the number of zeros. For example 6-0 (000000) is the smallest and 0 the thickest. Sizes 2-0 through 6-0 are most commonly used. Delicate tissue on areas such as the face and neck would be sutured with 5-0 to 6-0 suture material. These fine sutures would leave little scarring. Heavier sutures, such as 2-0, would be used for the chest or abdomen. The physician determines the type and gauge of sutures to be used. Table 4-2 summarizes suture uses, sizes, and types. Figure 4-19 illustrates different types of suture material.

Suture Needles

Suture needles are available in differing shapes depending on where they will be used. Needles have either a sharp cutting point, used for tissues that provide some resistance such as skin, or a round noncutting point used for more flexible tissue such as peritoneum. They are available in three shapes: straight, curved, or swagged.

The straight needle is used when the needle can be pushed and pulled through the tissue without the use of a needle holder. This type of needle will have an eye that needs to be threaded with the suture material. The suture material will then be double since it will enter the eye from one side and come out the other.

TABLE 4-2 **Suture Uses, Sizes, and Types**

Use	Gauge	Type of Material
Blood vessels	3-0 to 0	Chromic gut
	3-0	Cotton
	3-0 to 0	Silk
Eyelid	6-0 to 4-0	Silk
	6-0 to 5-0	Polyester
Skin	6-0 to 2-0	Nylon
	5-0 to 3-0	Polyethylene
	5-0 to 2-0	Stainless steel
Fascia	2-0 to 0	Chromic gut
	2-0 to 0	Silk
	2-0 to 0	Cotton
Muscle	3-0 to 0	Plain gut
	3-0 to 0	Chromic gut
	3-0 to 0	Silk

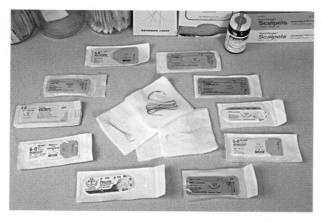

FIGURE 4-19

Types of suture material.

Curved needles allow the surgeon to go in and out of a tissue when there is not enough room to maneuver a straight needle. This type of needle requires a needle holder.

A swaged needle is one in which the needle and suture materials are combined in one length. They offer the advantage of not slipping off the needle since they are attached. A swaged needle pack will contain a label indicating the gauge, type, length of the suture material and the type of needle point (cutting or noncutting).

Other Wound Closure Materials

Other materials used for wound closure include sterile tapes, such as Steri-Strips (Figure 4-20). These sterile, nonallergenic tapes are available in a variety of widths. They are used instead of sutures when

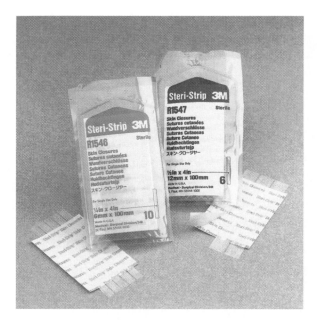

FIGURE 4-20

Steri-Strips from 3M.

not much tension will be applied to a wound, such as on a small facial cut. Sterile tapes must be applied by the physician since only a licensed physician can perform wound closure. The physician may delegate this task to another licensed professional, such as a physician's assistant (PA) or nurse (RN). Staples, made of stainless steel, are applied with a surgical stapler.

▶ SURGICAL ASSISTING

The medical assistant's role in surgical assisting varies depending on the type of office practice and the needs of the physician. For example, an eye surgeon who performs a large number of outpatient cataract operations may employ a full time **scrub assistant,** scrub tech, or O.R. tech, who will apply sterile gloves and hand instruments to the surgeon. In this case the medical assistant might act as the nonsterile assistant who positions the patient, uses transfer forceps to bring additional supplies as needed, holds the local anesthetic while the surgeon draws up the anesthetic, and applies dressings.

In many practices the medical assistant will scrub, apply sterile gloves, and act as the only assistant for the surgeon. A good assistant can help the procedure flow smoothly. The exact surgical tray setup and sequence of passing instruments will vary depending on the procedure and the surgeon's preferences.

A good assistant will anticipate the needs of the physician, use care in handing instruments, efficiently using care that an injury does not occur, and account for all materials used during the procedure. For example, if absorbent sponges are used to clean out the wound site during surgery, the assistant must maintain an accurate count to ensure that all sponges are removed before the patient's wound is closed.

The two types of assistants in the operating area are designated by the terms scrub and floater. The scrub assistant performs all procedures in sterile protective clothing using ster-

 Med Tip: Some physicians will have pictures on cards which demonstrate the setup and instrument packs they prefer.

Guidelines: Sterile Technique for Scrub Assistants

1. Always be aware of where your hands are since they should never touch an unsterile area. Immediately reglove if sterility is broken.

2. Arrange the surgical tray for efficiency closing all instruments that were left open during the autoclave process.

3. Close all instruments before passing them. Protect the surgeon from injury by handing needles with the point away from the physician, paying close attention to where scalpel blades and scissors' points are in relation to the physician's hands.

4. Anticipate the physician's needs by memorizing the types of instruments used in a procedure, and the order in which they are most often used. A card index with a list of the preferences for each procedure is useful for this purpose.

5. Do not release your grip on the instrument until you feel the physician take it away. This prevents an instrument falling to the floor and being damaged. In addition you may not have a duplicate of that particular instrument on your tray and it will cause a delay in the procedure.

6. Place the instrument with a firm "slap" into the physician's extended hand. Since he or she may not look up from the surgical site when their hand is extended, do not look away from the instrument until you feel it being taken from you. The handles should be placed into the physician's hands first.

7. If asked to provide retraction to open the incision area for better visualization, follow directions from the surgeon regarding the amount of pull needed. Move slowly and deliberately when retracting. Do not make abrupt, forceful moves.

8. If sutures are used to close the wound, be prepared to cut the suture material. The physician will pull both ends of the suture material together away from the wound. Cut both ends at the same time 1/8 to 1/4 inch above the knot.

9. Many requests for assistance will not be verbalized by the physician. It is important to pay attention and anticipate what instruments or assistance will be required next.

ile technique. Responsibilities include arranging the surgical tray to meet the physician's preferences, handing instruments, swabbing (sponging) bodily fluids away from the operative site, retracting the incision area, and cutting suture materials.

Figure 4-21 illustrates a medical assistant using proper technique when passing instruments to the physician. See the procedure for assisting the surgeon with a minor surgical procedure.

A float assistant provides the nonsterile needs during a surgical procedure and thus "floats" between the operating table, supplies, and equipment. One of the major roles of the float assistant is to monitor the patient by taking vital signs every 5-10 minutes.

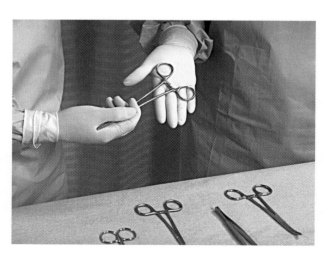

Med Tip: When practicing to assist as a scrub assistant, practice reaching for an instrument with your eyes closed. This is similar to the conditions under which the physician works since he or she does not look up from the operative site when reaching for instruments.

FIGURE 4-21

Medical assistant using proper technique when passing instruments to the physician.

Guidelines: Proper Technique for "Floating" Assistant During Surgical Procedure

1. Immediately report any unusual observations about the patient to the operating physician.

2. Use care not to touch the physician during any assisting since this will contaminate him or her and cause a delay in the procedure while the physician regloves (and regowns if necessary).

3. Provide additional medications such as local anesthetics that are needed during the procedure. This is done by following the correct procedure to identify the medication, clean top of vial/bottle with alcohol, hold vial/bottle upside down so that physician can insert sterile needle into vial without touching the contaminated outer surface, and keep the label in plain view for physician to read. Hold the vial firmly with both hands at your shoulder height for ease of withdrawal by the physician. Do not place the vial in front of your face. Note that the physician will have to use some force to be able to enter the vial with a needle.

4. Since the float assistant is unsterile, this person must perform all light adjustments, patient repositioning, chart notations made during the procedure, requisition forms, and specimen container labeling.

5. The float assistant can place additional sterile materials and instruments onto the sterile field by opening the packet without touching the sterile inside and gently "dropping" them onto the Mayo stand. The sterile scrub assistant or physician may remove them from the inside of the packet as the float holds firmly onto the outside.

6. When holding a container to receive a specimen, tilt the container slightly so the physician can place the specimen inside without touching the rim of the container.

A surgical setup for a typical minor surgical procedure would include:

- Local anesthetic materials
- 3 cc syringe with needle(s)
- Alcohol sponges to cleanse vial top
- Sterile gloves for surgeon
- 4 × 4 and 2 × 2 gauze sponges
- No. 3 scalpel blades and handle, extra scalpel blades (No. 10, 11, and 15)
- Curved iris scissors
- Tissue forceps
- Straight and curved mosquito forceps
- Straight and curved Kelly forceps
- Towel forceps
- Sterile drape towels
- Needle holder with mounted needle and suture materials
- Sterile specimen container with preservative solution

Figure 4-22 is an illustration of pouring sterile solution into a container and Figure 4-23 shows a sterile instrument setup.

▶ PREPARING THE PATIENT FOR MINOR SURGERY

For purposes of efficiency some of the preoperative patient preparation can take place before the patient arrives for the procedure. For example, patient education with an explanation of the procedure, preoperative and postoperative instructions, and laboratory testing can take place up to a week before the actual procedure.

Preoperative and postoperative instructions can be presented in a variety of formats including one-on-one discussion, videotapes, brochures, pamphlets, and models. These instructions need to be reinforced either through a telephone reminder, as with notification of the time to arrive for surgery, or through another explanation of the same material. It is especially important to provide

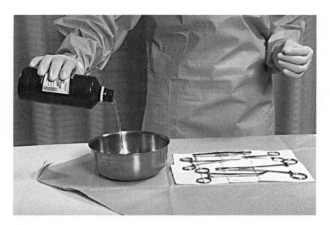

FIGURE 4-22

Pouring sterile solution into a container.

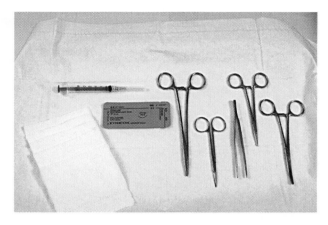

FIGURE 4-23

Sterile instrument setup.

postoperative instructions in a variety of formats since the patient may not be fully alert right after the surgery. Family members should be included in these explanations whenever practical.

Preoperative instructions might include an explanation of what laboratory testing is needed and when it is to be done, cleansing enemas, food and fluid restrictions, special bathing/skin cleansing preparations, and bedtime sedative use. At this time the patient can be instructed about when to call the physician postoperatively. The patient should be cautioned to call the medical office if they have any illness, such as a cold or fever, the day of surgery.

Patients should be told orally and in writing to have someone drive them to and from the surgical facility, especially if they will be given a general anesthetic. Questions should be encouraged. However, the medical assistant must refer all questions to the physician which relate to the risk of surgery or the possible outcomes.

 Med Tip: Ask the patient to restate the instructions if you are concerned that the patient does not understand. You can repeat specific instructions, clarifying the area(s) of confusion for the patient. Then chart, "patient states understanding of the procedure."

The patient's vital signs (blood pressure, temperature, pulse, and respirations) should be taken before the procedure.

INFORMED CONSENT

The patient must be provided an honest, thorough explanation of the surgical procedure including the benefits and risks. Any invasive procedure in which the body is entered with a scalpel, scissors, or other device requires written permission (consent) from the patient. Procedures in which a body cavity is entered for purposes of visualization, even though no incision is made, such as in bronchoscopy and cystoscopy, also require written consent.

The procedure, with all risks involved, must be explained by the physician. Every attempt must be made to determine if the patient actually understands the explanation given by the physician. The medical assistant can witness the patient's signing the consent form.

POSITIONING AND DRAPING

Instruct the patient to remove all clothing and put on a patient gown with the ties at the back, unless otherwise instructed. The patient is assisted onto the operating table and placed in the proper posi-

PROCEDURE: Assisting With Minor Surgery

**Terminal Performance
Competency:** Prepare all materials and equipment for immediate use in a surgical procedure using sterile technique.

Equipment and Supplies

Mayo stand

Side stand

Transfer forceps and container

Sharps container

Waste container/plastic bag

Biohazard waste container

Anesthetic

Alcohol swab

Sterile specimen container,
   depending on type
   of surgery

Sterile pack:

- Sterile gloves (2 pairs)
- Towel pack
- 4 × 4 sponge pack
- Patient drape
- Needle pack and
  suture materials

Instrument pack(s) including towel clamp pack

Syringe pack

Sterile basin pack (2)

Procedural Steps

1. Wash hands.
2. Open sterile tray packs on Mayo stand and side stand. Use sterile wrapper to create a sterile field. The wrapper will hang over the edges of the tray.
3. Use sterile transfer forceps to move instruments on tray or to place equipment from packets. Materials in peel-away packets should be flipped onto the tray.
4. Open sterile needle and syringe unit and drop gently onto sterile field. Use care not to reach over the sterile field.
5. Open sterile drape packs and towel clamp packs.
6. Open a set of sterile gloves for the physician.
7. After tray is ready with all equipment open and arranged, pull edge of sterile towel across the tray using sterile transfer forceps. **Rationale:** The sterile towel will provide a protective covering for the sterile tray until the procedure begins. The medical assistant should not leave the room once the tray is set up.

Operative Assist:

8. When the physician has donned the sterile gloves, remove the sterile towel covering the tray of instruments.

9. Remove the towel by standing to one side and grasp the two distal corners. Lift the towel toward you so that you do not reach over the unprotected sterile field.
10. Cleanse the vial of anesthetic with a sterile alcohol swab and hold it upside down in the palm of your hand with the label facing toward the physician. Hold it steady while the physician draws up the anesthetic.
11. Stand to one side of the patient and assist the physician as requested. Supply additional supplies as needed. *Note:* If you assist by handing instruments directly to the physician, you must perform a surgical scrub and wear a sterile gown and gloves.
12. Hold all containers for specimens, drainage, or contaminated 4 × 4s. Wear nonsterile gloves to protect yourself from contact with drainage.
13. Collect and place all soiled instruments in a basin out of the patient's view.
14. Place all soiled gauze sponges (4 × 4s) and dressings in a plastic bag. Do not allow wet items to remain on a sterile field.
15. Immediately label all specimens as they are obtained. Close the specimen container tightly.
16. Periodically reassure the patient by quietly asking how he or she is doing. Do not touch the patient with soiled gloves.
17. When procedure is complete, wash hands before assisting patient.
18. Allow the patient to rest and recover from the anesthetic. Periodically check the patient's vital signs according to office policy.
19. Provide clear oral and written postoperative instructions for the patient. Make sure the patient is stable before he or she leaves the office.
20. Send specimen(s) to the laboratory with requisition slip.
21. Clean, sanitize and sterilize the instruments. Clean and sanitize the room in preparation for the next patient.
22. Wash hands.

Charting Example

The physician will chart the details of the surgical procedure.

tion for the procedure by the medical assistant. Every attempt should be made to assure the patient's comfort since the patient may have to remain in one position for an extended period of time. General guidelines for positioning and draping are discussed in Chapter 5, Assisting with Physical Examinations.

ANESTHESIA

Anesthesia, the partial or complete loss of sensation, is used to block the pain of surgery. Anesthesia can also relax muscles, produce amnesia, calm anxiety, and cause sleep. Medical assistants do not administer anesthetics, but they should be familiar with them and their effects.

The two types of anesthetics are general or local (conduction). A general anesthetic depresses the central nervous system (CNS) to cause unconsciousness. It is generally administered through inhalation or intravenous injection (IV).

Inhalation types of anesthetics are in the form of gases or volatile liquids. In many cases, these are administered after a patient has received a sedative or narcotic to relieve pain or a tranquilizer to relieve anxiety. Sedatives and narcotics are usually administered intramuscularly before surgery. In some cases, they are administered by IV immediately before the general anesthetic is given.

Intravenous anesthetics (IV) are a type of hypnotic sedative that produce anesthesia, or sleep, when given in large doses. Sodium-Pentothal is an example of this type of anesthetic.

Precautions to be taken when administering an general anesthetic include:

- Administering the anesthetic on an empty stomach. This is to prevent vomiting and possible aspiration of vomitus into lungs resulting in pneumonia.
- Cautioning patients not to drive or engage in other activity that could result in harm from an impaired consciousness. General anesthetics can interfere with patient's alertness for 12 to 24 hours after surgery.
- Advising patients to avoid alcohol and depressant drugs 2-3 days before surgery and 1 day after surgery.

Local anesthetics provide loss of sensation in a particular location without overall loss of consciousness. A local anesthetic is also referred to as a conduction anesthetic. The conduction of pain transmission by way of the nervous system is blocked. Examples of this type of anesthetic are

- Topical and local infiltration which act on nerve endings.
- Nerve block which affects pain transmission along a single nerve.
- Regional block, spinal, epidural, or saddle blocks which affect a group of nerves.

A local infiltration anesthetic is injected directly into the tissue that will be operated upon. Examples of a "local" are lidocaine hydrochloride (Xylocaine) and procaine hydrochloride (Novocain). This type of anesthetic is used for such procedures as removal of skin growths, skin suturing and dental surgery. Local anesthesia takes from 5 to 15 minutes to become effective and lasts from 1 to 3 hours. An additional injection of anesthetic may have to be administered when the first has worn off.

Epinephrine, which is a vasoconstrictor causing superficial blood vessels to narrow, is often added to the local anesthetic when the physician is operating on the face and head. The addition of epinephrine allows for better visualization of the surgical site since bleeding is diminished. Epinephrine also causes local anesthetics to be absorbed by the body more slowly. This causes the anesthetic to have a longer lasting effect. Clearly mark anesthetics that have been prepared with the addition of epinephrine. Patients with heart problems could have a reaction to epinephrine causing tachycardia or irregularities.

Nerve blocks are administered by injection into a nerve adjacent to the operative site. This type of anesthetic is used for surgery on hands, fingers, and toes.

Topical anesthetics are local pain control medications that are applied

Med Tip: An emergency tray or cart containing drugs used to counteract shock and other emergencies should always be available in the medical office.

PROCEDURE: Assisting with Suturing

**Terminal Performance
Competency:** Assist with suture repair of an incision or laceration using sterile technique.

Equipment and Supplies

Mayo stand

Side stand

Anesthetic

Sterile transfer forceps

Sterile saline

Waste container/plastic bag

Biohazardous waste container

Sharps container

Sterile gloves (2 pairs)

Sterile pack(s):

- Patient drape
- Towel pack (four towels)
- 4 × 4 gauze sponge pack

Scalpel blades pack (No. 10 and 15)

Needle and syringe pack

Suture and needle pack
   (according to physician's preference)

Sterile basin (2)

Suture pack:

- Scalpel handle
- Needle holder
- Thumb forceps
- Two scissors
- Three hemostats

Procedural Steps

1. Use sterile scrub and gloving procedure.
2. Stand across from the physician.
3. Place two sponges ready for the physician near the wound site. *Rationale:* Physician will use sponges to clear drainage during initial inspection of the wound.
4. Assist by using additional sponges to keep wound dry.
5. Pass instruments, such as scissors, to physician using a firm "snap" of the handle into his or her hand. *Rationale:* The instrument should be firmly placed in the physician's hand without letting go until the physician has a firm grasp.
6. The blade is placed into the scalpel using a hemostat.
7. Hand the scalpel to the physician with blade edge down to avoid cutting the physician.
8. Continue to use sponges to keep the wound free of drainage.
9. Pass all instruments to the physician as requested. Try to anticipate the need for the next instruments, such as another hemostat or scissors for cutting suture.
10. Pass the toothed forceps to physician if laceration edges need to be grasped.
11. Mount the needle into the needle holder and pass as one unit to the physician using care to keep the suture within the sterile field. Pass the needle holder with the needle pointing outward. Hold the suture with the other hand and do not let go of it until the physician sees it.
12. Using the suture scissors prepare to cut the suture as directed by the physician (usually 1/8 to 1/4 inch from the knot).
13. Sponge the closed wound once with a sponge and discard.
14. Repeat this step with each suture.
15. Handle all soiled instruments after they are used by placing them back onto the sterile field if they will be used again, or discard into the instrument basin.
16. When procedure is complete, remove gloves and wash hands before assisting patient.
17. Allow the patient to rest and recover from the anesthetic. Periodically check the patient's vital signs according to office policy.
18. Provide clear oral and written postoperative instructions for the patient. Make sure the patient is stable before he or she leaves the office.
19. Clean, sanitize and sterilize the instruments. Clean and sanitize the room in preparation for the next patient.
20. Wash hands.

Charting example:
The physician will chart the details of the surgical procedure.

to the skin and produce a numbing effect. These can be applied by drop, spray, or swabbed. They are commonly used in eye procedures. An example of a spray anesthetic is ethyl chloride which produces a "freezing" effect on the skin. Benzocaine (Solarcaine) is another example of a topical anesthetic.

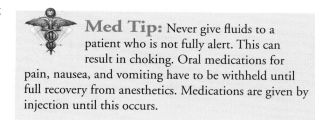

Med Tip: Never give fluids to a patient who is not fully alert. This can result in choking. Oral medications for pain, nausea, and vomiting have to be withheld until full recovery from anesthetics. Medications are given by injection until this occurs.

The effects of topical and other local anesthetics occur either immediately or within a few minutes. These effects wear off quickly. Large amounts of local anesthetic, beyond the normal dosages, are not recommended and may result in an adverse reaction in patients. Some patients are allergic to anesthetics and may slip into anaphylactic shock which requires emergency treatment.

Patients who receive a local anesthetic in their mouth or throat should be advised not to eat until the effects of the anesthetic wear off to prevent choking on food or burning the mouth. Table 4-3 contains examples of local anesthetics.

Both the strength and dosage of the anesthetic must be charted. Since only physicians or anesthesiologists can administer an anesthetic, only they can chart the administration. Either the medical assistant or the physician will draw up the local anesthetic. Using the correct procedure for drawing up medication as discussed in Chapter 7, the vial must be correctly identified and then wiped with an alcohol sponge. If the medical assistant draws up the medication then she or he must present both the syringe and the vial to the physician so that the label can be read by the physician. The anesthetic will be injected into the patient's prepared skin by the physician before the physician has donned gloves. This syringe is not placed onto the sterile field since it has been contaminated by the medical assistant's ungloved hands.

If the physician prefers to draw up the anesthetic, it can be done using a sterile syringe after he or she has applied gloves. The medical assistant will hold the vial securely while the physician withdraws the anesthetic without contaminating the needle. The outside of the vial cannot be touched by the physician's sterile gloved hand. This syringe can then be placed onto the sterile field.

Some physicians prefer to change the needle after drawing up the local anesthetic. For example, they may draw up the drug using a 21 gauge needle and then administer the solution using a 23 or 25 gauge needle.

PREPARATION OF PATIENT'S SKIN

While skin cannot be sterilized, it can be cleaned using medical aseptic technique. Careful cleansing of skin before performing a surgical procedure will reduce the number of microorganisms on the skin. This will reduce the chance of carrying infection producing microorganisms through the skin during the invasive procedure (incision into skin or entrance of a probe).

TABLE 4-3   Local Anesthetics

Anesthetic Agent	Use
Benzocaine	Topical use only
Chloroprocaine	Nerve block, epidural
Lidocaine (Xylocaine)	Infiltration or topical
Mepivacaine	Infiltration nerve block
Procaine (Novocain)	Infiltration; seldom used now
Tetracaine	Infiltration, topical nerve block, spinal

In some situations, the physician may order the surgical site to be shaved since bacteria can reside in hair. Care must be taken to avoid scraping or cutting the skin during the shaving process. The physician will order either a dry shave or a wet shave (moistening the skin with soap and water) according to the physician's preference. See procedure for skin preparation. Figure 4-24 illustrates preparation of the patient's skin for surgical procedures. See Figure 4-25 for an example of a dry skin prep tray.

▶ POSTOPERATIVE PATIENT CARE

Postoperative care includes caring for the patient during recovery from anesthesia, wound care, applying dressings, and patient instructions.

RECOVERY FROM ANESTHESIA

Patients must be observed carefully after surgery for signs of adverse reaction to the anesthetic, bleeding, and circulatory problems. The patient's vital signs (blood pressure, temperature, pulse, and respiration) should be monitored immediately after surgery and then every 15 minutes for the first hour.

Excessive disorientation and inability to arouse within a normal time for recovery should be reported immediately to the physician. The patient should be observed for nausea and/or vomiting. Medications may be ordered by the physician to counteract nausea and vomiting.

WOUND CARE

Any break in the skin, whether from an injury or a surgical incision, is referred to as a wound. A surgical procedure requiring an incision through the skin is considered an **invasive** procedure since the skin is entered and creates a wound. Wounds cause blood vessels to rupture and seep into tissues, which results in skin

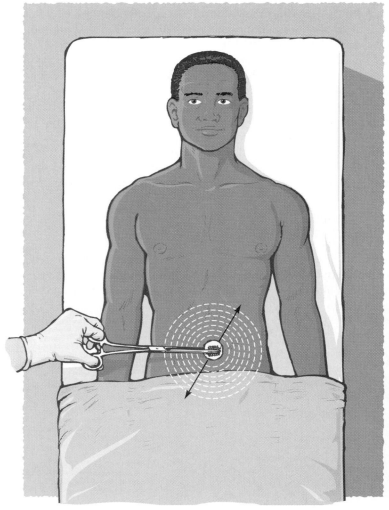

FIGURE 4-24

Preparing the patient's skin at the surgical site.

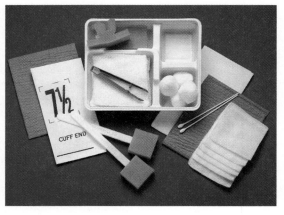

FIGURE 4-25

Dry skin prep tray.

PROCEDURE: Preparing the Patient's Skin for Surgical Procedures

**Terminal Performance
Competency:** To prepare patient's skin for surgical procedure using sterile scrub and shave.

Equipment and Supplies

Antiseptic germicidal soap

Sterile saline

Antiseptic such as betadine

Sterile applicators (8)

Mayo tray or side tray

Waste receptacle (may be included in sterile pack)

Hazardous waste container

Plastic bag for soiled dressings

Sterile Pack:

- Sterile gloves
- Towel pack (3-4 towels)
- Sterile basin pack (3 basins)
- Patient drape
- 4 × 4 gauze sponge pack (12-24 sponges)
- Shave prep kit

Note: This procedure follows a surgical hand scrub.

Procedural Steps

1. Wash hands
2. Assemble equipment by placing packs on Mayo stand or side tray and unwrapping outer wraps from all packs.
3. Identify patient and explain procedure.
4. Have patient remove appropriate clothing and gowning. Ask patient to void, if necessary.
5. Position and drape the patient to provide exposure of the operative site.
6. Unwrap the basin pack. Pour germicidal soap solution into one basin; sterile saline into the second basin; and antiseptic into the third. **Rationale:** Liquids are poured by holding the outer nonsterile surface of the containers before applying sterile gloves.
7. Wash using sterile scrub and apply sterile gloves.
8. Drape the skin with two towels placed 3-5 inches above and below the surgical site.
9. With a sterile gauze/sponge apply soapy solution to patient's skin. Use a circular motion starting at the site of proposed incision and move outward. Pass over each skin area only once. Place each used sponge into waste receptacle immediately. *Note:* Some physicians prefer the patient receive a dry shave.
10. Take a fresh sterile gauze/sponge for each cleansing wipe. Repeat this process until the area is com-

pletely washed. The last area cleansed will be the outer edges.

11. Rinse using sterile saline on clean gauze/sponge. Pat dry with dry gauze only on the area that has been washed. Avoid touching any other skin area. **Rationale:** The surrounding skin is considered contaminated since it has not been washed.
12. If shaving is ordered, then proceed with the following steps.
13. Apply soap solution to area. Remove razor from shave prep pack. Pull skin taut and shave surgical site in the direction in which the hair is growing. Rinse with saline solution using the single-pass, circular motion as before and pat dry. **Rationale:** Shaving against the direction of hair growth can irritate the skin. This skin breakdown will allow bacteria to enter.
14. Reapply soap solution to area and repeat the above process for the time according to office policy (around 5 minutes).
15. Pat dry the entire area with the third sterile towel.
16. Apply the antiseptic solution using two cotton applicators together in the same single-pass, circular motion.
17. Cover the prepared surgical site with the remaining sterile towel.
18. Properly dispose of gloves and soiled materials in biohazard bag/container.
19. To dispose of soiled dressings use following steps:
    a. Remove gloves.
    b. Place one hand into the empty plastic bag.
    c. Using the hand covered with the plastic bag, pick up all the soiled materials. With other hand pull the outside of the bag over the soiled dressings.
    d. Dispose of this bag in a hazardous waste bag/container.
20. Wash hands and document procedure.

Charting Example

3/12/XX Pt. arrived for removal and biopsy of growth on outer aspect of left forearm. Surgical site prepared using betadine. No cuts or lesions noted.   J. Wall, RMA

color changes. Typically, skin coloration during wound healing will change from erythema in a fresh wound to a greenish yellow color, during the healing process involving an oxidation of blood pigments. There are four types of wound classification:

- *Abrasion:*   Wound in which outer layers of skin are rubbed away due to scraping. Will generally heal without scarring.
- *Incision:*   Smooth cut resulting from a surgical scalpel or sharp material, such as razor or glass. May result in excessive bleeding if deep and scarring.
- *Laceration:*   Wound in which the edges are torn in an irregular shape. Can cause profuse bleeding and scarring.
- *Puncture:*   Wound made by a sharp pointed instrument such as a bullet, needle, nail, or splinter. External bleeding is usually minimal but infection may occur due to penetration with a contaminated object and there may be scarring.

Wound healing will pass through various stages, including inflammation, as the body starts to fight off potential infection. To prevent infection surgical wounds must be handled carefully. In most situations, a wound or surgical site will require a sterile dressing as protection against bacteria, trauma, to absorb any drainage, and to protect against motion damaging the suture site. The patient should be asked how long it has been since he or she received a tetanus shot. In the event that the shot was not received within the last ten years, the physician should be informed.

The size and shape of the dressing will depend on the size, location and amount of drainage from the wound. Sterile 4×4 inch gauze pads (called four by fours) are used for most dressings. If there is drainage expected from the wound, a prepared dressing such as Telfa may be used to prevent the dressing sticking to the wound. See Figure 4-26 for an example of a wound closure kit. The procedure for changing a sterile dressing follows.

A dressing is the application of a sterile covering over a surgical site or wound using surgical asepsis. Figure 4-27 illustrates classification of wound healing. A bandage is the application of covering over a nonsterile area using medical asepsis. Figure 4-28 shows various types of bandages.

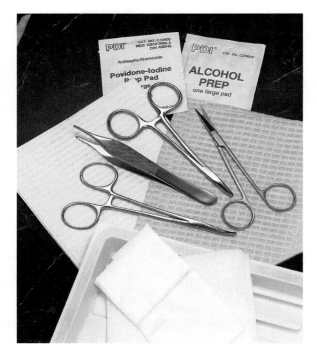

FIGURE 4-26

Wound closure kit.

First Intention

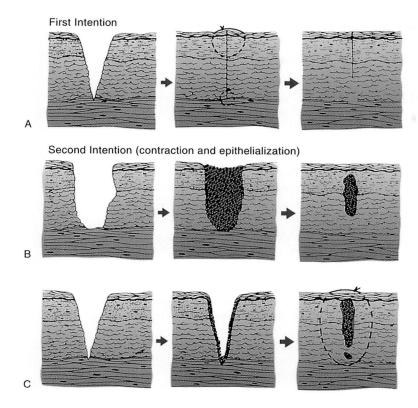

Second Intention (contraction and epithelialization)

A

B

C

FIGURE 4-27

Classification of wound healing: a) First intention: A clean incision is made with primary closure; there is minimal scarring. (B and C) Second intention: The wound is left open so that granulation can occur; a large scar results, b) or the wound is initially left open and later closed when there is no further evidence of infection c).

FIGURE 4-28

Various types of bandages.

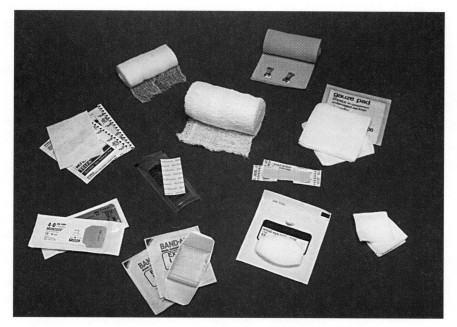

SUTURE REMOVAL

Sutures are inserted by the surgeon at the end of a procedure to hold tissues in alignment during the healing process. Sutures generally remain in place from 5-6 days and then have to be removed if they are nonabsorbable. If sutures remain in the body too long, they can cause skin irritation and

PROCEDURE: Changing a Sterile Dressing

Terminal Performance
Competency: Change a wound dressing using proper sterile technique.

Equipment and Supplies

- Disposable gloves
- Antiseptic solution
- Solution container
- Prepackaged dressing pack
- Thumb forceps
- Sterile cotton balls
- Sterile gloves
- Sterile dressing
- Adhesive tape
- Scissors, if necessary for tape
- Waste container/plastic bag
- Biohazardous waste container
- Mayo stand or side tray

Procedural Steps

1. Wash hands.
2. Assemble equipment using Mayo stand.
3. Prepare the sterile field using aseptic technique using prepackaged dressing packet. Use sterile transfer forceps to place additional sterile items onto the sterile field.
4. Explain procedure to patient.
5. Assist patient into comfortable position with area to be dressed resting on support, such as an examination table.
6. Apply nonsterile gloves.
7. Remove dressing from wound by loosening tape with gloved hands or forceps and pulling it from both sides toward the wound. Without passing the soiled dressing over the sterile field, place it into the soiled waste bag. Do not allow the dressing to touch the outside or edges of the bag.
8. Inspect the wound for signs of infection and inflammation. Note any discharge for type, amount and odor.
9. Discard gloves and contaminated forceps properly. Disposable gloves and forceps are placed in waste container. Reusable forceps are placed in basin for later cleaning.
10. Open sterile gloves and apply properly.
11. Drop antiseptic onto several cotton balls until they are moist but not saturated. Clean the wound by using sterile forceps to hold the cotton. Cleanse the wound moving from top to bottom of the wound once. Use a new cotton ball with antiseptic for each wipe. Move from the inside of the wound to the outside edges.
12. Pick up the sterile dressing with gloved hands and place over the wound.
13. Discard gloves and forceps.
14. Apply adhesive tape to hold dressing in place. Do not apply so tightly as to restrict circulation. The strips of tape should be long enough to hold the dressing in place. Do not wrap the tape entirely around an extremity or completely cover the dressing.
15. Instruct the patient on dressing care and follow-up appointment to see the physician.
16. Chart the procedure including date, time, location and condition of wound and instructions given to the patient.

Charting Example
2/14/XX 11:00 am. Drsg. change on Left anterior forearm. Moderate amt. serous drainage with slight erythema surrounding wound. Incision healing well with edges aligned. Cleansed with betadine. Sterile drsg. applied. Pt. instructed on wound care.   M. King, CMA

infection. The suture acts as a wick to carry bacteria through the skin and into the subcutaneous tissues. Suture removal times differ depending upon the site:

- Facial sutures may be removed after only 24 to 48 hours to prevent scarring.
- Head and neck sutures remain for 3-5 days.

- Abdominal sutures remain from 5 to 7 days.
- Sutures over weight bearing joints and large bones may remain 7 to 10 days.

The medical assistant prepares the patient for suture removal by removing the dressing, if one is present. Each edge of the dressing is removed by pulling toward the suture line. If the dressing is adhering to the suture line then a small amount of sterile saline or hydrogen peroxide can be used to moisten the dressing for ease in removing.

In some office practices and in some states, the medical assistant is able to remove sutures. The procedure should be explained to the patient reminding them that they may feel a pulling sensation. The skin is then thoroughly cleansed with an antiseptic such as alcohol or betadine solution. After opening the sterile suture packet and creating a sterile field with the wrapper, the knot of the suture is gently picked up using a thumb forceps. The suture is then cut with suture scissors below the knot as close to the skin as possible. The suture is removed by pulling the long remaining suture out. Suture material that is outside of the skin should not be pulled through the skin due to the danger of pulling infection along with it. Very little of the suture is actually pulled through the skin. Suture removal is illustrated in Figure 4-29. A disposable suture removal set is displayed in Figure 4-30.

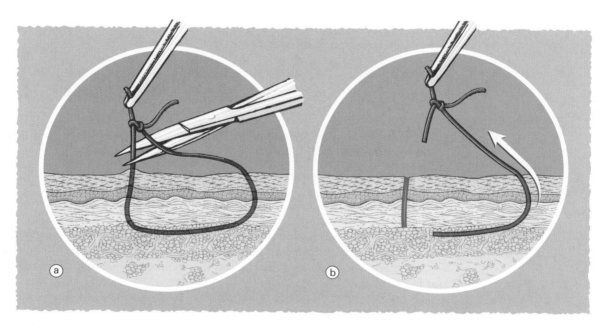

FIGURE 4-29

Removal of sutures.

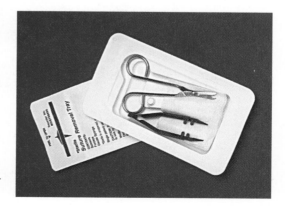

FIGURE 4-30

Disposable suture removal set.

▶ SURGICAL PROCEDURES PERFORMED IN THE MEDICAL OFFICE

Many minor surgical procedures can be performed efficiently in the physician's office. This saves the patient the time and expense of having to go into an ambulatory surgical facility or a hospital. The basic surgical setup is the standard setup with the addition of specific instruments for each procedure. Some of the minor procedures performed in the medical office include biopsy, cautery, colposcopy, cryosurgery, endocervical curettage, suture removal, removal of foreign bodies, incision and drainage, vasectomy, and removal of growths and tumors.

The medical assistant does not administer these procedures but must understand them and their effects so that he or she can assist the physician and the patient. A brief description of some of these procedures follows.

ELECTROSURGERY

Electrocautery, or cautery, is the use of high-frequency, alternating electric current to destroy, cut, or remove tissue. Electrocautery is also used to coagulate small blood vessels. Electrocautery has the advantage of sealing or cauterizing small blood vessels during a procedure such as small tumor removal, which results in reduced bleeding and cell loss. See Figure 4-31 for photo of a disposable cautery unit. Four types of currents are used in electrosurgery.

- *Electrocoagulation:* Destroys tissues and controls bleeding by coagulation.

- *Electrodessication:* Destroys tissue by creating a spark gap when the probe is inserted into unwanted tissue.

- *Electrofulguration:* Destroys tissue with a spark by holding the tip of the probe a short distance away from the unwanted tissue.

- *Electrosection:* Uses electric current to incise and excise the tissue.

Some physicians have miniature units called **hyfrecators.** The use of electrocautery is being replaced by the electrosurgical unit (ESU) and the ultrasonic surgical unit (USU).

The ESU is able to provide a more controlled, less damaging form of electric current through the use of a variety of attachments. For example, an incision can be made using ESU with a small electrode blade. The blade cauterizes as it cuts thus minimizing bleeding. Other attachments can be used to coagulate and suction.

The USU uses high-frequency sound waves to break apart calcified or sclerosed tissue so they can be removed in small segments. Some models have the ability to suction as they break apart and dissolve body calcifications. In some forms of electrosurgery, a local anesthetic may be administered.

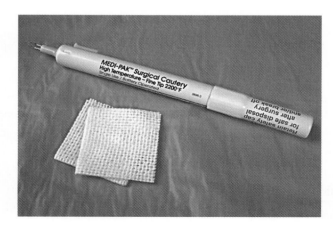

FIGURE 4-31

Disposable cautery unit.

COLPOSCOPY

Colposcopy is an examination of the vagina and cervix performed using a lighted instrument called a colposcope with the patient in the lithotomy position. The colposcope allows the physician to observe the tissues of this area in great detail through light and magnification. Abnormal areas of tissue or cells can then be removed for biopsy, or microscopic examination of cells for cancer. In some cases cryosurgery, using freezing temperatures to destroy cells, is then applied.

Colposcopy is performed

- If abnormal tissue development is observed by the physician during a routine pelvic examination.
- If Papanicoulaou (PAP) smear result is in abnormal range.
- For magnified visualization.
- To obtain a biopsy specimen.

If the physician is unable to visualize the entire cervical canal during the colposcopy, he or she may perform an endocervical curettage (ECC) to scrape endocervical cells from inside the cervical canal. These cells are then sent for further testing to determine any abnormality. (*Note:* Abnormal cell growth can be a sign of a pre-cancerous condition that, if untreated, could lead to the development of cancer.)

The patient may experience slight bleeding after this procedure if a biopsy is taken. Provide a perineal pad for the patient with instructions for home care. The patient should receive instructions to call the physician if there is abnormal pain or bleeding after this procedure.

CRYOSURGERY

Cryosurgery is used to treat cervical erosion and chronic cervicitis. This procedure is also referred to as cryocautery since the term "cautery" refers to a destruction of tissue. A colposcope is used to magnify the surface of the cervix and then a probe, capable of reaching freezing temperatures, is placed within the colposcope with the patient in the lithotomy position. This produces a freezing effect on tissues which destroys the abnormal cells.

The patient may experience mild cramping and a watery discharge after the procedure. The physician may advise her to take a mild analgesic, such as Tylenol. The patient should be advised against using a tampon which could irritate sensitive tissues for at least a month. Additional instruction should include instructions on reporting any unusual pain or foul discharge, abstaining from sexual intercourse for one month, and the time when she should return for a follow-up visit. The probe used in cryosurgery needs to be sterilized according to manufacturer's instructions immediately after use.

ENDOMETRIAL BIOPSY (EMB)

An endometrial biopsy (EMB) consists of using a curette or suction tool to remove uterine tissue for testing. EMB is performed for a variety of reasons including:

- To detect precancerous and cancerous conditions of the endometrial lining of the uterus.
- To detect inflammatory conditions.
- To determine if polyps are present.
- To assess abnormal uterine bleeding.
- To assess the effects of hormonal therapy.
- To screen for early detection of endometrial cancer (particularly if risk factors are present).

The American Cancer Society considers women with the following factors to be at high risk for endometrial cancer:

- Currently on estrogen therapy
- Obesity
- History of failure to ovulate
- History of infertility
- History of abnormal bleeding

An EMB is performed with the patient in the lithotomy position. The physician performs a bimanual examination of the uterus and administers a local anesthetic. A uterine sound is inserted into the uterus after the anesthetic has taken effect. The specimen is taken by means of a curette or with a suction device to aspirate a specimen. The specimen is sent to the laboratory in a container containing a 10% formalin preservative solution.

Provide a perineal pad for the patient with instructions for home care. The patient should receive instructions to call the physician if there is abnormal pain or bleeding after this procedure. She may experience mild cramping for which the physician may advise her to take a mild analgesic. She should be advised against using a tampon or douching for at least 72 hours.

INCISION & DRAINAGE (I & D)

Incision and drainage is performed to relieve the buildup of purulent (pus) material as a result of infection. The purulent discharge may need to be cultured to determine what microorganism is causing the infection, and thus, what antibiotic would be effective. The procedure is performed using sterile surgical technique. It should be remembered that the purulent material may be highly infectious. All soiled dressings and 4 × 4s should immediately be placed in a plastic waste container and then disposed of properly using OSHA guidelines.

A tray setup for an I & D would include:

- Scalpel handle and blades (No. 11)
- Curved iris scissors
- Tissue forceps
- Kelly hemostat
- Retractor
- Thumb dressing forceps
- 4 × 4 gauze squares

REMOVAL OF FOREIGN BODIES AND GROWTHS

A foreign body can include a variety of materials from a small splinter or fishhook to a large object, such as an arrow that is imbedded in tissue. Splinter forceps are needed on a tray for foreign body removal.

Growths include tumors, warts, moles, cysts. The most frequent growth removal procedure in the medical office is for cysts which are enclosed fluid-filled sacs. Some growths will be sent to the laboratory for biopsy testing depending upon the physician's instructions. The removal of a foreign body or neoplasm (growth) requires a surgical setup that includes:

- Thumb dressing forceps
- Retractor
- Scalpel handle and blades (No. 10 and 15)
- Curved tissue scissors
- Tissue forceps
- Hemostats
- Blunt probe
- Splinter forceps
- Needle holder
- Suture materials and needles
- Sterile 4 × 4 gauze

Figure 4-32 shows a surgical tray—biopsy removal.

VASECTOMY

The vasectomy procedure, tying and cutting of the vas deferens, on the male patient is a surgical procedure that is now commonly performed in the urologist's office. A vasectomy provides a permanent form of birth control for the male. As with any surgical procedure, a consent form needs to be signed

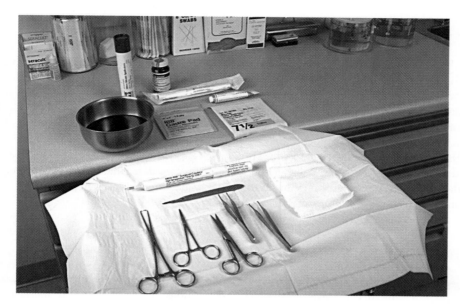

FIGURE 4-32

Surgical tray—biopsy removal.

and in the patient's record before beginning this irreversible procedure. The patient should be instructed to bring someone with them who can drive them home after the procedure. The patient will be uncomfortable for a short period of time (2-3 days). He should be given detailed instructions on home care including activity level and sexual intercourse. The instructions may vary somewhat from one urologist to another. A typical vasectomy tray will include:

- Scalpel handle and No. 15 blade
- Dressing forceps
- Towel clamp
- Straight and Curved Mosquito forceps
- Curved tissue scissors
- Tissue forceps
- Retractor
- Needle holder and suture material
- Suture scissors
- 4 × 4 gauze squares

LEGAL AND ETHICAL ISSUES

All patients must sign an informed consent form before any surgical procedure. This means that it is not enough to just tell the patient what procedure they are having done. The surgeon must also explain the risks, what might occur if nothing is done, and what other options are available. The medical assistant reinforces what the physician has explained and makes sure that there is a patient signature on the consent form before the procedure begins. If there is any doubt about the patient's ability to understand instructions, the medical assistant must bring this to the physician's attention. Preoperative and postoperative instructions should be read to the patient and clarified, if necessary.

Sterility during a surgical procedure cannot be compromised. The medical assistant has an ethical duty to provide the safest surgical environment possible for the patient.

Confidentiality relating to any surgical procedure a patient undergoes must be maintained. It is the physician's role to give the patient information about results of surgical procedures, biopsies, and tests.

Insurance information must be accurately documented. It is considered fraudulent to knowingly provide inaccurate information to an insurance company.

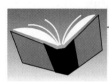

PATIENT EDUCATION

The medical assistant has a prominent role in educating the patient who will have a surgical procedure. Assisting the physician with obtaining the surgical consent is an opportunity to reinforce the physician's instructions. Explanations presented in easy to understand language can assure the patient will follow the correct steps of preparation.

Summary

Assisting with surgery includes maintaining aseptic technique, a thorough knowledge of gowning, gloving, surgical handwashing, setting up sterile instrument trays and passing equipment to the physician, packaging, and preparing the patient for the procedure. Assisting with surgical procedures carries with it a grave responsibility to maintain absolute sterile technique. The medical assistant incorporates a variety of clinical skills when assisting with a surgical procedure.

Competency Review

1. Define and spell the glossary terms for this chapter.

2. Perform handwashing using medical aseptic technique; using surgical aseptic technique.

3. Identify by name the pieces of equipment needed for:
   a. suture removal
   b. incision and drainage
   c. suture of laceration
   d. cervical biopsy
   e. removal of foreign body
   f. dressing change with wound culture
   g. endometrial biopsy

4. You have an open sore on your hand. What procedure should you follow when preparing to assist the surgeon?

ON THE JOB

Victor Krenz is assisting Dr. Connors with the fifth cataract surgical procedure for the day. The patient is Kathy Wall, a diabetic patient, whose condition has been stable enough for her to undergo a surgical procedure. Victor has performed a six minute surgical scrub on his hands before each of the five procedures. Dr. Connors indicates that he is in a hurry to get back to his office for a heavy afternoon schedule of patients. After both Dr. Connors and Victor are scrubbed and gowned and ready to begin the operation, Victor feels a slight prick on the tip of his gloved finger as he moves the sterile syringe and needle on the tray. Dr. Connors, who doesn't notice the acci-

dental needle prick to Victor's glove, states again what a hurry he is in to finish this procedure. Victor knows that if he has to change gloves it will delay the surgery. He also knows that his hands have had a surgical scrub five times that morning and they are clean.

What is your response?

1. Can Victor justify not changing into new gloves?

2. What could happen to Ms. Wall as a result of Victor's needle prick?

3. How should Victor handle this situation?

PREPARING FOR THE CERTIFICATION EXAM

Test Taking Tip — Be sure to eat breakfast or a light meal before taking a major examination, such as the CMA exam.

Examination Review Questions

1. Which of the following should NOT touch a sterile field?
   (A) 4 × 4s
   (B) transfer forceps
   (C) gloved hands
   (D) sterile specimen container
   (E) used instruments

2. The area that is considered sterile on a draped Mayo stand is
   (A) within a 2-inch border
   (B) outside a 2-inch border
   (C) within a 1-inch border
   (D) outside a 1-inch border
   (E) the entire drape is sterile

3. The portion of a hemostat located near the handle that protects it from slipping once it is closed is the
   (A) tooth   (D) lock
   (B) ratchet   (E) clamp
   (C) serrated tip

4. An instrument used by an obstetrician to measure an expectant mother's pelvis is the
   (A) curette
   (B) dilator
   (C) pelvimeter
   (D) vaginal speculum
   (E) none of the above

5. What is the correct method for shaving a surgical patient during the skin prep?
   (A) dry shave going with the grain
   (B) wet shave going against the grain
   (C) wet shave before preparing the patient's skin
   (D) wet shave going with the grain
   (E) dry shave after preparing the patient's skin

6. The surgical handwashing is performed
   (A) for 10 minutes using a clean hand brush
   (B) for 10 minutes using a sterile hand brush
   (C) by scrubbing for 2 minutes after removing rings
   (D) with a brush and disinfectant
   (E) using a germicidal soap

7. An example of a small gauge suture used for the skin is
   (A) stainless steel 5-0   (D) chromic gut 2-0
   (B) stainless steel 0   (E) nylon 2-0
   (C) plain gut 3-0

8. When applying sterile gloves
   (A) pick up the first glove under the cuff and pull over the other hand slowly
   (B) hold the gloves over the sink while you apply them since the sink is considered "clean"
   (C) place the fingers of the gloved hand under the cuff of the second glove, and then apply
   (D) leave the cuffs turned down after applying since this cuff will catch any spilled fluids
   (E) apply the gloves before setting up the equipment

9. When transferring sterile solutions to a sterile field
   (A) place the cap with outside edge facing up
   (B) place the cap with inside facing up
   (C) place the cap on the Mayo stand
   (D) pour the liquid by stabilizing the bottle on the edge of the basin
   (E) discard the liquid remaining in the bottle

10. A typical surgical setup consists of
    (A) scalpel, blades, trocar, probe, scope
    (B) scalpel, blades, hemostat, probe, scope
    (C) scalpel, blades, hemostat, scissors, suture
    (D) scalpel, blades, hemostat, scissors, suture, scope
    (E) scalpel, blades, scissors, suture, speculum

References

Fremgen, B. *Medical Terminology.* Upper Saddle River, NJ: Brady/Prentice Hall, 1997.

Fry, J., Higton, I., and Stephenson, J., *Colour Atlas of Minor Surgery in General Practice.* Boston: Kluwer Academic Publishers, 1990.

Groah, L. *Operating Room Nursing.* East Norwalk, CT: Appleton and Lange, 1990.

Nurse's Pocket Companion. Springhouse, PA: Springhouse Corporation, 1993.

Potter, P., Perry, P. *Fundamentals of Nursing—Concepts, Process and Practice,* 3rd ed. St. Louis: Mosby Year Book, 1993.

Reichert, M., Young, J. *Sterilization Technology in the Health Care Facility.* Gaithersburg, MD: Aspen, 1993.

Sheldon, H. *Boyd's Introduction to the Study of Disease.* Philadelphia: Lea and Febiger, 1992.

Taber's Cyclopedic Medical Dictionary, 18th edition. Philadelphia: F.A. Davis Company, 1997.

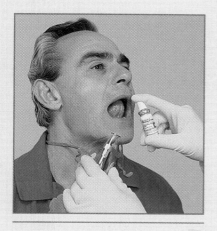

PHARMACOLOGY

OBJECTIVES

After completing this chapter, you should:

- Define and spell the glossary terms for this chapter.
- Differentiate between the legal (generic), commercial (trade) and chemical name for a drug.
- Know the precautions to be observed when administering drugs.
- Describe the drug reference books which should be in all physician's offices.
- List the "six rights" to medication administration.
- List the five schedules of the Controlled Substances Act.
- Know the conditions under which a medical assistant may administer medications.
- Cite the information that must be charted when administering a medication.

Glossary

addiction   An acquired physical and psychological dependence on a drug.

anaphylactic shock   A life-threatening reaction to certain foods, drugs, and insect bites in some people. This can cause respiratory distress, edema, rash, convulsions, and eventually unconsciousness and death if emergency treatment is not given.

broad-spectrum   The ability of a drug to be effective against a wide range of microorganisms.

Bureau of Narcotics and Dangerous Drugs (BNDD)   An agency of the federal government, used to enforce drug control.

chemotherapy   Use of chemicals, including drugs, to treat or control infections and diseases; commonly used to treat cancer by killing the cancer cells.

contraindicated   A condition in which the use of a drug should not be used.

dilute   To weaken the strength of a substance by the addition of something else.

drug tolerance   A decrease in susceptibility to a drug after the continued use of the drug.

Food and Drug Administration (FDA)   The official federal agency with responsibility for the regulation of food, drugs, cosmetics, and medical devices. It is a part of the US Department of Health and Human Services.

generic name   Common name by which a drug or product is known (for example, aspirin).

habituation   The development of an emotional dependence on a drug due to repeated use.

hemostatic   Any drug, medicine, or blood component that stops bleeding, such as vasopressin, vitamin K, or whole blood.

idiosyncrasy   An unusual or abnormal response to a drug or food by an individual.

parenteral   Medication route other than the alimentary canal (oral and rectal). Parenteral routes include subcutaneous, intravenous, and intramuscular.

pharmacist   A druggist or one who is licensed to prepare and dispense drugs.

pharmacology   The study of drugs, their origins, nature, properties and effects on the living organism.

Physician's Desk Reference (PDR)   A book used as a quick reference on drugs.

placebo   An inactive, harmless substance used to satisfy a patient's desire for medication. This is also used in research when given to a control group of patients in a study in which another group receives the actual drug. The effect of the placebo versus the drug is then observed.

prophylaxis   The prevention of disease. A medication, such as an antibiotic, can be used to prevent the occurrence of an infection prior to surgery (as opposed to antibiotics given to treat an infection).

side effect(s)   A response to a drug other than the effect desired.

toxicity   The extent or degree to which a substance is poisonous.

untoward effect   An undesirable side effect.

United States Pharmacopeia-National Formulary (USP-NF)   A drug book listing all the official drugs that are authorized for use in the United States. This is used in medical facilities and physicians' offices as a reference.

WARNING!

For all patient contact, adhere to Standard Precautions.
Wear protective equipment as indicated.

Pharmacology is the study of drugs, their origin, characteristics, and effects. The drugs used in the study of pharmacology are products of many different sources including: plants, animals, minerals, and synthetics.

Some drugs, such as vitamins, are naturally found in the foods we eat. Others, such as hormones, are obtained from animals. Penicillin and some of the other antibiotics are developed from molds which are a form of plant life. Many drugs, such as those used in **chemotherapy**, are synthetically formed by artificial means in the laboratory. Chemotherapy refers to the use of chemicals, including drugs, to treat or control infections and diseases. Chemotherapy is commonly used to treat cancer by killing the cancer cells.

Drugs prescribed to treat an infection are known as antibiotics; drugs prescribed or measures taken to prevent disease from occurring, for example drugs given to a patient prior to surgery, are prophylactics. **Prophylaxis** is prevention of disease through the prescribing of drugs and/or treatment.

Med Tip: The term drug and medication have the same meaning. However, the general public considers the term "drug" or "drugs" to mean a narcotic-type of medication. The term can also mean the use of illegal chemical substances. For purposes of medical terminology, the use of the word "drug" means a medication.

▶ DRUG NAMES

A drug may be known by as many as three different names: the **generic name**, the brand or trade name, and the chemical name. The generic term for a drug is the single name for identifying a drug. This is recognized by pharmaceutical companies and is considered the legal term for the drug. An example of a generic name for a drug would be tetracycline. The drug under the generic name can be manufactured by many companies which then place their own brand name on the drug.

Med Tip:

generic name	=	lower case	Example: acetaminophen
brand/trade name	=	Capitalized	Example: Tylenol

The brand or trade name is also referred to as the proprietary name. This is the commercial name that is patented by the pharmaceutical company that manufactures the drug. If the brand name is patented by the company, no other company can use that name for 17 years. Other drug companies can manufacture and patent the drug, but it must be under their own brand name. For example, Achromycin V, which is used to treat infection, is a brand name Lederle Laboratories uses for the generic drug, tetracycline. Tylenol is the brand name for acetaminophen. One drug can be manufactured by several companies under many brand names. Brand names are used by the pharmaceutical companies for advertising the drugs.

Generic drugs are usually priced lower than the brand name drug. However, not every drug is available generically and drug levels may not be as closely regulated in generic drugs as they are in brand name drugs. The physician can indicate on the prescription if the druggist may substitute a generic drug for a brand name. In some cases, the physician will prefer that a particular brand named drug be used if he or she believes it to be more effective than the generic drug.

The chemical name is the chemical formula for that particular drug. It is difficult for the lay person to comprehend and is used by the manufacturer and **pharmacists**. Pharmacists are licensed to prepare and dispense drugs. In the example above, the chemical name for Achromycin V is tetracycline hydrochloride (HCL). HCL after the term stands for the abbreviation for hydrochloride.

▶ REGULATIONS AND STANDARDS

The **Food and Drug Administration (FDA)**, a department within the Federal Department of Health and Human Services, ultimately enforces drug sales and distribution. The actual control of drugs is stipulated by the Federal Food, Drug, and Cosmetic Act of 1938. This act was initiated to ensure the safety of food, drugs, and cosmetics that are sold within the United States borders. The Controlled Substance Act of 1970 regulates the manufacture and distribution of the drugs which are capable of causing dependence and the **Bureau of Narcotics and Dangerous Drugs (BNDD)** is the agency of the federal government which is authorized to enforce drug control.

Med Tip: A physician can order a drug by either its generic or brand name. In general the generic drug is less expensive than the brand name drug. Many physicians will order the generic drug to save money for the patient. Never guess at the name of a drug if you are asked to interpret a physician's prescription. Always ask!

Med Tip: It is critical that patients receive the correct drug. Since it is not possible to list or remember all the drug names, you must acquire the habit of looking up any drug name you do not recognize in the *Physician's Desk Reference* (PDR). Every medical office or medical facility should have a copy of this book and update it each year.

▶ REFERENCES

There are two major resources for drug information and facts—the *Hospital Formulary* and the *Physician's Desk Reference* (PDR). The *Hospital Formulary* contains up-to-date information about drugs and their usage. It is published by the American Hospital Formulary Service and used extensively by pharmacists. The ***Physician's Desk Reference*** or *PDR* is an easy to use resource and should be in every physician's office or medical facility. The *PDR* is published by a private company and is sent free of charge to medical offices and hospitals. In addition to the well know book version, the *PDR* is also available on computer disk and CD-ROM. It lists drug products with addresses of manufacturers, generic and chemical name listings, and other valuable information.

Other books which are helpful include the ***United States Pharmacopeia-National Formulary (USP-NF)***. This is a drug book listing all the official drugs that are authorized for use in the United States.

▶ LEGAL CLASSIFICATION OF DRUGS

Drugs are classified as prescription and nonprescription drugs and controlled substances. A description of each of these categories follows. It is important for the medical assistant to be knowledgeable about these specific categories and to keep current with state and federal regulations that are published regarding a change of status of drugs, for example from "prescription" to "nonprescription."

PRESCRIPTION DRUGS

A prescription drug can only be ordered by a person who is licensed to dispense medications, such as physicians. These drugs must include on the label the words, "Caution: Federal Law prohibits dispensing without prescription." Antibiotics such as penicillin and heart medications such as digoxin are only available by prescription. A prescription is the written explanation to the pharmacist regarding the name of the medication, the dosage and the times of administration. A prescription can also be given verbally to the pharmacist by a licensed physician.

NONPRESCRIPTION DRUGS

A nonprescription drug is also referred to as an "over-the-counter" (OTC) drug. They are easily accessible in drug stores without a prescription. There are many medications or drugs that can be purchased without a prescription. Examples would include aspirin and antidiarrheal medications.

Some of these OTC drugs, for example cortisone ointments, required a prescription until recently. If taken incorrectly, some OTC drugs can be unsafe since they may react negatively with a prescription drug the patient is taking. For instance, aspirin taken along with an anticoagulant, such as Coumadin, can cause internal bleeding in some people. Antacids which are available as OTC drugs should not be taken with tetracycline since they interfere with the absorption of tetracycline into the body. Milk can have the same effect on tetracycline. It is best to allow the physician and the pharmacist to advise on the proper OTC drugs.

CONTROLLED SUBSTANCES

Certain drugs are controlled if they have a potential for **addiction** or abuse. The control of these drugs is enforced by the Drug Enforcement Agency (DEA). Controlled substances must be kept under lock and key. An accurate count of all narcotics is kept in a record called the "narcotic's log." The date and person to whom the drug was administered along with the signature of the person administering the drug are recorded. Most states do not allow medical assistants to administer narcotics.

The expiration dates of all medication in stock should be examined monthly. Do not place medications in waste containers. They are generally destroyed by pouring down a drain or flushing down a toilet. Two people should be present when controlled substances are destroyed. Both signatures are then placed on the narcotics log. Some more commonly controlled substances are:

- anabolic steroids
- APC with codeine
- butabarbital
- chloral hydrate

- cocaine
- codeine
- diazepam
- heroin

- LSD
- marijuana
- morphine

- opium
- phenobarbital
- secobarbital

The controlled drugs are classified into five schedules which indicate levels of abuse. The schedules are listed Schedule I through Schedule V. They are listed in Table 5-1.

▶ GENERAL CLASSES OF DRUGS

The classification of drugs relates to their action on the body. Table 5-2 presents a comprehensive list of names of drug classifications with descriptions of the use, or function, for each classification. Table 5-3 contains a similar list of drug classifications and provides specific examples of each drug type.

TABLE 5-1   Schedule for Controlled Substances

Level	Description	Comment
Schedule I	Highest potential for addiction and abuse. Not accepted for medical use. Example: Marijuana, heroin, and LSD	Not prescribed drugs.
Schedule II	High potential for addiction and abuse. Accepted for medical use in the US. Example: Codeine, cocaine, morphine, opium, and secobarbital	A DEA licensed physician must complete the required triplicate prescription forms entirely written in his or her own handwriting. The prescription must be filled within seven days and it may not be refilled. In an emergency, the physician may order a limited amount of the drug by telephone. These drugs must be stored under lock and key if they are kept on the office premises. The law requires that a dispensing record of these drugs be kept on file for two years.
Schedule III	Moderate to low potential for addiction and abuse. Example: Butabarbital, anabolic steroids, and APC with codeine	A DEA number is not required to write a prescription for these drugs but the physician must hand write the order. Five refills are allowed during a six month period and must be indicated on the prescription form. Only the physician can give telephone orders to the pharmacist for these drugs.
Schedule IV	Lower potential for addiction and abuse than Schedule III drugs. Example: Chloral hydrate, Phenobarbital, and diazepam	A medical assistant may write the prescription order for the physician, but it must be signed by the physician. Five refills are allowed over a six month period of time.
Schedule V	Low potential for addiction and abuse. Example: Low-strength codeine combined with other drugs to form cough suppressant	Inventory records must be maintained on these drugs also.

TABLE 5-2   Drug Classification Names and Descriptions of Use

Name	Use
adrenergic	Increases the rate and strength of the heart muscle. Acts as a vasoconstrictor, dilates bronchi, dilates pupils and relaxes muscular walls. Used to treat asthma, bronchitis and allergies.
adrenergic blocking agent	Increases peripheral circulation, decreases blood pressure and vasodilation. Used to treat hypertension.
analgesic	Relieves pain without the loss of consciousness. These may be either narcotic or non-narcotic. Narcotic drugs are derived from the opium poppy and act upon the brain to cause pain relief and drowsiness. For example, morphine.
anesthetic	Produces a lack of feeling which may be of local or general effect depending on the type of administration.
antacid	Neutralizes acid in the stomach.
antianxiety	Relieves or reduces anxiety and muscle tension. These are used to treat panic disorders, anxiety, and insomnia.
antiarrhythmic	Controls cardiac arrhythmias by altering nerve impulses within the heart.
antibiotic	Destroys or prohibits the growth of microorganisms. These are used to treat bacterial infections. They have not been found to be effective in treating viral infections. Antibiotics must be taken regularly for a specified time period to be effective.
anticoagulant	Prevents or delays blood clotting. Also referred to as blood thinners. These may be administered by intravenous injection, such as with the drug heparin. Oral drugs, such as warfarin, cannot be taken along with aspirin since the interaction between the two medications could cause internal bleeding.
anticonvulsant	Prevents or relieves convulsions. Drugs such as phenobarbital reduce excessive stimulation in the brain to control seizures and other symptoms of epilepsy.
antidepressant	Prevents or relieves the symptoms of depression. These drugs are also used in the prevention of migraine headaches.
antidiabetic	Drugs that control diabetes by regulating the level of glucose in the blood and the metabolism of carbohydrates and fat.
antidiarrheal	Prevents or relieves diarrhea.
antidote	Counteracts the effects of poisons.
antiemetic	Controls nausea and vomiting. These generally act upon the vomiting center in the brain.
antifungal	Kills fungus.
antihelminthic	Kills parasitic worms.
antihistamine	Counteracts histamine and controls allergic reactions.
antihypertensive	Prevents or controls high blood pressure. Some of these drugs act to block nerve impulses that cause arteries to constrict and thus increase the blood pressure. Other drugs slow the heart rate and decrease its force of contraction. Still others may reduce the amount of the hormone aldosterone in the blood that is causing the blood pressure to rise.
anti-inflammatory	Counteracts inflammation.
antineoplastic	Kills normal and abnormal cancerous cells by interfering with cell reproduction.
antipruritics	Relieves itching.
antipyretic	Reduces fever.
antiseptic	Prevents the growth of microorganisms.

Name	Use
antitussive	Controls or relieves coughing. Codeine is an ingredient in many prescription cough medicines. It acts upon the brain to control coughing.
astringent	A substance that has a constricting or binding effect by coagulating proteins on a cell's surface. This may be used to stop hemorrhage.
bronchodilator	Dilates or opens the bronchi (airways in the lungs) to improve breathing.
cardiogenic	Strengthens the heart muscle.
cathartic	Causes bowel movements to occur. These drugs may have a strong purging action and can become habit forming.
contraceptive	Used to prevent conception.
decongestant	Reduces nasal congestion and swelling.
diuretic	Increases the excretion of urine which promotes the loss of water and salt from the body. This can assist in lowering blood pressure, therefore, these drugs are used to treat hypertension. Potassium in the body may be depleted with continued use of diuretics. Potassium-rich foods, such as bananas, kiwi, and orange juice along with medications for potassium deficiency, can help correct this deficiency.
emetic	Induces vomiting.
estrogen	A hormone used to replace estrogen lost during menopause. Estrogen is responsible for the development of secondary sexual characteristics and is produced by the ovaries.
expectorant	Assists in the removal of secretions from the bronchopulmonary membranes.
hemostatic	Controls bleeding.
hypnotic	Produces sleep or hypnosis.
hypoglycemic	Lowers blood glucose level.
immunosuppressive	Suppresses the body's natural immune response to an antigen. This is used to control autoimmune diseases such as multiple sclerosis and rheumatoid arthritis.
laxative	Used to promote normal bowel function.
miotic	Constricts the pupils of the eye.
muscle relaxant	Produces the relaxation of skeletal muscle.
mydriatic	Dilates the pupils of the eye.
narcotic	Produces sleep or stupor. In moderate doses this drug will depress the central nervous system and relieve pain. In excessive doses it will cause stupor, coma and even death. Can become habit-forming (addictive).
purgative	Stimulates bowel movements.
psychedelic	Drugs such as lysergic acid diethylamide (LSD) that can produce visual hallucinations.
sedative	Produces relaxation without causing sleep.
stimulant	Speeds up the heart and respiratory system. Used to increase alertness.
tranquilizer	Used to reduce mental anxiety and tensions.
vaccine	Given to promote resistance (immunity) to infectious diseases.
vasodilator	Produces a relaxation of blood vessels to lower blood pressure.
vasopressor	Produces the contraction of muscles in the capillaries and arteries which elevates the blood pressure.
vitamin	Organic substances found naturally in foods that are essential for normal metabolism. Most have been produced synthetically to be taken in pill form.

TABLE 5-3   Classification of Drugs by Type or Usage With Examples

Type/Usage	Example
adrenergic	Isuprel (isoproterenol)
	Sudafed (pseudoephedrine hydrochloride HCL)
adrenergic blocking agent	Aldomet (methyldopa)
	Inderal (propranolol HCL)
analgesic	Advil (ibuprofen)
	Acetophen (aspirin)
	Darvon (propoxyphene HCL)
	Dilaudid (hydromorphine HCL)
	Demerol (meperidine HCL)
	Talwin (pentazocine HCL)
	Tylenol (acetaminophen)
anesthetic	Carbocaine (mepivacaine HCL)
	Novocaine (procaine HCL)
	Nupercaine (dibucaine HCL)
	Xylocaine (lidocaine HCL)
antacid	Milk of Magnesia (magnesia magma)
	Mylanta (aluminum hydroxide)
	Maalox (aluminum hydroxide)
antianxiety	Valium (diazepam)
antiarrhythmic	Digoxin (digoxin)
	Norpace (disopyramide)
	Pronestyl (procainamide HCL)
antibiotic	
Aminogylcosides	Garamycin (gentamicin sulfate)
	Kantrex (kanamycin)
	Mycifradin Sulfate (neomycin sulfate)
	Nebcin (tobramycin sulfate)
	Neobiotic (neomycin sulfate)
Cephalosporins	Ancef (cefazolin sodium)
	Anspor (cephradine)

(Continued)

Type/Usage	Example
Cephalosporins	Ceclor (cefaclor)
	Duricef (cefadroxil)
	Keflix (cephalexin)
	Keflin (cephalothin sodium)
Penicillins	Amoxil (amoxicillin)
	Bicillin (penicillin G potassium)
	Duracillin (penicillin G procaine)
	Polycillin (ampicillin)
Tetracyclines	Acromycin (tetracycline HCL)
	Declomycin (democlocycline)
	Terramycin (oxytetracycline)
	Vibramycin (doxycycline Hyclate)
anticholinergic	Atropine (atropine sulfate)
	Banthine (methantheline bromide)
	Donnatol (belladonna)
anticoagulant	Coumadin (warfarin sodium)
anticonvulsant	Dilantin (phenytoin sodium)
	Phenobarbital (phenobarbitol)
antidepressant	Elavil (amitriptyline HCL)
antidiabetic	Insulin and oral medications: Precose and Metformin
antidiarrheal	Kaopectate (kaolin and pectin mixture)
	Lomotil (diphenoxylate)
antiemetics	Atarax (hydroxyzine HCL)
	Compazine (prochlorperazine)
	Dramamine (dimenhydrinate)
	Phenergan (promethazine HCL)
antifungal	Mycostatin (nystatin)
antihelminthics	Vermox (mebendazole)
antihistamine	Adrenalin (epinephrine)
	Benadryl (diphenhydramine)

(Continued on next page)

TABLE 5-3   Classification of Drugs by Type or Usage With Examples

Type/Usage	Example
antihistamine	Chlor-Trimeton (chlorapheneramine maleate)
	Dimetane (brompheniramine maleate)
antihypertensives	Aldomet (methyldopa)
	Catapres (clonidine HCL)
	Lopressor (metoprolol tartrate)
	Minipress (prazosin HCL)
anti-inflammatory	Aspirin (acetylsalisylic acid)
	Indocin (indomethacin)
	Motrin (naprosyn)
	Nalfon (fenoprofen calcium)
	Naproxen (naprosyn)
antineoplastic	Cytoxan (cyclophosphamide)
	Fluorouracil (5FU)
	Adriamycin (doxorubicin HCL)
antipruritic	Calamine lotion (calamine)
	Hydrocortone (hydrocortisone sodium phosphate)
antipyretic	Advil (ibuprofen)
	Aspirin (acetylsalicylic acid)
	Tylenol (acetaminophen)
antiseptic	Cidex (glutarldehyde)
	pHisoHex (hexachlorophene)
antitussive	Codeine (codeine phosphate)
bronchodilator	Alupent (metaproterenol sulfate)
	Brethine (terbutaline sulfate)
	Isuprel (isoproterenol HCL)
	Theolair (theophylline)
contraceptive	Ortho-Novum 10/11-21 (estrogen with progestogen)
	Enovid-E 21 (estrogen with progestogen)
decongestant	Neo-Synephrine (phenylephrine HCL)
	Sudafed (pseudoephedrine HCL)
diuretic	Diuril (chlorothiazide)

(Continued)

Type/Usage	Example
diuretic	Hygroton (chlorthalidone)
	Lasix (furosemide)
emetic	Ipecac syrup
estrogen	Estrace (estrogen)
expectorant	Robitussin (guaifenesin)
hormone	Testosterone
	Premarin, estrogen
hypnotic	Seconal (secobarbital)
hypoglycemic	Precose (oral)
	Metformin (oral)
laxative	Dulcolax (bisacodyl)
muscle relaxant	Valium (diazepam)
	Robaxin (methocarbamol)
narcotic	Demerol (meperidine HCL)
	Percodan
purgative	Ex-Lax (phenolphthalein)
psychedelic	LSD (lysergic acid diethylamide)
sedative and hypnotic	Amytal (amobarbital)
	Butisol (butabarbital sodium)
	Nembutal Sodium (phenobarbital)
	Seconal Sodium (secobarbital sodium)
	Valium (diazepam)
stimulant	Dexedrine (dextroamphetamine sulfate)
tranquilizer	Haldol (haloperidol)
vasodilator	Isordil (isorbide dinitrate)
	Nitro-bid (nitroglycerin)
	Nitrostat (nitroglycerin)
vasopressor	Levophed (norepinephrine)
vitamin	Vitamin A
	Vitamin C
	Vitamin D
	Vitamin K

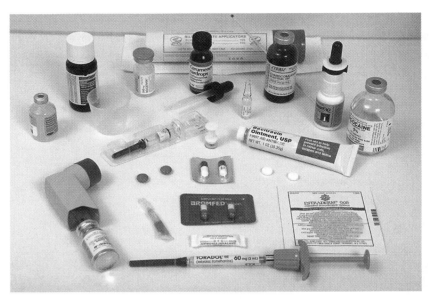

FIGURE 5-1

Different types of medication require different routes of administration.

▶ ROUTES AND METHODS OF DRUG ADMINISTRATION

The method by which a drug is introduced into the body is referred to as the route of administration (Figure 5-1). In general the routes of administration are

1. *Oral:* This method includes all drugs that are given by mouth. The advantages are ease of administration and a slow rate of absorption via stomach and intestinal wall. The disadvantages include slowness of absorption and destroying of some chemical compounds by gastric juices. In addition, some medications, such as aspirin, can have a corrosive action on the stomach lining.
2. *Sublingual:* These are drugs that are held under the tongue and not swallowed. The medication is absorbed as the saliva dissolves it. Nitroglycerin to treat angina or chest pain is administered by this route.
3. *Parenteral:* This is an invasive method of administering drugs since it requires the skin to be punctured by a needle. The needle with syringe attached is introduced either under the skin, into a muscle, vein, or body cavity. Table 5-4 lists the methods for parenteral administration and provides a description of each method.

TABLE 5-4   Methods for Parenteral Administration of Drugs

Method	Description
Intradermal	A very shallow injection just within the top layer of skin. This is a method commonly used in skin testing for allergies and tuberculosis.
Subcutaneous (SC)	An injection under the skin and fat layers. The middle of the upper, outer arm is usually used.
Intramuscular (IM)	An injection directly into the muscle of the buttocks or upper arm (deltoid). This method is used when there is a large amount of medication or it is irritating.
Intravenous (IV)	An injection into the veins. This route can be set up so that there is a continuous administration of medication, usually post-op a major surgery or during a major procedure.
Intrathecal	Injection into the meninges space surrounding the brain and spinal cord.
Intracavity	Injection into a body cavity such as the peritoneal and chest cavity.

Additional methods (other than parenteral) for administering medication are given in Table 5-5. Drugs must be administered by a particular route in order to be effective. Sometimes there is a variety of routes by which a drug can be administered. For instance, the female hormone estrogen can be administered orally in the form of a pill or topically in the form of a skin patch. Table 5-6 lists numerous forms in which medications are prepared and routes through which they are administered.

▶ FREQUENTLY ADMINISTERED DRUGS

New drugs are constantly being developed, researched, tested, and distributed by the pharmaceutical (drug) companies. As a result, **broad spectrum antibiotics**, that have the ability to be effective against a wide range of microorganisms, are frequently prescribed instead of a less-complex drug that targets more specific microorganisms.

TABLE 5-5 Non-parenteral Methods for Administering Drugs

Method	Description
Rectal	The drug is introduced directly into the rectal cavity in the form of suppositories or solution. Drugs may have to be administered by this route if the patient is unable to take them by mouth due to nausea, vomiting, and surgery of the mouth.
Inhalation	This category of drugs includes those that are inhaled directly into the nose and mouth. Aerosol sprays are administered by this route.
Topical	These drugs are applied directly to the skin or mucous membranes. They are distributed in ointment, cream or lotion form. These drugs are used to treat skin infections and eruptions. Transdermal patches, for example nicotrol, estraderm, and nitoderm.
Vaginal	Vaginal tablets and suppositories are used to treat vaginal yeast infections and other irritations.
Eye drops	Drugs placed into the eye to control eye pressure in glaucoma. Used during eye examinations to dilate the pupil of the eye for better examination of the interior of the eye. Also used to treat infections.
Ear drops	Drugs placed directly into the ear canal for the purpose of relieving pain or treating infection.
Buccal	Drugs, such as nitroglycerin for anginal pain, which are placed under the lip or between the cheek and gum.

TABLE 5-6 Routes of Drug Administration

Form	Route	Form	Route
aerosol	Inhalation	**pills**	Oral
caplets	Oral	**powders**	Topical
capsules	Oral	**skin patch**	Topical
elixir	Oral	**spansules**	Oral
liniment	Topical	**spray**	Oral, topical
lotion	Topical	**suppository**	Rectal, vaginal
lozenges	Oral	**syrup**	Oral
ointment	Topical	**tablet**	Oral

Fifty of the most frequently dispensed drugs as listed in the *American Druggist* are noted in Table 5-7 along with the classification or group to which each belongs. The drugs are listed by brand name.

▶ SIDE EFFECTS OF MEDICATIONS

In addition to the desirable effects for which drugs are prescribed, there are undesirable **side effects** for all medications. In some cases these side effects can be lethal for the patient, so it is important to take these **untoward** (undesirable) **effects** seriously.

TABLE 5-7 Frequently Administered Drugs

Brand Name	Type	Brand Name	Type
1. Amoxil	antibiotic	26. Lopressor	beta-blocker
2. Lanoxin	cardiotonic	27. Lasix	diuretic
3. Zantac	antiulcer	28. Voltaren	nonsteroidal anti-inflammatory
4. Xanax	tranquilizer		
5. Premarin	hormone (estrogen)	29. Darvocet-N	analgesic (narcotic)
6. Cardizem	cardiotonic	30. Dilantin	anticonvulsant
7. Ceclor	antibiotic	31. Monistat	antibiotic (antifungal)
8. Synthroid	hormone (thyroid)	32. Augmentin	antibiotic (pencillin)
9. Seldane	antihistamine	33. Micronase	oral hypoglycemic agent
10. Tenormin	beta-blocker	34. Feldene	nonsteroidal anti-inflammatory
11. Vasotec	antihypertensive		
12. Tagamet	antiulcer	35. Micro-K	potassium supplement
13. Naprosyn	nonsteroidal anti-inflammatory	36. Provera	hormone (progestin)
		37. Motrin	nonsteroidal anti-inflammatory
14. Capoten	antihypertensive		
15. Ortho-Novum 7/7/7	synthetic hormone	38. Mevacor	cholesterol-lowering
16. Dyazid	diuretic	39. Triphasil	synthetic hormone
17. Ortho-Novum	synthetic hormone	40. Prozac	antidepressant
18. Proventil	bronchodilator	41. Lo/Ovral	synthetic hormone
19. Tylenol with codeine	analgesic (narcotic)	42. Valium	tranquilizer
		43. Retin-A	antiacne
20. Procardia	calcium channel blocker	44. Cipro	antibiotic
21. Calan	calcium channel blocker	45. E-Mycin	antibiotic
		46. Maxzide	diuretic
22. Ventolin	bronchodilator	47. Coumadin	anticoagulant
23. Inderal	beta-blocker	48. Carafate	antiulcer
24. Halcion	sedative	49. Timoptic	beta-blocker
25. Theo-Dur	bronchodilator	50. Slow-K	potassium supplement

Some side effects are as simple as an individual patient's **idiosyncrasy** or reaction to the medication. See Table 5-8 for some medications that have a negative interaction with food products. In some cases, the effects are quite obvious, for example a rash, indicating an allergy to a medication. In other cases, the side effects are hidden and may require laboratory testing to detect. Some specific side effects to drugs include:

1. **Anaphylactic shock** is a life-threatening reaction in some people to a drug, food, or insect bite. This can cause severe respiratory distress, edema, convulsions, unconsciousness, and even death if untreated.
2. **Drug tolerance** that results in a decrease of a drug's effectiveness, may result after a continued use of the drug, such as in the case of an antibiotic. Another drug to which the patient has not yet developed a tolerance, will have to be prescribed. This is a problem when antibiotics are over prescribed for ailments, such as colds, which will clear up naturally. An increase in the dosage of a drug beyond the recommended amount may result in a condition known as **toxicity** from that drug.

TABLE 5-8   Drug-Food Interactions

Drug	Negative Reaction to Food
Accutane	Dairy products and food increase absorption.
Achromycin V	Dairy products and food interfere with absorption of tetracycline.
Apresoline	Food increases the plasma levels of the drug.
Antihypertensive drugs	Licorice decreases effect.
Hismanal	Food reduces absorption by 60%.
Bacampicillin HCL	Food decreases drug absorption.
Caffeine	Caffeine-containing beverages and food may cause irritability, nervousness, sleeplessness and rapid heartbeat.
Calcium gluconate	Cereals, bran, rhubarb, and spinach interfere with calcium absorption.
Capoten	Food reduces drug absorption by 30% to 40%.
Ceftin	Food increases drug absorption.
Coumadin	Diet high in vitamin K decreases prothrombin time.
Declomycin	Dairy products and food interfere with absorption.
Dicumarol	Diet high in vitamin K decreases prothrombin time.
Digoxin	Food high in bran fiber reduces availability of drug.
Erythromycin	Food interferes with absorption.
Feosol	Dairy products and eggs inhibit iron absorption.
Ibuprofen	Food reduces rate of absorption.
Inderal	Food increases availability of drug.
Monopril	Food slows rate of absorption.
Pepcid	Food increases availability of drug.
Plendil	Grapefruit juice doubles the concentration.
Procardia XL	Food alters rate of absorption.
Sinemet	High protein diet impairs absorption.
Synthroid	Soybean formula (in infants) causes excessive stools.
Xylocaine	Food enhances danger of aspiration due to topical anesthesia which may impair swallowing.

3. Habituation, or dependence on a drug, may develop to habit-forming drugs, such as laxatives and narcotics.

In general, unexpected side effects range from a rash and/or itching to drowsiness, runny nose, constipation, dizziness, headache, temporary ringing in the ears (tinnitus), blurred vision, loss of appetite, nausea, and vomiting.

The patient should be instructed to call the physician if these side effects are persistent or troublesome (Figure 5-2). The physician may adjust the medication dosage or change to a similar medication with fewer side effects. In all cases, patients should be instructed not to adjust the dosage themselves or stop taking the medication without consulting the physician. A **placebo**, which is an inactive harmless substance, such as a sugar pill, may occasionally be used by a physician to satisfy a patient's desire for unnecessary medication.

▶ DRUG USE DURING PREGNANCY

Since the thalidomide tragedy during the 1950's when thousands of malformed babies were born after their mothers took this sedative during pregnancy, there has been better research and testing of drugs. Today most drugs carry special warnings concerning medication use during pregnancy either on the label or in the enclosed literature insert.

There are very few drugs that are approved for use during pregnancy. Even aspirin carries its dangers. Therefore it is especially important for women of child-bearing age to be warned about the risks. Fetal development during the first trimester is particularly at risk.

A woman should be asked for the date of her last menstrual period and whether she could be pregnant before she is administered any medication. Women should be cautioned to advise their physicians when there is a possibility of pregnancy.

DRUG USE AND THE BREAST FEEDING MOTHER

Medications that a nursing mother takes do appear in breast milk. She should be instructed to breast feed before taking any medication since the blood levels are highest immediately after ingestion.

With a physician's permission, there are some medications, such as medication to control epilepsy, that the nursing mother can continue to take. However, there are medications which are **contraindicated.** This means the medications are so dangerous for the infant that the mother must stop breast feeding and place her baby on bottle feedings while she is taking any of these medications. These contraindicated medications include:

- Tetracyclines
- Chloramphenicol
- Sulfonamides (during the first 2 weeks postpartum)
- Oral anticoagulants
- Iodine-containing drugs
- Antineoplastics

A nursing mother should avoid taking any medication without talking to her physician first.

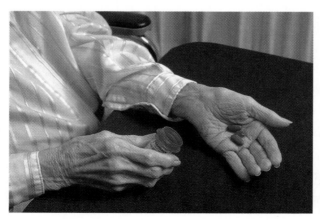

FIGURE 5-2

Older adults may need special assistance with medications.

▶ HOW TO READ A PRESCRIPTION

A prescription is not difficult to read once you understand the symbols that are used. Symbols and abbreviations based on Latin and Greek words are used in order to save time for the physician. For example, the abbreviation "po" meaning "to be taken by mouth" comes from the Latin words *per os* which mean by mouth. There are seven main parts to a prescription:

1. Patient's name, address, age (if a child), and date appear on the top line.
2. The superscription, consisting of the symbol Rx from the Latin term *recipe,* means "take thou." This symbol is usually preprinted on the prescription form.
3. The inscription specifies the name of the drug, actual ingredients, and the amount per dose.
4. The subscription tells the pharmacist how to mix the drug and the number of doses to supply to the patient.
5. The signa (Sig.) from the Latin term *signa,* means "mark." The instructions that should be given to the patient are stated here.
6. The physician's name, address, telephone number and DEA number. In some cases, all except the signature are printed at the top of each prescription blank. A prescription becomes a legal document when signed by the physician.
7. And finally, the number of times that the prescription can be refilled.

Figure 5-4 is an example of a prescription. In this example, the physician has ordered the medication Estrace which is a form of the hormone estrogen. The prescription tells the pharmacist to give 100 (dtd C) tablets, and orders a 1 mg dosage which is to be taken once a day (1 q am). The instruction to the pharmacist is to refill the prescription 3 times and not to substitute with another (generic) medication.

On some prescriptions, the physician will give a "prn" refill order meaning that the prescription can be refilled as needed. The physician will fill in the name, address, age of the patient and date. The physician must also sign his or her name at the bottom of the prescription. A blank prescription cannot be handed to a patient. Be sure that prescription blanks are not left out but in a secure place.

The physician's instructions to the patient will be placed on the label. The pharmacist will also include instructions about the medication and alert the patient to side effects of the medication

Guidelines: Administration of Medications

1. Medications/drugs can only be administered to a patient under the supervision of a licensed physician. To do otherwise is considered "practicing medicine without a license." The medication order must be written and signed on the patient's medical record by the physician.
2. The medical assistant acts as the liaison or intermediary between the physician and the patient. Some of the duties include ordering, storing, rotating, and checking expiration dates on medications.
3. Medications must be checked three times before administration.

The "Three Befores" are:

- Before medication is removed from the medication cabinet
- Before medication is poured or drawn up into a syringe
- Before medication is returned to the cabinet

4. Medications cannot be returned to the container once they have been removed. If they are not administered, they must be discarded.
5. Remember the "six rights" for administering medications (Figure 5-3).

The "Six Rights" are:

- Right patient
- Right medication
- Right dosage
- Right route
- Right time
- Right documentation

(Continued on next page)

Guidelines: Administration of Medications (*continued*)

6. Keep a record of all allergies on the patient's medical record. Often these allergies are noted on the front of the medical record as well as within the medical record.
7. The documentation on the patient's medical record must include the following:
   a. Name of the medication
   b. Dosage
   c. Route of administration
   d. Date of administration
   e. Site of administration
   f. Signature of the person administering the medication along with initials designating the person's status, for example CMA, RMA
8. All narcotics must be recorded into a record maintained for that purpose. This is referred to as "logging a narcotic." Every narcotic must be accounted for.
9. Be careful that you administer the medication by the correct route. Methods of administration include:
   a. Oral (by mouth)
   b. Sublingual (under the tongue)
   c. Buccal (in the cheek)
   d. Rectal (inserted into the anal cavity)
   e. Vaginal (inserted into vaginal canal)
   f. Parenteral (by injection)
   g. Topical (applied to the skin)
   h. Inhalation (by breathing the medication)
   Medical assistants do not administer medications by the following routes:
   a. Intrathecal (into the meninges space)
   b. Intracavity (into a body cavity)
   c. Intravenous (IV) (into a vein)
10. Medication labels should be clean and readable. If they become soiled, unreadable, or fall off the container they must be discarded.
11. If you are not familiar with a particular medication, you must look it up in the PDR. Never violate this rule.
12. Know the side effects for the medication you are administering.
13. Always advise the patient to take the complete number of dosages ordered in the prescription. This is especially important when using antibiotics.
14. Advise the patient to only use medication for the member of the family or person it was prescribed for.

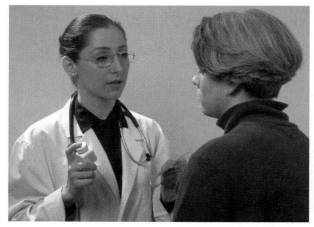

FIGURE 5-3

Remember the "Six Rights" when administering medications.

that the patient may experience. These side effects may need to be reported to the physician. In addition, any special instructions regarding the medication (for example "take with meals" or "do not take along with dairy products") will also be supplied by the pharmacist. The label on the medication container must always be checked to match the prescription. If in doubt always question the pharmacist (Figure 5-5).

Some prescriptions can be filled by telephone. At such times, the patient's record should be pulled for the physician and the refill order or new medications prescribed should be documented.

▶ ABBREVIATIONS USED IN PHARMACOLOGY

Medical abbreviations are used extensively in pharmacology. The general public cannot usually decipher prescriptions due to the use of medical abbreviations. You will have to assist your patients with their questions.

Med Tip: Many abbreviations have multiple meanings such as "od" which can mean either once a day (od) or right eye (OD) depending on whether the letters are small or capitalized. Care must be taken when reading abbreviations since some may be written too quickly making them difficult to decipher. Never create your own abbreviations. Some of the most common abbreviations used in pharmacology are listed in Table 5-9.

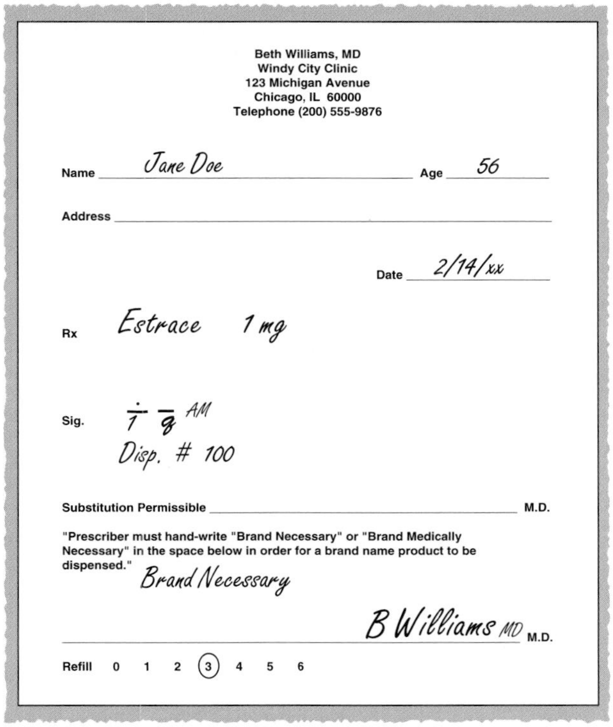

Beth Williams, MD
Windy City Clinic
123 Michigan Avenue
Chicago, IL 60000
Telephone (200) 555-9876

Name _Jane Doe_ Age _56_

Address _____

Date _2/14/xx_

Rx _Estrace   1 mg_

Sig. _1̇ ℥ AM_
Disp. # 100

Substitution Permissible _____ M.D.

"Prescriber must hand-write "Brand Necessary" or "Brand Medically Necessary" in the space below in order for a brand name product to be dispensed." _Brand Necessary_

B Williams MD M.D.

Refill 0 1 2 ③ 4 5 6

FIGURE 5-4

Sample prescription.

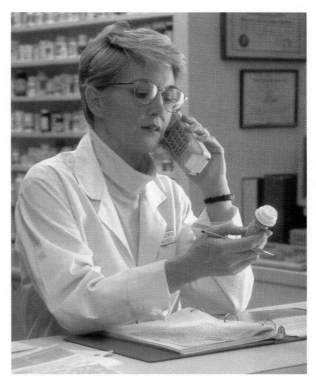

FIGURE 5-5

Speak with the pharmacist about any questions you have about prescription medications.

TABLE 5-9   **Common Abbreviations Used in Pharmacology**

Abbreviation	Meaning	Abbreviation	Meaning
@	At	ext	Extract/external
a	Before	Fe	Iron
aa	Of each	fl	Fluid
ac	Before meals	G	Gauge
AD	Right ear	gal	Gallon
ad lib	As desired	g	Gram
alt dieb	Alternate days	gr	Grain
alt hor	Alternate hours	gt	One drop
alt noc	Alternate nights	gtt	Two or more drops
am, AM	Morning	H	Hour/hypodermic
amt	Amount	hs	Hour of sleep
ante	Before	IM	Intramuscular
aq	Aqueous (water)	inj	Injection
AS	Left ear	IV	Intravenous
AU	Both ears	k	Potassium
Ba	Barium	kg	Kilogram
bid	Twice a day	L	Liter
C	100	L	Left
c̄	With	liq	Liquid
cap(s)	Capsule(s)	M ft	Make
cc	Cubic centimeter	mug	Microgram
d	Day	mg	Milligram
DC, disc	Discontinue	mL	Milliliter
d/c, DISC	Discontinue	mitt#	Give this number
disp	Dispense	mm	Millimeter
dil	**Dilute**	noct	Night
dtd#	Give this number	non rep	Do not repeat
Dx	Diagnosis	NPO	Nothing by mouth
dr	Dram	NS	Normal saline
elix	Elixir	noc	Night
emul	Emulsion	O	Pint
et	And	od	Once a day/daily

Abbreviation	Meaning	Abbreviation	Meaning
OD	Right eye	s or ṡ	Without
o m	Every morning	SC	Subcutaneous
OS	Left eye	SOB	Shortness of breath
OU	Both eyes	Subc, SubQ	Subcutaneous
OTC	Over the counter	Sig.	Label as follows/directions
oz or ℥	Ounce	sl	Under the tongue
pc	After meals	sol	Solution
per	With	ss or s̄s̄	One-half
PM	Evening	stat	At once/immediately
po	By mouth	subling	Sublingual
prn	As needed	suppos	Suppository
pt	Pint	susp	Suspension
pulv	Powder	syr	Syrup
q	Every	T, tbsp	Tablespoon
q2h	Every two hours	tab	Tablet
qam	Every morning	tid	Three times a day
qd	Once a day/every day	tinc/tr	Tincture
qh	Every hour	top	Apply topically
qhs	Every night	tsp	Teaspoon
qid	Four times a day	u	Unit
qm	Every morning	ung	Ointment
qod	Every other day	UT	Under the tongue
®	Right	ut dict, UD	As directed
Rx	Take	wt	Weight

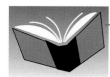

LEGAL AND ETHICAL ISSUES

You must always remember that even though you work under the supervision of a physician as a medical assistant, nevertheless, you are still legally and ethically responsible for your own actions. The physician must report any known patient drug abuse. As the medical assistant, you may be the first person to become aware of a patient's problem. It is therefore your ethical responsibility to inform the physician.

You have a responsibility for maintaining accurate records for all narcotic use. State laws regarding what a medical assistant may and may not do vary from state to state. You must become familiar with the laws in your own state. In addition, careful triple-checking of all medications before administering them, remaining current on all medications which are prescribed in your office, and remembering the "six rights" of drug administration will help to protect you legally and ethically. Never administer a medication with which you are unfamiliar.

PATIENT EDUCATION

Patient education is especially important when working with medications. Instructions regarding the type of medication prescribed, dosage, side effects, and reaction with foods must be clearly explained. You may have to develop teaching materials and aids, such as a written schedule indicating when medications should be taken, to assist patients who have difficulty remembering.

It is the medical assistant's responsibility to keep the physician informed of all medications patients have indicated they are taking, as well as any allergies the patients may have to specific medications. Patients have to be instructed to throw out all out-dated medications. Patients must be warned to keep medications out of the reach of children, and, of course, never to share their medicines with others.

Summary

The medical assistant works directly under the supervision of the physician. This relationship needs to be well understood with regard to medication administration. The medical assistant must know the legalities concerning the limitations of his or her credentials. A medical assistant may administer medications only when they have been prescribed and documented on the patient's medical record by a licensed physician. At no time can the medical assistant prescribe even the simplest of drugs, for example an aspirin. A medical assistant can lose his or her certification for "practicing medicine without a license."

In addition to knowing how drugs are classified—prescription, nonprescription, and controlled substances—the medical assistant must have a thorough knowledge of dosage, abbreviations, and side effects relating to medications. In whatever situation you work, be sure to follow the federal, state, and local regulations regarding the administration, storage, inventory, and dispensing of drugs.

Competency Review

1. Define and spell the glossary terms for this chapter.
2. Name the governmental agency which enforces drug sales and distribution.
3. Describe the differences between the legal, commercial, and chemical names for a drug.
4. List 10 of the 14 precautions to observe when administering medications.
5. Name a reference book that is one of the most frequently used sources of information when administering medications in the physician's office.
6. Name the federal act that controls the use of drugs causing dependency.
7. List the "six rights" to medication administration.
8. Discuss the "three befores" that must take place before dispensing medication.
9. Describe what you would do when a patient indicates a drug allergy.
10. State under what conditions a medical assistant may administer a medication.
11. Define "logging a narcotic."
12. List the information that must be charted when administering a medication.
13. Explain the functions of the following types of medication: diuretic, bronchodilator, antiemetic, hypnotic, sedative, anti-inflammatory agent, vasodilator, anti-convulsive, anesthetic, analgesic, antacid, antibiotic, anticoagulant, antihistamine.
14. Write out the following prescription instructions:
    a. Pravachol, 20 mg., Sig. i qd @ noc, dtd 30, refill 3x, no sub.
    b. Lanoxin 0.125 mg., Sig. iii stat, then ii a AM, dtd C, refills prn.
    c. Synthroid 0.075 mg., Sig. i qd, C, refill x4.
    d. Norvasc 5 mg., i q am, dtd 60, refillable.

PREPARING FOR THE CERTIFICATION EXAM

Test Taking Tip — Wear a watch when you study for an exam or take a test. Pace yourself so that you can work quickly not spending too much time on any one question.

Examination Review Questions

1. The chemical name for the OTC medication Aleve is
   (A) acetaminophen
   (B) naproxen sodium
   (C) Naprosyn
   (D) Tylenol
   (E) Aldomet

2. According to the Drug Enforcement Agency, controlled substances
   (A) can be addictive
   (B) may have the potential for abuse by a patient
   (C) must be kept under a lock and key
   (D) (the dispensation of) must be recorded in a narcotic's log
   (E) all of the above

3. An example of a Schedule IV drug is
   (A) Xanax
   (B) morphine
   (C) Vicodin
   (D) MS Contin
   (E) Tylenol with codeine

4. Capoten, which is an ACE inhibitor, is classified as an
   (A) antibiotic
   (B) anti-inflammatory
   (C) antipruritic
   (D) antihypertensive
   (E) antipyretic

5. Which of the following is a method for the administration of a drug by means of an injection under the skin and fat layers?
   (A) intradermal
   (B) intramuscular
   (C) subcutaneous
   (D) intravenous
   (E) intrathecal

6. A non-parenteral method for administering drugs would be
   (A) inhalation
   (B) topical
   (C) vaginal
   (D) buccal
   (E) all of the above

7. The "Six Rights" a medical assistant must observe when administering medications include the right medication, documentation, and
   (A) time
   (B) route
   (C) dosage
   (D) patient
   (E) all of the above

8. Which, if any, of the following routes of administration may not be used by a medical assistant?
   (A) ID
   (B) IV
   (C) IM
   (D) Z-track IM
   (E) SC

9. Which part of a prescription precedes the instructions that should be given to the patient?
   (A) Sig.
   (B) Rx
   (C) superscription
   (D) inscription
   (E) subscription

10. A common abbreviation, used in pharmacology, that means "as needed" is
    (A) aa
    (B) ac
    (C) prn
    (D) ante
    (E) NS

ON THE JOB

Dr. Waring is in solo practice. When she is on vacation, she arranges for Dr. Dumphey to cover her patients. Dr. Dumphey's medical assistant, Theresa, has just received a call from a patient of Dr. Waring's.

The patient is an elderly woman, with multiple medical problems, who is experiencing what may be a reaction to a medication that Dr. Waring prescribed 2 days ago for bronchitis. Her symptoms include nausea, upset stomach, dizziness, headache, rash on her chest, and extreme exhaustion. Theresa senses that the patient may be exhibiting some disorientation to time and place as it is difficult to elicit consistent responses from her regarding her medications.

The patient is reporting to Theresa that the newest medication she has been taking is Bioxin. The other medications she says she takes include Prinivil, Cardizem CD, Premarin, Prilosec, Robaxin, Zocor, Prozac, Ambien, Fosamax, Seldane and aspirin. The patient does not know the dosage of any of these medications, but is willing to "open up her bag of medicine" and read each prescription label to Theresa. What should Theresa do?

What is your response?

1. Does Theresa have an obligation, as Dr. Dumphey's medical assistant, to handle this situation with this patient or should Dr. Waring simply be notified?
2. Is this an emergency situation, or potential emergency situation and, if so, what should Theresa do immediately?
3. Since the patient seems disoriented, should Theresa even trust in what the patient is reporting? Would it be appropriate for Theresa to speak to a member of Theresa's family, perhaps, in this regard?
4. Should Theresa have the patient read the label of each of her medications?
5. Consider the newly prescribed medication, Bioxin, that the patient is taking. Could this medication cause the adverse reaction that the patient is reporting?
6. Given the other medications that the patient is reporting taking, could Bioxin be interacting with any of them and, therefore, causing an adverse reaction?

References

Anderson, K., and Anderson, L. *Mosby's Pocket Dictionary of Medicine, Nursing, & Allied Health.* Chicago: Mosby, 1994.

Bledsoe, B., Clayden, D. and Papa, F. *Prehospital Emergency Pharmacology,* 4th ed. Upper Saddle River, NJ: Brady/Prentice Hall, 1996.

Hemby, M. *Medical Assisting Review.* Upper Saddle River, NJ: Brady/Prentice Hall, 1995.

Hitner, H. and Nagle, B. *Basic Pharmacology for Health Occupations,* 3rd ed. New York: Glencoe, 1994.

Levine, G. *Pocket Guide to Commonly Prescribed Drugs.* Stamford, CT: Appelton & Lange, 1996.

Lewis, M. and Tamparo, C. *Medical Law, Ethics, and Bioethics in the Medical Office.* Philadelphia: F.A. Davis Company, 1993.

Moore, H. and Best, G. *Drug Calculations.* Upper Saddle River, NJ: Prentice Hall, 1995.

Nurse's Pocket Companion. Springhouse, PA: Springhouse Corporation, 1993.

Physicians' Desk Reference, 44th ed. Oradell, NJ: Medical Economics, l990.

Prescription Drugs. Lincolnwood, IL: Publications International, Ltd., 1995.

Professional Guide to Drugs. Horsham, PA: Intermed Communications, Inc., 1991.

Schwinghammer, T. *Pharmacology: A Patient Focused Approach.* Stamford, CT: Appelton & Lange, 1997.

Spratto, G. and Woods, A. *Nurse's Drug Reference.* Boston: Delmar, 1997.

Stringer, J. *Basic Concepts in Pharmacology.* St. Louis: McGraw-Hill, 1996.

Taber's Cyclopedic Medical Dictionary, 18th ed. Philadelphia, F.A. Davis Company, 1997.

Watts, E. *Pharmacology for Medical Assistants.* Upper Saddle River, NJ: Prentice Hall, 1987.

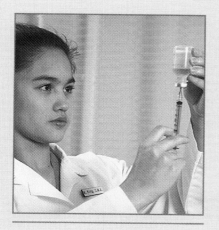

ADMINISTERING MEDICATIONS

- Weights and Measures
- Drug Calculation
- Administration Procedures: OSHA Standards
- Parenteral Medication Administration
- Injectable Drugs Used in the Medical Office
- Charting Medications
- Legal and Ethical Issues
- Patient Education

OBJECTIVES

After completing this chapter, you should:

- Define and spell the glossary terms for this chapter.
- State the difference between the apothecary and the metric systems.
- Correctly calculate medication dosage using mathematical equivalents.
- State four rules for calculating pediatric dosage.
- Describe the OSHA standards relating to needle sticks.
- Correctly describe the procedure for the administration of oral medications.
- Correctly describe the procedure for the administration of parenteral medications.
- List the standard needle lengths and gauges.
- List and define the four sites for intramuscular injections (IM).
- State the rationale for using the Z-track injection method.
- State the names of ten drugs commonly found in the medical office.
- List the precautions used when administering an injection to an infant or small child.

CLINICAL PERFORMANCE OBJECTIVES

After completing this chapter, you should perform the following tasks:

- Correctly calculate drug dosage.
- Prepare a medication for injection using the correct sterile technique.
- Correctly inject medication into the deltoid, gluteus medius, and vastus lateralis muscles using the proper needle and syringe.
- Correctly inject medication using the subcutaneous route of administration.
- Correctly administer an intradermal injection using the proper needle and syringe.
- Correctly administer a medication using the Z-track method.
- Instruct a patient on the use of vaginal medications.
- Instruct the patient on the use of rectal medications.

Glossary

apothecary system   A system of weights and measures, used by physicians and pharmacists, that is based on these basic units of measurements: grain (gr.), gram (g), and dram (℥), for example. This system has been replaced by the metric system whenever possible.

handbreadth   Use the size and surface of one's hand to measure distance on a patient for injection purposes.

metric system   A system of weights and measures based upon the meter as the unit of measurement. This system uses the decimal system.

untoward effect   An unexpected or adverse reaction of a patient to a medication.

WARNING!

For all patient contact, adhere to Standard Precautions. Wear protective equipment as indicated.

One of the most important functions for the medical assistant is administering medications. Pharmacology and drug therapy involve the skills and expertise of many health care professionals including the physician, pharmacist, nurse, and medical assistant. The role of the medical assistant in administering the correct medication at the correct time and in the proper amount is a critical part of the process. Before proceeding with this chapter, review the "three befores" and the "six rights" of drug administration discussed in Chapter 5.

▶ WEIGHTS AND MEASURES

Two systems of weights and measurements are used to calculate dosages: apothecary and metric. The medical assistant must be familiar with both systems since drugs may be ordered in one system but contain a label in another system. You will have to be able to easily convert from one system to another. In addition, there are common household measurements, such as teaspoon (t) and tablespoon (T), which are used even though they are not considered medical measurement units. These household measures are useful when instructing patients.

THE APOTHECARY SYSTEM

The **apothecary system** is considered to be the oldest system of measurement. Dry weight equivalent is 1 grain = 1 gram of wheat. The basic units of weight are grain (gr), gram (g), dram (℥), ounce (℥), and pound (lb). Fluid measurements using the apothecary system are called minims (mn), fluid dram (fl ℥), fluid ounce (fl ℥), pint (pt), quart (qt), and gallon (c). Some of common household measures, for example pint, quart, and gallon, are based on the apothecary system.

Roman numerals are used when numbering in this system. For example, 3 grains would be gr iii and 4 ounces would be ℥ iv. The apothecary system also uses fractions such as 1/4, 1/2, 2/3. Therefore three-fourths of a grain would be gr 3/4. The unit of measurement (gr) is placed before the dosage in the apothecary system.

THE METRIC SYSTEM

The **metric system** is used more widely for prescriptions. This system of measurement is based on the decimal system. This means that all the numbers are derived by either multiplying or dividing by the power of 10. In the metric system, the liter (l) means volume, gram (g) stands for weight, and meter (m) represents length. See Table 6-1 for common abbreviations for weights and measures.

TABLE 6-1   Common Abbreviations for Weights and Measures

Apothecary System			Metric System	
Symbol/Abbreviation		**Meaning**	**Symbol/Abbreviation Weights**	**Meaning**
gtt	drop	drop	mg	milligram
m	Min	minim	gm	gram
ʒ	dr	dram	**Symbol/Abbreviation Volume**	
	f dr	fluid dram		**Meaning**
ʒ	oz	ounce	L	liter
	fl oz	fluid ounce	mL	milliliter
O	pt	pint	cc	cubic centimeter
C	gal	gallon		
	gr	grain		

Guidelines: Conversion Within the Metric System

1. There is no change necessary to change milliliters into cubic centimeters. They are equal to each other.
2. To change grams to milligrams, multiply grams by 1000 or move the decimal point 3 places to the RIGHT.
3. To change milligrams to grams, divide milligrams by 1000 or move the decimal point 3 places to the LEFT.
4. To convert liters to milliliters, multiply liters by 1000 or move the decimal point 3 places to the RIGHT.
5. To convert milliliters to liters, divide milliliters by 1000 or move the decimal point 3 places to the LEFT.

When using the metric system, the dosage is written as a decimal with the unit of measurement (such as mL) following.

See Table 6-2 for commonly used equivalents.

Table 6-3 lists some common household measures.

For a comparison of the three systems for liquid measurements see Table 6-4.

▶ DRUG CALCULATION

Med Tip: By placing the greater than (>) or less than (<) signs between the units, you can see which way to move the decimal point.

Some offices and clinics keep a supply of medications which are referred to as stock medications. The physician may order a medication dosage for a patient that is different from the dosage of the medication you keep in stock.

You may have a conversion chart to use when calculating the correct dosage from a stock dosage. However, it is necessary for you to know how to arrive at the correct calculation of a dose so that you can double-check for accuracy.

Calculating the correct amount of drug to give a patient depends on many factors including patient's age, weight, and current state of health. In addition, you will need to know what other

TABLE 6-2   Commonly Used Equivalents for the Apothecary and Metric Systems

Measure Apothecary	Equivalent Metric
1 gr	65 mg or 0.065 g
5 gr	325 mg or 0.33 g
10 gr	650 mg or 0.67 g
15 or 16 gr	1 g
15 or 16 m	1.00 mL or cc
1 dram	4 mL
1 oz	30 cc, 30 mL, 8 tsp, 8 drams, 3 tbsp
1 lb	450 g
1 lb	0.4536 kg
1 minim (m)	0.06 mL
4 m	0.25 mL
Liquid Measure	
1 fl dr	4 mL
2 fl dr	8 mL
2.5 fl dr	10 mL
4 fl dr	15 mL
1 fl oz	30 mL
3.5 fl oz	100 mL
7 fl oz	200 mL
1 pt	500 mL
1 qt	1000 mL
60 gtts	4 mL

medications the patient is taking since some drugs will be either weakened or strengthened in combination with other drugs.

After receiving the medication order from the physician, the medical assistant should check to see if the order and the medication label are written in the same system of measurement. In other words, is everything in the metric system or in the apothecary system? If a combination of the two systems has been used (for example, physician's order is written in the metric system and the medication label is in the apothecary system), you will have to use a conversion chart as in Tables 6-2 and 6-4.

Dosages can be calculated using either the formula method or by ratios. Both methods will be explained in this chapter. You should use the method that is easiest for you.

TABLE 6-3   **Common Household Measures**

Measure	Equivalent
60 gtts. (drops)	1 teaspoon (tsp.)
3 tsp	1 Tablespoon (T.)
2 T	1 oz
4 oz	1 small juice glass
8 oz	1 cup (C) or glass
16 T. or 8 oz	1 C
2 Cups	1 pint (pt)
2 pints	1 quart (qt)
4 quarts	1 gallon

TABLE 6-4   **Comparison of Household/Apothecary/Metric Liquid Measurements**

Household	Apothecary	Metric
1 drop	1 minim (m)	0.06 mL
1 tsp.	1 fl dr (fl ℨ)	4-5 mL
1 T	4 fl dr (fl ℨ)	15-16 mL
2 T	1 fl oz (fl ℥)	30-32 mL
1 cup or glass	8 fl oz (fl ℥)	250 mL
2 cups or glasses	16 fl oz/ 1 pt	500 mL
4 cups or glasses	1 qt	1000 mL = approximately 1 liter

REVIEW OF MATH PRINCIPLES

In order to understand the methods used for drug calculations, you must refresh your memory concerning mathematics. Remember that there is a relationship between fractions, ratios, percentages, and decimals. Refer to Table 6-5 for examples of some mathematical equivalents.

TABLE 6-5   **Example of Mathematical Equivalents**

Fraction	Ratio	Percent	Decimal
1/4	1:4	25%	.25
1/2	1:2	50%	.50
2/3	2:3	66%	.66
3/4	3:4	75%	.75
7/8	7:8	88%	.88
1/100	1:100	1%	.01
1/200	1:200	.5%	.005
1/1000	1:1000	.1%	.001

For example, the fraction 1/2 is the same as the ratio 1:2 (one-to-two). A ratio is another way of expressing a fraction. This is also the same as the percentage 50% and the decimal .50.

Using ratios is one method for calculating the correct drug dosage from a stock dosage. We would compare the amount of drug the physician ordered to the amount we have on hand (stock medications).

To determine a percentage from a fraction, divide the numerator (top number) by the denominator (bottom number). The decimal number that results can then be converted into a percentage by moving the decimal point two spaces to the right.

For example:
1/2 = 1 ÷ 2 = .50
.50 = 50.0% or 50%

When you have two ratios to compare, you then have a proportion. A proportion resulting from the fraction 1/2 or ratio 1:2 could be 10/20 = 1/2 or 10:20 :: 1:2. The proportion is read as 10 divided by 20 equals 1 divided by 2, or ten is to twenty as one is to two. Even though the numbers may be larger, the actual proportions or relationship to each other is the same. If you know three numbers in the above equation (10/20 = 1/2 or 10:20 :: 1:2), you can solve for the fourth, or unknown quantity by using mathematic principles. We use the symbol x for the unknown quantity. For example: 10/20 = 1/x

Cross-multiply to find the unknown quantity. To cross-multiply means to multiply the top number against the opposite bottom number. Therefore 10 × x = 1 × 20. Restate this to 10x = 20. Since we want to find the value of x, we need to have it stand alone. If we divide both sides of the equation by the same number, we can have x stand alone. Therefore, 10x ÷ 10 = 1x or x. Next divide the other side of the equation by 10. 20 ÷ 10 = 2. This means that x = 2.

$$\frac{10}{20} \diagtimes \frac{1}{x} = 10 \times x = 20 \times 1$$

$$10x = 20$$

$$\frac{10x}{10} = \frac{20}{10}$$

$$1x = 2$$

$$x = 2$$

Another method is to convert $\dfrac{10}{20} = \dfrac{1}{x}$ into the ratio 10:20 :: 1:x.

Then, multiply the extremes (two outer numbers 10 and x) by each other and the means (the two inner numbers 20 and 1) to solve for *x* (the unknown).

10 : 20 :: 1 : x
10 × x = 20 × 1
10x = 20
20 ÷ 10 = 2
2 = x
2 cc = x

To prove this answer is correct multiply the extremes and multiply the means. If the answer is correct, they will be equal.

10 : 20 :: 1 : 2
10 × 2 = 20 × 1
20 = 20 Proven

Problem: Physician's order is to give 80 mg of Lasix. The supply on hand states that there is 40 mg/cc.

80 mg : x cc :: 40 mg : 1 cc
80 × 1 = 40 × x
80 = 40x
x = 2 cc

2 cc of Lasix needs to be administered to give an 80 mg dose using the Lasix in stock (40 mg/cc).

CALCULATING DOSAGES

Using the concepts about ratios you have just reviewed, it is possible to calculate dosages using a formula. To find an amount of a drug that is needed to administer set up the following formula (proportion).

Calculation Formula:

$$\frac{\text{available strength}}{\text{ordered strength}} = \frac{\text{available amount}}{\text{amount to give}}$$

- Available strength = The potency (strength) of the drug you have in stock.
- Available amount = (What actually contains the drug.)

For instance, a vial marked 1000 mg/cc. means that in every 1 cc. of liquid there is contained 1000 mg of medication. An oral pill that contains 10 gr. means that 10 grains of medication are in every pill.

- Ordered strength = The potency or strength the physician has ordered in this prescription.
- Amount to give = This is the unknown amount (x) or the amount that you will be solving the problem to find.

Using this formula we can solve the following problem.

Physician's order: Give 500 mg of a drug.
Available: A vial which contains 1000 mg/cc.

Calculation Formula:

$$\frac{\text{available strength}}{\text{ordered strength}} = \frac{\text{available amount}}{\text{amount to give}}$$

Strength of the drug in the vial = 1000 mg/cc.
Available amount = 1 cc
Ordered Strength = 500 mg
Amount to give = x

$$\frac{1000 \text{ mg}}{500 \text{ mg}} = \frac{1 \text{ cc}}{x}$$
$$1000 \times x = 500 \times 1$$
$$1000x = 500$$
$$\frac{1000x}{1000} = \frac{500}{1000}$$
$$1x = 5/10 = 1/2 \text{ cc} = 0.5 \text{ cc}$$

You would fill the syringe with 0.5 cc of liquid to give you the physician's order of 500 mg of medication. To solve a problem using other forms of medication, such as tablets, use the same formula.

Physician's order: Give 10 grains of medication.
Available: Tablets containing 2.5 grains each.

Calculation Formula:

$$\frac{\text{available strength}}{\text{ordered strength}} = \frac{\text{available amount}}{\text{amount to give}} =$$

HAVE/WANT

2.5 gr = 1 tablet
10 gr x (no. of tablets)
2.5 × x = 10 × 1
2.5x = 10
$$\frac{2.5x}{2.5} = \frac{10}{2.5}$$
1x = 4 tablets

Another formula that is frequently used is D/H × Quantity.

D = Desired or ordered dose
H = Supply on hand or available supply
Q = Quantity available

Problem: The physician ordered Penicillin 250 mg. The bottle from the supply you have in stock is labeled "Penicillin 500 mg per cc."

Solution: Set up the formula

$$\frac{\text{Desired}}{\text{Hand}} \times \text{Quantity}$$

The physician's order is placed in the Desired (D) space and the supply you have on hand is placed in the Hand (H) space. The quantity per cc is placed in the Quantity (Q) space.

$$\frac{D}{H} \times Q = \frac{250}{500} \times 1$$

Divide 250 by 500 $\times \frac{1}{1} = 0.5$ cc.

The answer is 0.5 cc or 1/2 a cc.

RULES FOR CONVERSION

Remember that in converting from one system to another the equivalencies are only going to be approximate. It may be necessary to round off the amounts. A simplified list of conversions that you may wish to memorize is found in Table 6-6. It is based on Table 6-2.

CALCULATING PEDIATRIC DOSES

Adult medications are generally not suitable for children even if the dosage is changed. However, there are situations when only an adult dose is available. In that event, a child's—pediatric—dosage can be calculated using the adult dosage as the base.

Determining the correct dosage for a child is the responsibility of the physician. You may be asked to assist by performing the calculations. However, this can only be done under the supervision of the physician.

TABLE 6-6   Conversion List

Apothecary	Metric
15 or 16 minims (m)	1 mL or 1 cc
1 fluid dr	4 mL or cc
1 fluid oz	30 mL or cc
1 quart	1000 mL or cc
1/60 grain	1 milligram (mg)
1 grain	0.065 gram
15 grains	1 gram
2.2 pounds	1 kilogram

Med Tip: Remember that when converting a larger unit to a smaller unit, you multiply. When converting a smaller unit to a larger unit, you divide.

Guidelines: Conversion

1. To change grains to grams, divide by 15.
2. To change ounces to cubic centimeters (cc's), multiply by 30.
3. To change grains to milligrams (mg), multiply by 60. (Only use this rule when you have less than one grain.)
4. To change kilograms to pounds, multiply by 2.2.
5. To change cubic centimeters (cc's) to ounces, divide by 30.
6. To change drams to milliliters (mL), multiply by 4.
7. To change cubic centimeters (cc) or milliliters (mL) to minims, multiply by 15 or 16.
8. To change minims to cubic centimeter's (cc's), divide by 15 or 16.
9. To convert drams to grams, multiply by 4.

There are several rules or "laws" for calculating pediatric dosage which bear the names of the person who developed the rule. These include Clark's Rule, Fried's Law, Young's Law, and West's Nomogram.

Clark's Rule

Clark's Rule is based on the weight of the child. Many physicians favor using this rule since children's weight at a particular age can vary greatly from one child to another. The formula for Clark's Rule is:

Pediatric dose =
$$\frac{\text{child's weight in pounds}}{150 \text{ pounds}} \times \text{adult dose}$$

To use Clark's Rule divide the weight of the child by 150 pounds. Multiply this number by the adult dose to arrive at the pediatric dosage. For example: Penicillin is ordered for a child weighing 35 pounds. The average dose for an adult is 360 mg. How many mg. will the child receive?

$$\frac{35}{150} \times 360 \text{ mg} = 83.9 \text{ mg}$$

To convert the mg into cc's use the $\frac{D}{H} \times Q$ formula.

Fried's Law

Fried's law applies to children under the age of one year. The principle is based on the age of the child in months as compared to a child who is 12 1/2 years old. Fried's assumption is that a 12 1/2 year old child could take an adult dose. The formula for using Fried's Law is:

$$\text{Pediatric dose} = \frac{\text{child's age in months}}{150 \text{ months}} \times \text{adult dose}$$

First, convert 12 1/2 years into months (150 months) since the calculation will be done using months of age as the base. Then, take the patient's age in months and divide it by 150. Multiply this number by the adult dose of the medication to determine what the appropriate pediatric dose would be.

Physician's order:
Child's age: 6 months
Pediatric Dose:

Young's Rule

Young's Rule is used for children who are over 1 year of age. The formula for Young's Rule is:

$$\text{Pediatric dose} = \frac{\text{child's age in years}}{\text{child's age in years} + 12} \times \text{adult dose}$$

To use this formula divide the child's age in years by the same number plus 12. Multiply this number by the adult dose to determine the correct pediatric dosage.

Problem: An adult dose of Phenobarbitol is 30 mg. What would it be for a four year old child?

Solution: $\frac{4}{4 + 12} \times 30 \text{ mg} = 7.5 \text{ mg}$

West's Nomogram

The West's Nomogram is considered the most accurate of all the methods. This method is preferred for sick and underweight children. The nomogram can be used for both infants and children. The nomogram chart is found in pediatrician's offices, medical textbooks and dictionaries.

West's Nomogram is the preferred method of most physicians for calculating pediatric dosage since it is based on a calculation of the child's body surface area (height and weight). The body surface area (BSA) is expressed in square meters (m^2). The nomogram chart has three columns (see Figure 6-1). To calculate the child's BSA a straight line is drawn from the patient's height in

FIGURE 6-1
_____

Nomogram Chart.

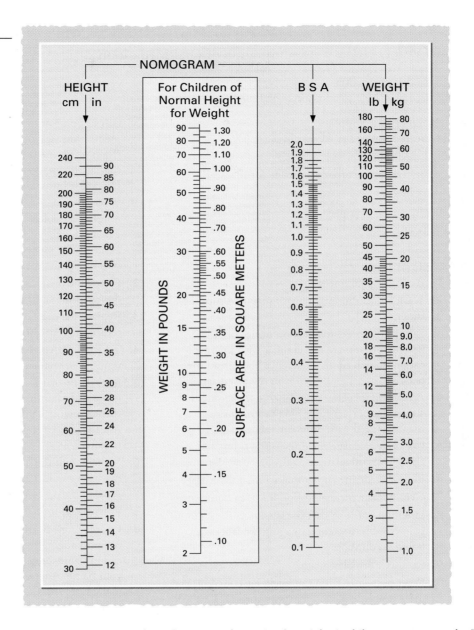

inches or centimeters across the columns to the patient's weight in kilograms or pounds. This straight line will intersect on the BSA column. The reading at this point of intersection will give the BSA average. Once the BSA average is found, then a calculation using the formula below is done to calculate the child's dose. The formula for using West's Nomogram is:

$$\text{Pediatric dose} = \frac{\text{basic surface area of child}}{1.73 \text{ square meters}} \times \text{adult dose}$$

To use this formula you must use West's Nomogram chart. The basic surface area (BSA) for the child has been calculated on the chart. Find the child's weight and height on the chart. Lay a ruler or a paper's sharp edge across the chart and find the point of intersection where the child's weight and height intercept the BSA. Take this calculation and divide it by 1.73 square meters. Then, multiply this number by the adult dose to find the pediatric dosage.

PROCEDURE: Administration of Oral Medication

Terminal Performance
Competency: Able to administer oral medication without error.

Equipment and Supplies
Medication order signed by physician
Oral medication
Calibrated paper cup or receptacle for medication
Water in glass
Patient instruction sheet
Biohazard waste container
Pen

Procedural Steps

1. Assemble equipment.
2. Wash hands thoroughly with soap and running water.
3. Select the correct medication using the "three befores." If you are not familiar with the medication, look it up in a reference book, read the package insert, and/or consult the physician.
4. Always double-check the label to make sure the strength is correct since medications are manufactured with different strengths.
5. Correctly calculate the dosage in writing. Double-check your calculations with someone else.
6. Place a medicine cup/container on a flat surface.
7. Gently shake the medication if it is in liquid form.
8. Hold the bottle so that the label is in the palm of your hand to prevent damaging the label with liquid medication.
9. Re-check the label again.
10. Remove the cap from the medicine container and place it upside down on a clean surface. This will keep a clean area on the inside of the cap which can then be replaced on the bottle.
11A. *Liquid medication:* Hold the calibrated medicine cup at eye level and pour the medication into the cup stopping at the correct dosage line. Pour the medication away from the label side of the bottle. If too much medication is poured into the calibrated cup, do not return it to the bottle. Discard it into a sink.
11B. *Tablet or capsule medication:* Shake out the correct number of tablets or pills into the bottle cap. Then place them in the medicine cup. If you accidentally pour out an extra tablet, do not return it to the medication bottle. Discard it.
12. Check the medication again to make sure the dosage is the same as the medication order.
13. Replace the cap on the medication bottle and return the bottle to the storage shelf.
14. Take the prepared medication and a glass of water to the patient.
15. Identify the patient both by stating his or her name and examining any printed identification such as a wrist name band or medical record. Ask the patient if he or she has any allergies (Figure 6-2).
16. Remain with the patient until the medication has been swallowed.
17. Provide the patient with written follow-up instructions if further medication is to be taken.
18. Chart the medication administration on the correct patient's record noting the time, medication name, dosage, route (oral procedure), and your name. After giving the medication to the patient, it is best to have the patient wait in the office for 30 minutes.

Charting Example

2/14/XX	1 PM	ASA, 500 mg, po.
		N. Young, RMA

► ADMINISTRATION PROCEDURES: OSHA STANDARDS

The Occupational Safety and Health Administration (OSHA) has established guidelines for disposal of contaminated needles and syringes. In addition, OSHA's bloodborne pathogens standard has provisions for medical follow-up procedures that health care workers must take if they have experienced a puncture with a contaminated needle.

If a medical assistant is accidentally stuck with a contaminated needle, a physician must be notified immediately. Exposure to contaminated needles carries with it a risk of infection from the

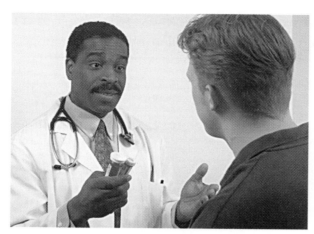

FIGURE 6-2

Provide patient instruction as needed.

hepatitis B virus (HBV) or the human immunodeficiency virus (HIV) which causes acquired immune deficiency syndrome (AIDS). There is a greater incidence of acquiring hepatitis from a contaminated needle stick than AIDS.

Immediate reporting of needle sticks is important so that early testing and action can begin. It can also assist employers in determining how to prevent other such occurrences in the future. It is the responsibility of the employer to provide free medical evaluation and treatment for employees who experience a contaminated needle stick while on the job.

 Med Tip: Remember that *all* needles are considered contaminated.

According to law all medical offices must have a rigid, locked safety container labeled with an international biohazard sticker for the disposal of sharps. When this waste container is 2/3 to 3/4 full, it is to be removed and properly disposed of using a waste removal service which will incinerate the contents or by autoclaving.

Refer to the procedures for oral, buccal, and sublingual administration of medication when administering medication by any of these routes.

Another method for administering oral medications is via an inhaler or nebulizer which discharges the medication into the respiratory track. See Figure 6-3 for an example of a nebulizer with a medication inhaler.

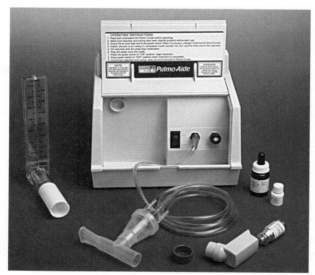

FIGURE 6-3

A nebulizer with a medication inhaler.

PROCEDURE: Administration of Sublingual or Buccal Medication

Terminal Performance
Competency: Be able to administer without error a medication to a patient under the tongue or between the cheek and gum as ordered by the physician.

Equipment and Supplies
   Medication order signed by physician on the patient's medical record
   Oral medication
   Paper cup or receptacle for medication
   Patient instruction sheet
   Biohazard waste container
   Pen

Procedural Steps
   1. Assemble equipment.
   2. Wash hands thoroughly with soap and running water.
   3. Select the correct medication using the "three befores."
If you are not familiar with the medication look it up in a reference book, read the package insert and/or consult the physician.
   4. Always *double-check* the label to make sure the strength is correct since medications are manufactured with different strengths.
   5. Correctly calculate the dosage in writing. Double-check your calculations.
   6. Place a medicine cup/container on a flat surface.
   7. Shake the tablet ordered into the bottle cap and then into a medication container.
   8. *Check the dosage again* against the medication order.
   9. Replace the cap on the medication bottle and return the bottle to the storage shelf after reading the label again.

   10. Identify the patient both by stating his or her name and examining any printed identification, such as a wrist name band or medical record. Ask the patient if he or she has any allergies.
   11A. *Sublingual medication:* Have the patient place the tablet under the tongue. Instruct the patient not to swallow until the tablet has dissolved.
   11B. *Buccal medication:* Have the patient place the tablet between the cheek and gum area. Instruct the patient not to swallow until the tablet is dissoled.
   12. Tell the patient not to take fluids until the tablet is dissolved.
   13. Remain with the patient until the medication has dissolved.
   14. Provide the patient with written follow-up instructions if further medication is to be taken.
   15. Chart the medication administration on the correct patient's record noting the time, medication name, dosage, route, and your name. After giving the medication to the patient, it is best to have the patient wait in the office for 30 minutes.

Charting Example
2/14/XX   9 AM Nitroglycerin tab 1,
(gr. 1/100) subling., P = 60
                                    N. Young, RMA

The procedure for insertion of a rectal or vaginal suppository provides instruction for administering (inserting) medication into the rectum or vagina.

▶ PARENTERAL MEDICATION ADMINISTRATION

The term parenteral means to administer medication by injection. The advantages to using the parenteral route for medication administration include (1) fast absorption of the medication into the system, (2) introduction of medications into the system which cannot otherwise be absorbed through the digestive system, and (3) ability to administer medication to the patient whose condition will not tolerate oral medications.

PROCEDURE: Administration (Insertion) of a Rectal or Vaginal Suppository

Terminal Performance
Competency: Be able to insert a suppository without error as ordered by the physician.

Equipment and Supplies
Medication order signed by physician
Lubricant
Water
Biohazard waste container
Patient instructions
Vaginal suppository and supplies:
 Vaginal suppository or cream
 Sterile gloves
 Sanitary napkin
Rectal suppository and supplies:
 Rectal suppository
 Nonsterile gloves
 4 × 4 gauze square
Pen

Procedural Steps
1. Assemble equipment.
2. Wash hands thoroughly with soap and running water.
3. Select the correct medication using the "three befores."

If you are not familiar with the medication, look it up in a reference book, read the package insert and/or consult the physician.

4. Always double-check the label to make sure the strength is correct since medications are manufactured with different strengths.
5. Correctly calculate the dosage in writing. Double-check your calculations with someone else.
6. Check the dosage again against the medication order.
7. Replace the cap on the medication bottle and return the bottle to the storage shelf or refrigerator after reading the label again.
8. Identify the patient both by stating his or her name and examining any printed identification, such as a wrist name band or medical record. Ask the patient if he or she has any allergies.
9. Give patient a gown or sheet. Have the patient remove all clothing from the waist down.
10A. *Rectal suppository:* Have the patient lie on left side, if possible, with top leg bent. Drape a sheet over the patient. Put on nonsterile gloves. Open the suppository wrapper and place suppository on a gauze square. Moisten the suppository with a small amount of lubricant or water. With one hand separate the buttocks. Pick up the suppository with the other hand. Ask the patient to breathe slowly as you insert the suppository from 1 to 1 1/2 inches through the rectal sphincter. Hold the buttocks together and instruct the patient not to bear down or push out the suppository. Wipe the anal area with the gauze and discard gauze into a biohazard waste container. Have the patient remain in the side position for around 20 minutes until the suppository melts.

10B. *Vaginal suppository:* Have the patient assume the dorsal recumbent position with legs apart. Drape the patient. Open the sterile glove pack on a flat surface leaving the gloves in place. Use the inside of the glove wrapper as a sterile field. Peel open the suppository container and drop the suppository onto the inside of the glove wrapper. If an applicator is provided drop it onto the sterile surface also. Glove using sterile technique. With one gloved hand separate the labia minora and hold it in place. Using the other hand insert the suppository one finger length into the vagina. If an applicator is used, place the suppository into the applicator and insert it in a downward direction. Instruct the patient to remain in this position for at least 10 minutes for the suppository to dissolve. Place applicator into the glove wrapper. Remove one glove by pulling inside out from the cuff. With the remaining gloved hand, roll the contaminated wrapper and contents. Hold these waste items as you remove the remaining glove over them. Dispose of all materials into a biohazard waste container. Give the patient a sanitary napkin.

11. Remain with the patient until the medication has dissolved.
12. Provide the patient with written follow-up instructions if further medication is to be taken.
13. Chart the medication administration on the patient's record noting the time, medication name, dosage, injection site, route and your name.

Charting Example
2/26/XX   9 AM   Ducolax 15 mg. Rectal supp.
                       M. King, CMA

The disadvantages include (1) inability to remove the medication once it has been injected, (2) potential for infection via the needle, and (3) trauma to tissue from the needle and harsh medications.

The routes for injection include intradermal (ID), subcutaneous (subq), and intramuscular (IM). The Z-track method is also used for intramusular injections. A fourth route for the administration of parenteral medications is by intravenous (IV) fluids. Medical assistants do not administer medications by this route. Figure 6-4 illustrates the angle of needle insertion for these four types of injections.

EQUIPMENT USED FOR MEDICATION ADMINISTRATION

Equipment for dispensing parenteral medications will vary slightly from office to office. Generally you will need to make sure that you have the correct needle gauge, needle length, syringe size and type.

Needle Gauge

Gauge of the needle refers to the actual width of the needle. The gauge ranges from size 14 (largest) to 28 (smallest). The most common gauges for subcutaneous (subq) injections are 25 and 26. Large gauge needles (20-23) are used for intramuscular (IM) injections when a thick or viscous medication, such as penicillin, is administered. You will not generally use a needle larger than a 20 gauge when administering medications. These larger gauge needles are used for venipuncture and blood transfusions. Smaller gauge needles (27-28) are used when a small needle opening is needed. This smaller size is used for giving intradermal (ID) injections when a small amount of medication is placed within the top layer of the skin.

Med Tip: Remember the smaller the number the larger the needle opening. Carefully select the correct gauge needle for the type of injection to be administered. A large gauge needle can cause tissue damage and pain for the patient if used for anything other than an intramuscular injection.

Needle Length

In addition to the size of the needle opening (gauge), the length of the needle is important. Needle sizes vary from 3/8 inch to 4 inches in length. The length of needle selected depends upon the route used and the area of the body to be injected. See Figure 6-5 for an example of a hypodermic needle.

The 3/8 inch needle is used for intradermal injections when a very short needle is needed to insert within the skin. Subcutaneous needles are 1/2 or 5/8 inches in length. A longer needle is not necessary or advised since a longer needle could be inserted beyond the subcutaneous layer. A longer (1-inch, 1 1/2 inch, 2 inch, or 3 inch) needle is used for injection into a muscle. The actual length used would depend on the size and weight of the patient and the muscle that is used.

Med Tip: The correct needle length is extremely important since you will be placing the entire needle, up to 1/8 inch of the hub, into the patient. If the needle is too long there is a danger of touching the patient's bone.

Syringes

Syringes come in a variety of sizes. They are selected based on the type and the amount of medication to be dispensed. The U 100 syringe is the most commonly used insulin syringe. Figures 6-6 A-D show different types of syringes.

The smallest syringe is the tuberculin syringe. It is a long narrow syringe holding only 1 cc (mL) of medication. The tuberculin syringe is calibrated in one hundredths (1/100) of a milliliter and minims. It is used for tuberculosis testing and when small amounts of medication are needed, such as in skin testing for allergies.

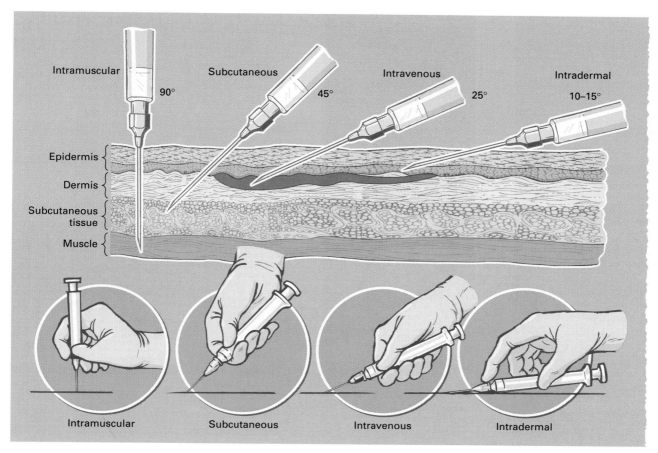

FIGURE 6-4

Angle of needle insertion for four types of injection.

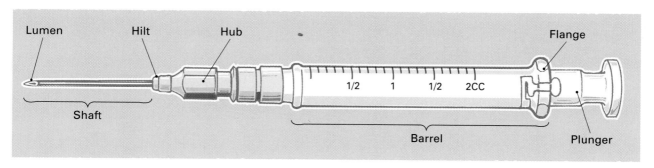

FIGURE 6-5

A hypodermic needle.

The insulin syringe is a small syringe that is calibrated into "Units (U)" especially for the administration of insulin. Since insulin is administered by its concentration of insulin rather than by cubic centimeters the calibrations are in units.

Larger syringes are available that hold 2 cc (mL), 3 cc (mL), 5 cc (mL), 10 cc (mL), and up to 60 cc (mL) of medication. The most commonly used syringe is the 3 cc (mL) size which is calibrated in tenths of a mL (cc) and minims. Table 6-7 provides a summary of needle and syringe sizes.

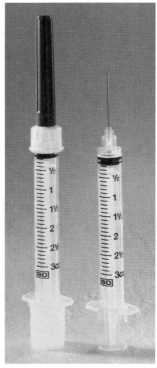

FIGURE 6-6 A

Med-Saver syringe.

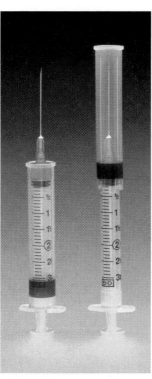

FIGURE 6-6 B

Safety-Lok syringe.

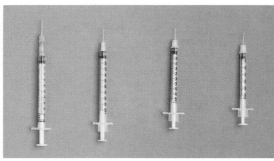

FIGURE 6-6 C

Insulin syringes.

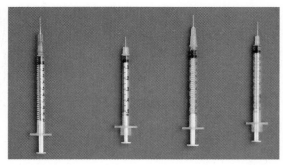

FIGURE 6-6 D

Tuberculin syringes.

TABLE 6-7   **Summary of Needle and Syringe Sizes**

Route	Gauge	Length	Syringe to Use
Intradermal (ID)	27-28	3/8 inch	tuberculin
Subcutaneous (subq)	25-26	1/2, 5/8 inch	tuberculin; 2 cc; or insulin
Intramuscular (IM)	20-23	1-3 inch	2-5 cc
Deltoid (IM)	25	1/2 inch	2 cc
Vastus lateralis	25	5/8 inch	2 cc

Disposable syringes with needles attached come in peel-apart paper wrappers. There is a rigid sheath which protects the needle. Once the sheath protecting the needle has been removed it should not be replaced using your hands since an accidental needle stick can occur. See Figure 6-7 for an example of a biohazard sharps container.

Using a Prefilled Cartridge Injection System

Some drug manufacturers package medications in single-dose glass cartridges which can be placed into a special cartridge holder. You can use the cartridge holder over and over again. The advantage to this system is that the dose is already correctly drawn into the cartridge which eliminates the need

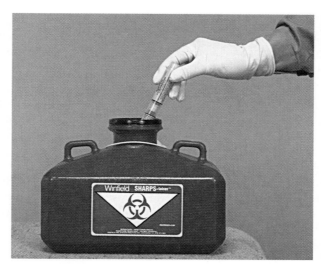

FIGURE 6-7

Biohazard sharps container.

Med Tip: Never put the syringe and needle down on any surface after completing the injection. A portable biohazard sharps container should be within reach so that the needle can immediately be discarded. The most critical time for a needle stick incident is immediately *after* the injection.

to withdraw medication from a vial or bottle. The cartridge holder is sturdy and long-lasting. This system can save money for the office. See Figure 6-8 for an illustration of the Tubex cartridge system. The Medi-jector needle-free insulin delivery system is illustrated in Figure 6-9.

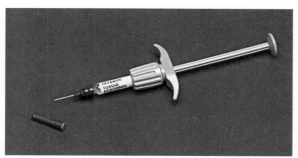

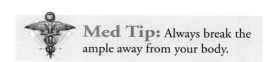

Med Tip: Always break the ample away from your body.

FIGURE 6-8

Tubex cartridge system.

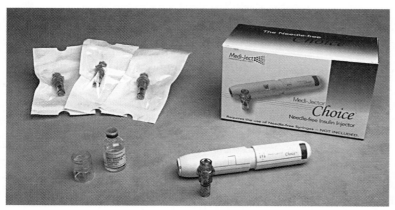

FIGURE 6-9

Medi-jector needle-free insulin delivery system.

Ampule

An ampule is a small sealed glass tube which contains medication. An ampule generally contains a single dose of liquid medication and is packed in a storage container to prevent breakage. There is generally an indentation in the neck of the ampule which is the weak point.

Single-dose and Multi-dose Vials

Single-dose and multi-dose vials (bottles) containing fluid medication are small bottles with rubber stoppers on the top. The rubber stopper on the top of the vial allows you to enter the vial with a needle and syringe to withdraw more than one dose.

The single-dose vial is meant to be discarded after withdrawing one dose. Both types of vials will contain instructions concerning the total amount of fluid in the vial. In addition, the instruction will state what the dosage is in each cc of fluid. It is good practice to review the procedure for withdrawing medication from a single-dose and a multi-dose vial before performing the procedure.

SITES FOR INTRAMUSCULAR INJECTIONS

An intramuscular (IM) injection can be administered in one of four major sites. These sites or muscles are the deltoid, vastus lateralis, dorsogluteal, and ventrogluteal. A description of each muscle follows, including the location of the muscle and the medication circumstance to which the muscle is best suited.

PROCEDURE: Using an Ampule

Terminal Performance
Competency: Be able to correctly open and withdraw medication from an ampule.

Equipment and Supplies
  Ampule containing medication
  Soap
  Alcohol sponge
  Needle
  Syringe
  Hazard waste container
  Pen

Procedural Steps
1. Do not open the ampule until you are ready to withdraw the fluid. *Note:* Always follow the "three befores" when checking medications against the medication order.
2. Thoroughly wash hands with soap and running water.
3. Snap your thumb and middle finger gently against the tip of the ampule to move all the medication away from the neck and into the bottom of the ampule. (Figure 6-10 illustrates breaking a glass ampule.)
4. Clean the neck of the ampule using an alcohol swab.
5. Use gauze between ampule and thumbs when breaking ampule. Using one hand to hold the bottom of the vial, snap the top off with the other hand using a gauze square to prevent a cut when the glass neck breaks.
6. If the top of the ampule does not snap off easily, you may have to use a file to create a cut or "score" the ampule at the neck. The glass ampule should then break easily at this point.
7. Insert a needle (attached to a syringe) into the ampule and withdraw the fluid without touching the sides of the ampule.
8. Withdraw all the medication from the ampule. It may be necessary to tip the ampule slightly to withdraw all the fluid.
9. Discard the broken ampule into a hazard waste container.

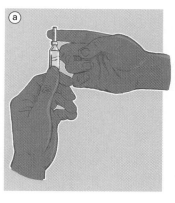
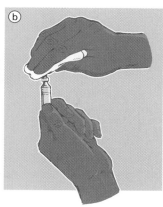
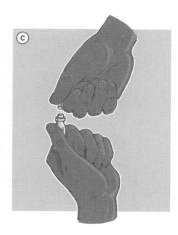

FIGURE 6-10

Breaking a glass ampule containing medication.

PROCEDURE: Withdrawing Medication From a Single-dose and Multi-dose Vial

Terminal Performance

Competency: Be able to correctly withdraw medication from a single-dose and a multi-dose vial.

Equipment and Supplies

Disposable gloves	Syringe
Biohazard waste container	Alcohol sponge
Biohazard sharps container	Medication vial
Soap	Pen
Needle	

Procedural Steps

1. Check the medication using the "three befores" technique before beginning. Compare the medication vial (bottle) against the physician's order.

2. Select the correct syringe and needle depending on the type of medication and location for the injection site.

3. Thoroughly wash hands with soap and running water.

4. Roll the medication vial between your hands to mix any medication that has settled on the bottom.

5. Wipe the rubber stopper with an alcohol sponge firmly in a circular motion. Then set the vial on a clean surface while you prepare the syringe.

6. Remove the protective cap from the needle on the syringe. Maintain the sterility of the inner surface of the protective cap since it will be needed to cover the needle again after you have filled the syringe. Figure 6-11 A-E shows the steps involved in filling a syringe.

7. Withdraw the syringe plunger and allow air to enter the syringe in an amount equal to the amount of medication to be withdrawn. Since the vials are vacuum sealed, this will allow for easier withdrawal of fluid.

8. Turning the vial upside down at eye level, using care not to touch the rubber stopper, insert the needle into the rubber stopper and inject the air into the vial. Be extremely cautious concerning contamination as you enter the multiple-dose bottle. *Rationale:* There is an increased danger of contamination since the multiple-dose vial may be entered more than once by several people.

9. Keeping the upside down vial at eye level, slowly withdraw the correct amount of fluid medication. *Rationale:* Rapid withdrawal of fluid may cause air bubbles to form in the syringe.

10. While the needle is still in the vial, check to make sure that the dosage is accurate. Any air bubbles in the syringe will give you an inaccurate dose since they take up the space needed for medication. To remove air bubbles, flick your fingers against the side of the syringe until the air bubbles go back into the tip of the syringe. Expel these bubbles back into the vial and withdraw more medication until the dosage is accurate.

11. Remove needle from vial.

12. If you have accidentally withdrawn too much fluid then discard the excess fluid by shooting it into a sink or waste receptacle. Never return medications to the vial or bottle from which they came.

13. Check the medication vial after you have withdrawn the dosage to make sure you are correct. This is the last step of the "three befores" for checking medications. Also, check to see if the multi-dose vial needs to be refrigerated after opening.

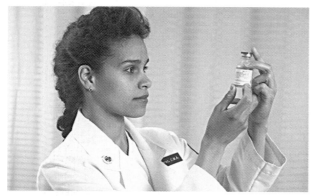

FIGURE 6-11 A

Read the label on the medication bottle.

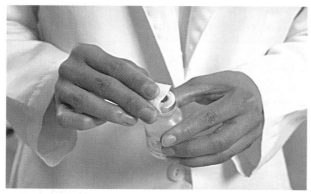

FIGURE 6-11 B

Clean the top of the bottle.

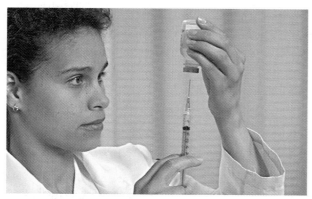

FIGURE 6-11 C

Invert bottle and inject the same amount of air into the bottle as amount of medication to be withdrawn.

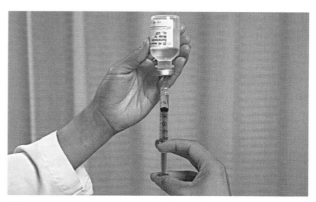

FIGURE 6-11 D

Keeping the bottle inverted, draw the correct amount of medication into the syringe.

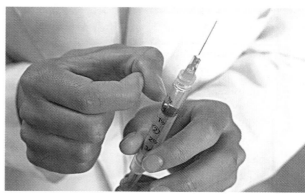

FIGURE 6-11 E

Remove the needle from the bottle and expel the air or tap out the air bubbles.

Deltoid Muscle

The deltoid muscle is located at the top of the arm on the upper, outer surface. This is a small muscle mass which is not a good site for a large amount of medication. This muscle is commonly used for injections such as tetanus boosters in adults. The deltoid muscle can be used for older children, but it should not be used for infants and small children since the muscle is not well-developed.

The deltoid muscle is found by measuring two fingerbreadths below the acromion process of the shoulder. The back surface of the arm should be avoided since the major blood vessels and nerves in the upper arm are located in the posterior portion of the arm. A 23-gauge, 1-inch needle is most commonly used for injection into this site. Use a 25 gauge, 5/8 inch needle for a small arm.

Vastus Lateralis Muscle

The vastus lateralis, or thigh muscle, is located on the upper outer thigh and is part of the quadriceps muscle group. This site is considered to be the safest site for an intramuscular (IM) injection since there are fewer major blood vessels located there. The vastus lateralis muscle lies below the greater trochanter of the femur and within the upper lateral quadrant of the thigh (Figure 6-12).

This muscle is well developed in the infant and is recommended by the American Academy of Pediatrics as the preferred site for all infants and children. Children's immunization are commonly administered into the vastus lateralis muscle in the thigh. Table 6-8 gives a recommended schedule of children's immunizations.

Med Tip: Remember: once you have withdrawn medication into a syringe, there is no way to tell by simply looking if it is the correct medication. You must double check the medication vial after you withdraw the needle from it and before you put the vial away.

In the adult, the vastus lateralis extends from the middle of the anterior (front) thigh to the middle of the lateral thigh. The measurement at the top is one **handbreadth** below the greater trochanter and one handbreadth above the knee. A handbreadth is measured using the size and surface of the hand. The patient may be either in a sitting or supine position.

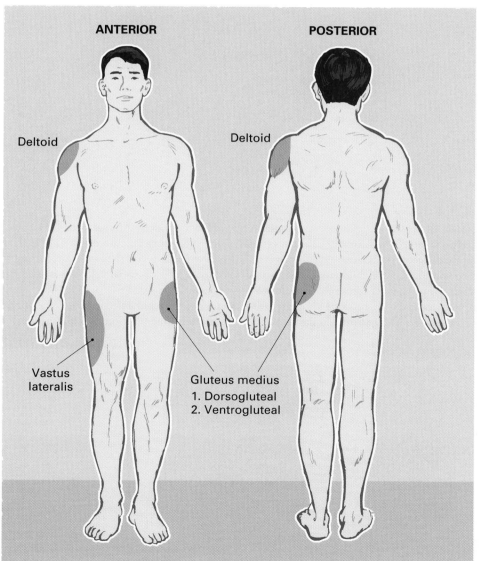

ANTERIOR   POSTERIOR

Deltoid   Deltoid

Vastus
lateralis

Gluteus medius
1. Dorsogluteal
2. Ventrogluteal

FIGURE 6-12

Sites for intramuscular injections.

TABLE 6-8   Schedule of Child Immunizations

Age	Immunizations
Birth	HBV (hepatitis B) #1
2 months	DPT (Diptheria, pertussis, tetanus) #1
	Oral Polio #1
	HBV #2
	Hib (*Haemophilus influenzae*) #1
4-5 months	DPT #2
	Oral Polio #2
	Hib #2
6 months	DPT #3
	Oral Polio #3
	HBV #3
1 year	MMR (Measles, Mumps, Rubella)
	TB test
1 1/2 year	DPT Booster
	Oral Polio Booster
	Rubeola (measles) one dose only
4-6 years	DPT Booster
	Oral Polio Booster

Dorsogluteal (Gluteus Medius) Muscle

The dorsogluteal muscle is the muscle most commonly used when a deep intramuscular (IM) injection is needed for injecting irritating or viscous (thick) medications such as antibiotics. Since there is a danger of damage to the sciatic nerve in this area, many physicians prefer the vastus lateralis muscle be used for adults' and children's intramuscular injections. The vastus lateralis site is used for infants since their gluteus medius muscle is not well-developed.

This injection needs to be done carefully using landmarks to avoid injecting near the sciatic nerve (Figure 6-13). The patient should be asked to lie in the prone position. Ask the patient to

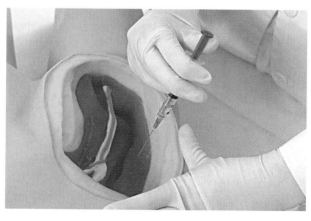

FIGURE 6-13

Care must always be taken to avoid injecting too close to the sciatic nerve.

point his or her toes inward which will cause the muscles to relax. To avoid the sciatic nerve draw an imaginary line from the greater trochanter of the femur to the posterior superior iliac spine. You can feel these bone prominences on the patient. Give the injection above and lateral to the imaginary line. See Figure 6-14 for an illustration of the needle position for an IM injection. You can also divide the buttocks into four imaginary quadrants and inject into the upper outer quadrant (Figure 6-15).

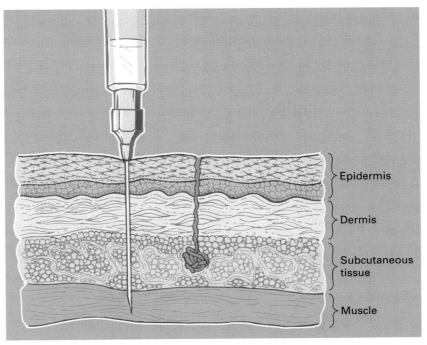

FIGURE 6-14

Needle position for an intramuscular injection.

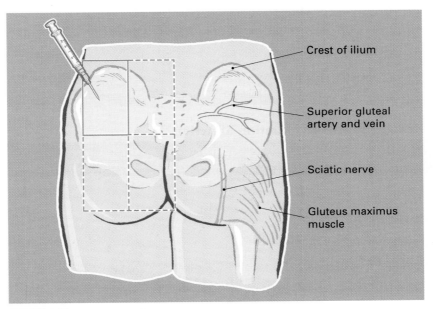

FIGURE 6-15

Injecting the upper outer quadrant of the buttocks.

Ventrogluteal (Gluteus Medius) Muscle

The ventrogluteal site is considered safer than the dorsogluteal site since the gluteus medius muscle does not contain major nerves and blood vessels. This site is considered to be safe for infants, children, and adults.

When injecting into the left side of the patient, the site is located by placing the palm of the right hand on the greater trochanter and the index finger on the anterior superior iliac crest. Next, stretch the index finger as far as possible along the iliac crest. Then, spread the middle finger away from your index finger. The injection is made in the V that is formed by middle and index fingers (Figure 6-16). Always use the hand opposite the patient's side, for example your left hand and patient's right gluteus medius, when using this method to determine the injection location.

SITES FOR SUBCUTANEOUS INJECTION

The subcutaneous injection is given just under (sub) the skin (cutaneous). The injection is given into adipose tissue rather than into muscle. This method is ideal when a small dose of a non-irritating medications, such as in immunizations, insulin, and analgesics, are given. Table 6-9 lists insulin types

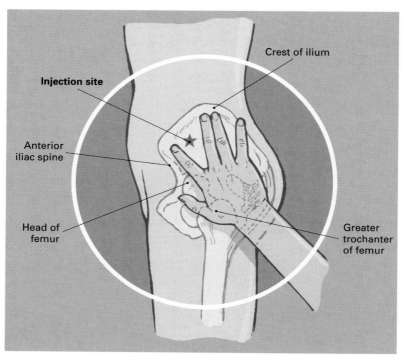

FIGURE 6-16

Injecting the ventrogluteal muscle.

TABLE 6-9   Insulin Types and Duration of Action

Insulin Name	Type	Common Name	Action Onset	Action Peak	Action Duration
Crystalline	Rapid action	Regular	1 hour	2-4 hr	6-8 hr
Semilente	Rapid	Regular	1 hour	4-10 hr	12-16 hr
Humulin-R	Rapid	—	15 min	1 hr	6-8 hr
Isophane	Intermediate	NPH	2-4 hr	6-15 hr	24-48 hr
Insulin Zinc Suspension	Intermediate	Lente	2-4 hr	6-15 hr	24-48 hr
Humulin-N	Intermediate	—	1 hr	4 hr	24 hr
Protamine Zinc	Slow action	PZI	3-6 hr	12-20 hr	24-36 hr
Ultralente	Slow	PZI	8 hr	12-24 hr	36 hr +

and duration of action. The deltoid area and upper back are commonly used. However, when the injection is self-administered by the patient, other sites are commonly used, such as the thighs and abdomen. See Figure 6-17 for an illustration of the sites for subcutaneous injection.

The subcutaneous injection is usually administered at a 45-degree angle with the exception of insulin and heparin which are given at a 90-degree angle (Figure 6-18). When a medication is frequently administered, for example insulin, the sites must be rotated. A record of the rotation sites is kept in the patient's medical record. The patients must also be instructed on how to maintain their own rotation at home. See Figure 6-19 for an example of rotation sites.

When allergy medication is administered, the patient should be asked to remain in the office for an additional 30 minutes following the injection, in case the patient has a reaction to the medication.

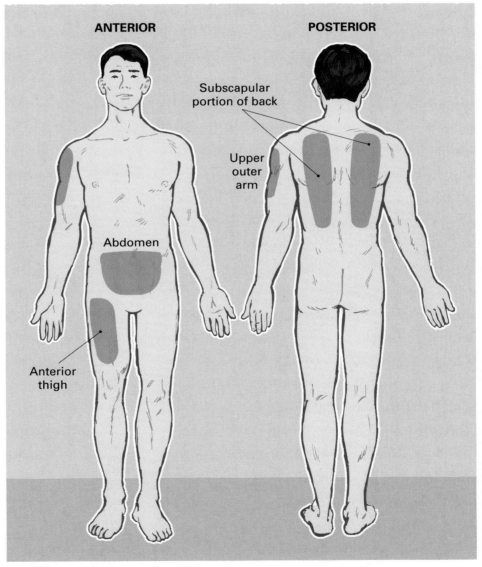

FIGURE 6-17

Sites for subcutaneous injection.

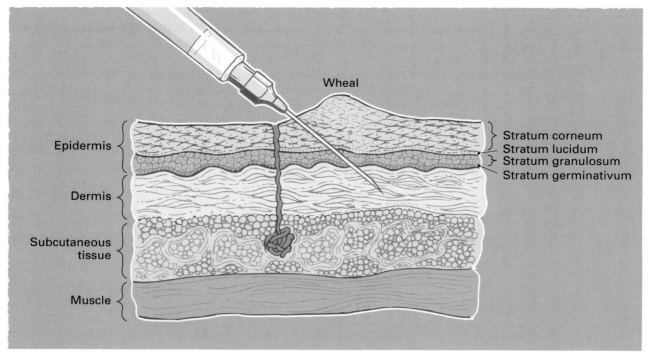

Wheal

Epidermis {

Stratum corneum
Stratum lucidum
Stratum granulosum
Stratum germinativum

Dermis {

Subcutaneous
tissue {

Muscle {

FIGURE 6-18

Needle position during subcutaneous injections.

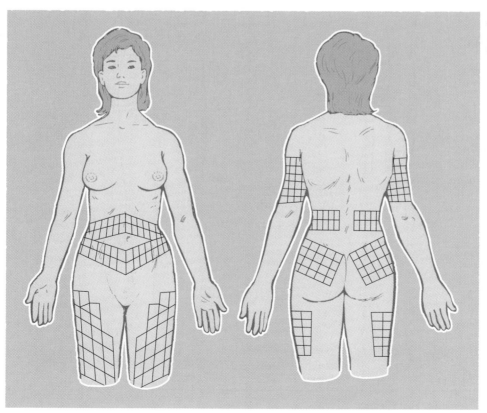

FIGURE 6-19

Rotation sites for administering insulin.

PROCEDURE: Administration of Parenteral (Subcutaneous (SC) or Intramuscular (IM) Injection)

Terminal Performance

Competency: Be able to administer SC and IM injections without error.

Equipment and Supplies

Medication order signed by physician

Vial of medication

Nonsterile gloves

Alcohol sponges

Biohazard sharps container

Biohazard waste container

Subcutaneous injection: 25-gauge, 5/8-inch needle for small arm; 23-gauge, 1-inch needle for average arm

Disposable 3-mL syringe

Intramuscular injection: 22g, 1 1/2-inch needle

Disposable 3-mL syringe

Pen

Procedural Steps

1. Thoroughly wash hands with soap and running water.
2. Apply nonsterile gloves and follow universal blood and body-fluid precautions.
3. Select the correct medication using the "three befores."

Note: Always double-check the label to make sure the strength is correct since medications are manufactured with different strengths, for example 250 mg/cc and 500 mg/cc.

4. Gently roll the medication between your hands to mix any medication that may have settled. Refrigerated medication can be rolled between your hands to warm it slightly.
5. Prepare the syringe using the correct technique. Carefully carry the covered needle and syringe to the patient.
6. Identify the patient both by stating his or her name and examining any printed identification, such as a wrist name band or medical record. Ask the patient if he or she has any allergies.
7. Position the patient depending on the site you are using.
8. Using a circular motion clean the patient's skin with an alcohol sponge. Wipe the skin with a sweeping motion from the center of the area outward. This prevents recontamination of the injection site by the alcohol sponge. Figure 6-20 illustrates the sites for administering an injection.
9. Once again check the medication dosage against the patient's order to determine if this is the correct time to administer the dose (one of the "six rights").
10. Remove the protective covering from the needle using care not to touch the needle. If you accidentally touch the needle, excuse yourself to the patient, then return to the preparation area and change the needle on the syringe. If you are using a self-contained syringe and needle unit that does not come apart, discard the entire syringe with the medication and start the process over again. ***Rationale:*** A contaminated needle can cause a severe infection in an already ill patient. Remember: the patient's safety is your first priority.
11. When you are prepared to administer the injection, place a new alcohol sponge or a cotton ball between two fingers of your nondominant hand so that you can easily grasp it when you are through with the injection.
12. Firmly grasp the syringe in your predominant hand similar to the way a pencil is held.
13A. *To administer a subcutaneous injection:* With your nondominant hand, pick up the skin at the injection site and form a small mass of tissue. This will aid in the needle entering only the subcutaneous tissue.
13B. *To administer an intramuscular injection:* With your nondominant hand stretch the skin tightly where you will insert the needle. Pulling the skin taut allows the needle to enter the skin more easily. (If the patient is thin or a child you would pinch the muscle into a bundle and squeeze as the needle is inserted. In this way you would avoid going deeper than the muscle and touching a bone.)
14. Grasping the syringe in a dart-like fashion insert the entire needle with one swift movement.
15A. *For subcutaneous injection:* Insert into the subcutaneous tissue at a 45-degree angle.

(Continued)

PROCEDURE: Administration of Parenteral (Subcutaneous (SC) or Intramuscular (IM) Injection) *(Continued)*

15B. *For intramuscular injection:* Insert needle directly into the muscle at a 90-degree angle. ***Rationale:*** The selection of the correct size needle is important since you will be inserting the entire needle into the patient.

16. Do not move the needle once you have inserted it. If the needle is pushed in further, contaminants are carried into the skin from the exposed needle.

17. Aspirate to determine if you have entered a blood vessel. To do this pull back slightly on the plunger with the hand holding the syringe while holding the needle steady in the muscle. If blood appears in the hub area of the syringe it means that you are in a blood vessel. You will then have to withdraw the needle using correct technique and discard the syringe containing the blood and medication. Begin the procedure again with step 1 and fresh supplies. ***Rationale:*** You may not administer a subcutaneous or intramuscular injection intravenously into a blood vessel.

18. If you do not see a return of blood in the syringe when you aspirate, slowly inject the medication without moving the needle. Do not move the needle until you have completed injecting all the medication. See Figure 6-21 for illustrations of intramuscular injection. *Note:* Insert and withdraw the needle quickly to minimize pain *but* administer the medication slowly.

19. Taking the alcohol sponge (or cotton ball) from between the last two fingers of your nondominant hand place it over the area containing the needle. Withdraw the needle at the same angle you used for insertion using care not to stick yourself with the needle.

20. With one hand place the sponge firmly over the injection site. With the other hand discard the needle in a biohazard sharps container.

21. You may gently massage the injection site to assist absorption and ease pain for the patient.

22. Make sure the patient is safe before leaving him or her unattended. Observe the patient for any untoward effect of the medication for at least 15 minutes.

23. Correctly dispose of all materials.

24. Remove gloves into biohazard bag and wash your hands.

25. Chart the medication administration on the patient's record noting the time, medication name, dosage, injection site, route, lot # on immunizations, and your name.

Charting Example

2/14/XX   1:30 PM   Penicillin G. procaine, 600,000 unit   IM Right gluteus.

M. King, CMA

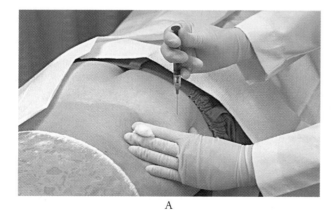

A

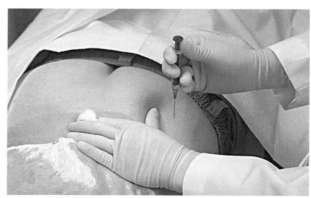

B

FIGURE 6-20 A-F

Sites for administering medication.

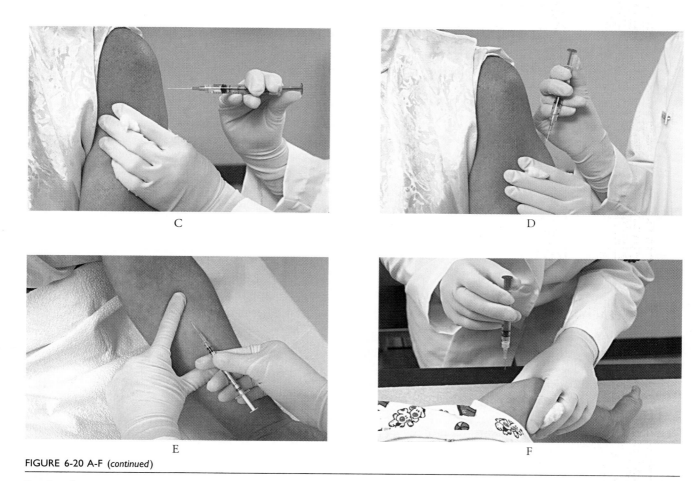

C

D

E

F

FIGURE 6-20 A-F (*continued*)

Sites for administering medication.

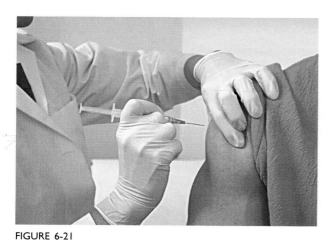

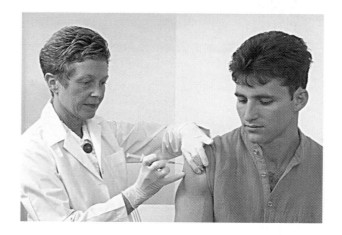

FIGURE 6-21

Intramuscular injections.

PROCEDURE: Administration of a Z-track Injection

Terminal Performance

Competency: Be able to administer Z-track injection using proper technique without error.

Equipment and Supplies

Alcohol sponges
Biohazard sharps container
Biohazard waste container
Disposable gloves
Medication order signed by the physician
Pen
Sterile needle and syringe
Vial of medication

Procedural Steps

Follow steps **1** through **15** of the procedure for administration of an intramuscular injection.

16. After withdrawing the medication from the vial, change to a fresh needle. This will eliminate any irritating medication that may be within the needle from coming into contact with the patient's tissue until the needle is placed into the muscle layer.

17. When ready to administer the medication, pull the skin of the buttock to one side and hold it in place with your nondominant hand. You may wish to use a dry gauze sponge if the skin is slippery.

18. With your dominant hand and using a dart-like grip on the syringe, insert the needle up to the hub quickly into the gluteus medius muscle. Do not move the needle once it is in place.

19. While still maintaining a firm hold on the taut skin with your nondominant hand, pull back on the plunger of the syringe to check for a blood return with the fingers of the hand holding the syringe. To do this simply move your fingers up the syringe, while keeping the needle steady within the patient's buttocks, until your thumb and index finger reach the top of the plunger. If blood appears in the hub of the syringe, then using correct technique, withdraw the syringe, discard, and begin with step 1 again.

20. If there is no return of blood, then very slowly inject the medication into the muscle.

21. Wait several seconds after injecting the medication before you withdraw the needle. Cover the area with the alcohol sponge and withdraw the needle at the same angle of insertion. Wait at least 10 seconds before releasing the skin being held by the nondominant hand.

22. Do not massage the area. Observe the patient for at least 15 minutes for any untoward reaction. You may advise the patient to walk around to assist in the absorption process of the medication.

23. Correctly dispose of all materials.

24. Remove gloves and wash your hands.

25. Chart the medication administration on the patient's record noting the time, medication name, dosage, injection site, route and your name.

Charting Example

2/14/XX   3:30 PM   Iron dextran, 50 mg-Z-track into left gluteus. No C/O pain.

                        N. Young, RMA

PARENTERAL INJECTIONS: INTRAMUSCULAR (IM) AND SUBCUTANEOUS (SC)

The basic procedure for parenteral injections is similar for both intramuscular and subcutaneous injections. The administration sites and needle gauge and lengths differ. Follow this procedure when administering subcutaneous and intramuscular injections.

Intramuscular Injections: Z-track

The Z-track method for injecting medications into the muscle is used for irritating medications, for example ferrous sulfate (iron). This method involves pulling aside the skin, injecting the medication, and then allowing the skin to move back over the injection site. This will help to prevent irritating medications from causing tissue damage by seeping from the muscle into the subcutaneous tissue. See Figure 6-22 for illustration of Z-track injection.

The Z-tract method is only used for injections into the gluteus medius muscle of the buttocks. Do not massage the area over the injection site after withdrawing the needle. Advise the patient to walk around which will encourage absorption of the medication. Chart whether the injection was administered into the right or left buttock so that you know to rotate to the other side when you give the next injection. Tell the patient not to rub the area.

INTRADERMAL INJECTION

The intradermal injection is commonly used for allergy skin testing in which a minute amount of material is injected within the top layer of skin to determine a patient's sensitivity. Since just the top level of skin is entered, a small "wheal" or bubble which contains the injection fluid appears on the skin. Don't rub the area after giving the injection.

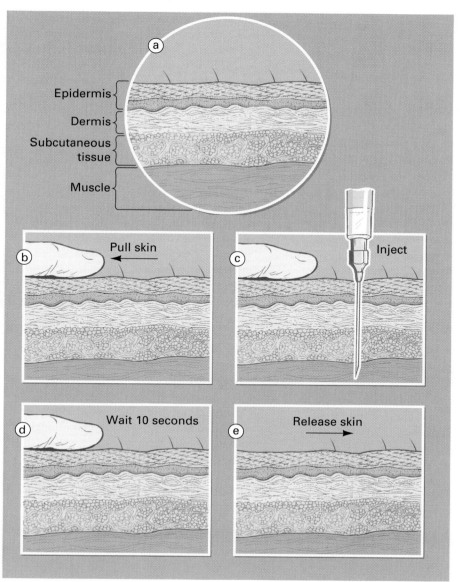

FIGURE 6-22

An example of the Z-track method of injection.

PROCEDURE: Administration of an Intradermal Injection

Terminal Performance

Competency: Be able to correctly administer an intradermal injection without error as ordered by the physician.

Equipment and Supplies
Disposable gloves
Biohazard sharps container
Alcohol sponges
Sterile needle
Sterile syringe
Vial of medication
Medication order signed by physician
Pen

Procedural Steps

I. Preparation:

1. Thoroughly wash hands with soap and running water.
2. Apply nonsterile gloves and follow universal blood and body-fluid precautions.
3. Select the correct medication using the "three befores."
   Always double-check the label to make sure the strength is correct since medications are manufactured with different strengths, for example 1:10, 1:100, or 1:1000 dilutions.
4. Gently roll the medication between your hands to mix any medication that may have settled. Refrigerated medication can be rolled between your hands to warm it slightly.
5. Prepare the syringe using the correct technique. Carefully carry the covered needle and syringe to the patient.
6. Identify the patient both by stating his or her name and examining any printed identification such as a wrist name band or medical record.
7. Select the proper site (center of forearm, upper chest or upper back). See Figure 6-23 for intradermal skin injection sites.
8. Using a circular motion clean the patient's skin with an alcohol sponge. Wipe the skin with a sweeping motion from the center of the area outward. This prevents recontamination of the injection site by the alcohol sponge.

9. Allow time for the antiseptic on the sponge to dry to reduce the possibility of it reacting with the medication.
10. Once again check the medication dosage against the patient's order to determine if this is the correct time to administer the dose (one of the "six rights").
11. Remove the protective covering from the needle using care not to touch the needle. If you accidentally touch the needle then excuse yourself to the patient. Return to your preparation area and change the needle on the syringe. If you are using a self-contained syringe and needle unit that does not come apart, you will have to discard the entire syringe with the medication and start the process over again. (Remember: The patient's safety is your first priority. A contaminated needle can cause a severe infection in an already ill patient.)

II. Injection:

12. Hold the syringe between the first two fingers and thumb of your dominant hand with the palm down and the bevel of the needle up. Figure 6-24 A-F illustrates the steps used to administer an intradermal skin test.
13. Hold the skin taut with the fingers of your nondominant hand. If you are using the center of the forearm, then place the nondominant hand under the patient's arm and pull the skin taut. This will allow the needle to slip into the skin more easily.
14. Using a 15-degree angle insert the needle through the skin to about 1/8 inch. The bevel of the needle will be facing upward and covered with skin. The needle will still show through the skin. Do not aspirate.
15. Slowly inject the medication beneath the surface of the skin. A small elevation of skin (wheal) will occur where you have injected the medication.

PROCEDURE   *(Continued)*

16. Quickly withdraw the needle. With the other hand discard the needle into the biohazard sharps container.

III. Patient follow-up:

17. Do not massage the area.
18. Make sure the patient is safe before leaving him or her unattended. Observe the patient for any **untoward effect**, such as an allergic reaction to the medication, for at least 20 to 30 minutes. Tell the patient not to rub the area.
19. Correctly dispose of all materials.

20. Remove gloves and wash your hands.
21. Chart the medication administration on the patient's record noting the time, medication name, dosage, injection site, route, appearance of the intradermal site after injection and your name.

Charting Example

2/14/XX   10 AM   Mantoux (PPP) tuberculin test, 0.10 mL ID Right anterior forearm. Instructed to return on 2/16 to have test read.

M. King, CMA

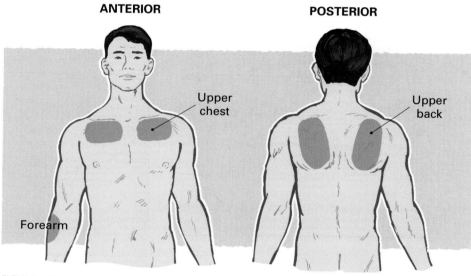

ANTERIOR   **POSTERIOR**

Upper chest   Upper back

Forearm

FIGURE 6-23

Intradermal skin injection sites.

The intradermal injection is also the method of administration for the tuberculosis (TB) test. The TB test is "read" 48 hours after it has been administered. Reading consists of a medical professional examining the injection site for any signs of reaction, such as elevated wheal or redness, to the tuberculin material.

▶ INJECTABLE DRUGS USED IN THE MEDICAL OFFICE

Many physician's offices and clinics keep a stock of injectables locked in the medication cabinet. Table 6-10 lists some of the most commonly stocked injectable drugs. The emergency medications which are found at the end of the list may be kept in an emergency cart or special locked cabinet. See Figure 6-25 for examples of injectable drugs.

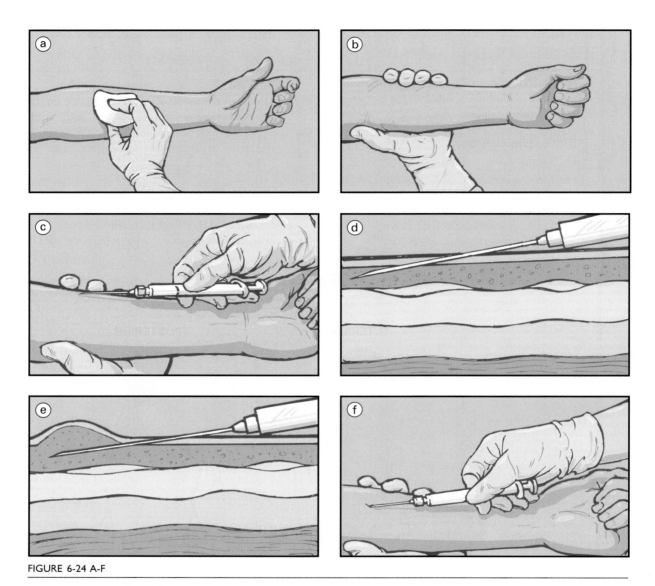

FIGURE 6-24 A-F

Administering an intradermal skin test.

GIVING INJECTIONS TO INFANTS AND CHILDREN

Be sure to obtain the parent's permission before giving any child an injection. If the physician has examined the child and then ordered the injection while the parent is present and not objecting, this constitutes permission.

A child should be told that he or she is going to receive some medicine that will help them. Tell the child honestly that there will be a slight sting but it will be over soon. A child who can count may find that by counting slowly to ten, the procedure will go more quickly. Some children like to have a small bandage applied after they have received an injection.

When giving an infant or child an injection be sure to have another adult (assistant or parent) restrain the child. If the child were to suddenly move while the needle is in their body severe damage could occur. It is extremely difficult for one person to restrain an uncooperative child while giving an injection. Always get help before you begin. If the parent seems to be disturbed by the procedure, then ask the parent to wait outside.

The preferred site for an infant's or child's injection is in the vastus lateralis muscle of the thigh (top of the thigh). In the case of an infant, you may find it is possible to secure the baby by placing

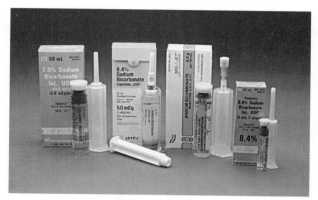

A

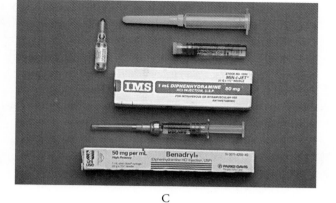

C

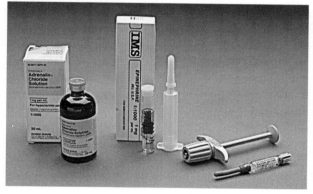

B

D

FIGURE 6-25

Injectable drugs.

your nondominant arm across the baby or use a papoose type of wrapping while you inject into his or her thigh.

The areas to avoid are: buttocks and deltoid muscle. The buttocks is avoided in infants since the sciatic nerve is quite large and could be entered accidentally. The gluteus medius is underdeveloped in children until they begin to walk. Similarly, the deltoid muscle is not well-developed in babies.

► CHARTING MEDICATIONS

Parenteral medications are charted using the same documentation as for oral medications: name of medication, dosage, route, date, site, and signature of person administering the medication. It is also necessary to document that you have provided instructions to the patient regarding follow-up care. Examples of charting follow.

9/10/XX 9:00 AM, nitroglycerin, I tab. sublingually. Written instructions given to pt. Precautions explained. Told to call progress in to office at 1:00 PM today.   M. Richards, CMA.

1/19/XX   11:00 AM, Monistat-3, 200 mg. Vaginal. Pt. given written instructions for follow-up care.   M. Richards, CMA.

10/10/XX 1:00 PM Mantoux test, 0.1 mL. Tuberculin Purified Protein Derivative, L forearm, ID, Small wheal noted. Pt. instructed not to rub or cover the area and to return for reading in 48 hours. M. Richards, CMA.

TABLE 6-10   Injectable Drugs Commonly in Stock in the Medical Office

Name Generic	Trade Name	Route	Usage
Amitriptyline HCL	Elavil	IM	Depression
Bropheniramine maleate	Dimetane	IM/SC	Allergy
Chlorpromazine HCL	Thorazine	IM	Psychosis
Diazepam	Valium	IM	Anxiety
Dimenhydrinate	Dramamine	IM	Nausea/Vomiting
Diphenhydramine	Benadryl	IM	Allergic reaction
Diphtheria, tetanus toxoid	Same name	IM	Immunization active vaccine
Furosemide	Lasix	IM	Edema
Gentamicin sulfate	Garamycin	IM	Infection
Heparin sodium	Same name	SC	Prevent clotting
Hydromorphine HCL	Dilaudid	SC/IM	Severe pain
Lidocaine HCL 1%, 2%	Xylocaine	SC	Anesthetic for minor surgery
Prochlorperazine	Compazine	IM	Psychosis
Promethazine HCL	Phenergan	IM	Nausea/Vomiting
Sodium Chloride with benzyl alcohol 0.9%	Sodium Chloride Bacteriostatic		Diluent for injection
Tetanus & diphtheria toxoids	Same name	IM	Immunization active vaccine
Tetanus antitoxin	Same name	IM	Prevention passive vaccine
Tetanus immune globulin	Hyper-Tet	IM	Prevention passive vaccine
Tetanus toxoid	Same name	IM	Immunization active vaccine
Tuberculin protein derivative	Tine test	ID	Tuberculin testing
Water for injection	Same name		Diluent for injection
Emergency Drugs Bretylium Tostlate	Bretylol	IV	Arrhythmia
Epinephrine		IV SC	Cardiac arrest Allergic reaction
Norepinephrine	Levophed	IV	Hypotension
Sodium Bicarbonate		IV	Acidosis
Electrolytes/Ringer's 1000 cc		IV	Dehydration

ID = intradermal; IM = intramuscular; SC = subcutaneous; IV = intravenous (*Note:* Only physician and nurse may administer intravenous medications.)

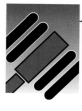

LEGAL AND ETHICAL ISSUES

The medical assistant must use careful aseptic technique when administering injections to patients. There is a danger of pain and infection for the patient with improperly administered drugs. There is also the danger of liability for both the physician and medical assistant. The ethical issue of always placing the patients needs first is of paramount importance when administering medications.

Verbal orders, in which the medication order is told to the MA, must be recorded and then signed by the physician and the medical assistant. No medication can be administered to a patient without the written order of a physician. The medical assistant must be willing to say, "I'm sorry, but I'm not allowed to perform that procedure without the doctor's order."

The medical assistant must constantly seek clarification on orders and dosage calculations. A thorough knowledge of drug interactions and side effects is necessary before dispensing any medication. The medical assistant has a responsibility to look up any unfamiliar medication. Failure to do so puts the physician and the medical assistant in jeopardy. Do not perform the administration of a medication with which you are unfamiliar. Never give a parenteral injection if you have not been trained in the procedure.

Pediatric medication administration is especially susceptible to liability since even a small error can result in major problems for the child. All calculations should be reviewed and double-checked with the physician or a nurse.

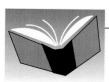

PATIENT EDUCATION

The physician will be the first to discuss medications with the patient. It is the medical assistant's responsibility to reinforce what the physician has explained. Some clarification of what the physician has said may be needed. It is especially important that the patients know why they are taking medications. Do not assume anything when teaching about medication administration. There is a risk that the patient will not take the medication or will take it incorrectly if the patient did not understand the explanation.

Medication names, dosages, expected results, and side effects have to be carefully explained in language the patient will understand. The inserts that are placed into sample drug packets can be helpful to patients. However, they may need to be interpreted for the patient. You may have to provide simple line drawings for patients who are hearing impaired or cannot

understand your verbal explanation. This instruction should be documented.

Patients may not understand the metric or the apothecary systems for calculating dosage. It is important for the medical assistant to easily move between the metric, apothecary, and household systems of measure, in order to be able to explain medication dosage in terms of household measures, if necessary.

Special emphasis must be placed on the need to take all the medication that is prescribed. For example, antibiotics must be taken for the entire length of time or they will be ineffective and the infection may reoccur. In many cases, dietary instructions will be needed along with an explanation of drug administration. For example, a patient who is taking a diuretic should know that it depletes sodium which may require the need for extra potassium. This can be replenished with foods, such as bananas and kiwis.

Summary

The medical assistant must be able to calculate dosages correctly since any error has the potential to be fatal to the patient. Also, observing the "three befores" before dispensing medication and the "six rights" before administering medication, can help to reduce errors. Any errors must be immediately reported in order for the physician to handle the situation. Failure to report an error compounds the seriousness of the error.

Thorough preparation of the patient who is to receive an

injection can help to eliminate unnecessary pain. Injections are always given under the supervision of a physician. This means that in addition to writing the order for the medication, the physician must be physically present in the facility when you are administering the drug. This can be critical when giving allergy tests or medications since a minute amount of medication can cause a life-threatening allergic response in a sensitive patient.

Competency Review

1. Define and spell the glossary terms for this chapter.
2. What are the "six rights" for drug administration?
3. State what you would do if Mrs. Lopez, age 88, refuses to cooperate while receiving an injection.
4. State what you would do if Billy Mendez, age three, refuses to cooperate while receiving a tetanus shot.
5. State what you would do if you have drawn up a narcotic that is not needed.
6. State what you would do if you see a small amount of blood appear in the syringe as you withdraw the plunger.

PREPARING FOR THE CERTIFICATION EXAM

Test Taking Tip — Move quickly through the exam so that you have time to review your answers. One of the most common examination errors is to misread a question. You will need time to double-check that you haven't missed a key word, such as "always," "never," or "except."

Examination Review Questions

1. The two systems of weights and measurements that are used to calculate medication dosages are
   - (A) metric and apothecary
   - (B) metric and pounds
   - (C) metric and ounces
   - (D) apothecary and pounds
   - (E) apothecary and ounces

2. Cubic centimeters are equal to
   - (A) ounces
   - (B) grams
   - (C) drams
   - (D) milliliters
   - (E) millimeters

3. In liquid measures, one fluid ounce is equal to
   - (A) 1 mL
   - (B) 10 mL
   - (C) 30 mL
   - (D) 100 cc
   - (E) 30 cc

4. In regard to medication, available strength refers to
   - (A) what actually contains the medication
   - (B) the potency of the medication in stock
   - (C) the potency the physician has ordered
   - (D) the amount of medication that should be administered
   - (E) the calculated strength

5. According to the rules for converting from one system of measurement to another, to change
   - (A) grains to milligrams, multiply by 60
   - (B) grains to grams, multiply by 15
   - (C) cc's to ounces, divide by 50
   - (D) cc's to mL, divide by 15
   - (E) drams to grams, multiply by 2

6. What is the preferred method of most physicians for calculating pediatric dosages?
   - (A) Young's Rule
   - (B) Fried's Law

   - (C) West's Nomogram
   - (D) Clark's Rule
   - (E) none of the above

7. When administering oral or sublingual medication
   - (A) assemble all of the equipment and use aseptic technique
   - (B) select the correct medication using the "three befores"
   - (C) double-check the label on the medication
   - (D) A and B
   - (E) A, B, and C

8. In regard to the administration of parenteral medication, a smaller gauge needle is used for which type of injection?
   - (A) intramuscular
   - (B) Z-track
   - (C) subcutaneous
   - (D) intradermal
   - (E) intravenous

9. Since the entire needle, up to the hub, must go into the patient, what length needle should be used for an intradermal injection?
   - (A) 3/8 inch
   - (B) 4/8 inch
   - (C) 5/8 inch
   - (D) 6/8 inch
   - (E) 1 inch

10. Which site, because there are fewer major blood vessels, is considered the safest for an intramuscular injection?
    - (A) vastus lateralis
    - (B) deltoid
    - (C) dorsogluteal
    - (D) ventrogluteal
    - (E) gluteus medius

Section Three
CERTIFICATION EXAM PREPARATION

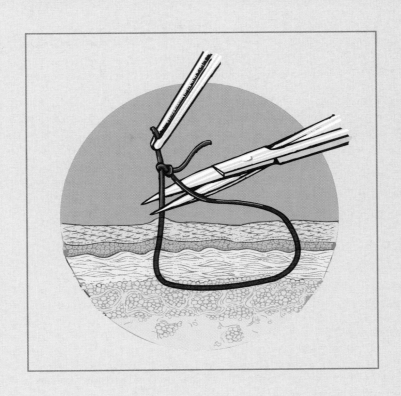

▶ CHAPTER 7, PART ONE: INFECTION CONTROL: ASEPSIS

1. What famous surgeon discovered that germs could be killed using carbolic acid and would clean surgical wounds by spraying the surrounding tissue with carbolic acid?

    (A) Louis Pasteur   **(D)** Robert Koch

    (B) Joseph Lister   **(E)** Andreas Vesalius

    (C) Ignaz Semmelweiss

    (B)   is correct.

    (A)   Louis Pasteur was a French chemist who discovered that many diseases are caused by bacteria that could be killed by excess heat. He also perfected a treatment that prevented rabies and discovered a means for controlling anthrax; he is known as the father of bacteriology and for the process of pasteurization.

    (C)   Ignaz Semmelweiss taught his medical students to wash their hands before delivering babies, which dramatically decreased the deaths from childbed fever in new mothers.

    (D)   Robert Koch, a German physician, developed the culture plate method for isolation of bacteria, discovered the cause of cholera, and isolated the tuberculin bacteria.

    (E)   Andreas Vesalius, a Belgium anatomist, is known as the father of modern anatomy.

2. What physician perfected the treatment for rabies?

    (A) Louis Pasteur   **(D)** Robert Koch

    (B) Joseph Lister   **(E)** Andreas Vesalius

    (C) Ignaz Semmelweiss

    (A)   is correct.

3. What man is known as the father of modern anatomy?

    (A) Louis Pasteur   **(D)** Robert Koch

    (B) Joseph Lister   **(E)** Andreas Vesalius

    (C) Ignaz Semmelweiss

    (E)   is correct.

4. This is a thick-walled reproductive cell so strong that it can withstand exposure to many harmful chemicals and extreme temperatures. It is known as a/an

    (A) spore   **(D)** anaerobe

    (B) normal flora   **(E)** nosocomial

    (C) aerobe

    (A)   is correct. A spore can withstand exposure to chemicals and extreme temperatures. A spore is the dormant stage of some bacteria.

    (B)   Normal flora are microorganisms that normally reside within certain areas of the body. Their function is to protect the body from harmful microorganisms. They are nonpathogenic if they stay within the region of the body where they normally reside.

    (C)   Aerobes are pathogens that thrive in oxygen-rich environments.

    (D)   Anaerobes are pathogens that thrive in oxygen-free environments.

    (E)   Nosocomial refers to an infection that is acquired after a person has entered a hospital.

5. What microorganisms are harmless to certain areas of the body in which they reside and work to protect the body from pathogenic microorganisms?

    (A) spore   **(D)** anaerobes

    (B) normal flora   **(E)** nosocomial

    (C) aerobe

    (B) is correct. Normal flora are microorganisms that are harmless to certain areas of the body in which they reside and protect the body from pathogenic microorganisms.

6. Pathogens that grow in oxygen-rich environments are known as

    (A) spores   **(D)** anaerobes

    (B) normal flora   **(E)** nosocomial

    (C) aerobes

    (C) is correct. Aerobes are pathogens that grow in oxygen-rich environments.

7. In order for the chain of infection to occur, a pathogen must find a means of exit from its reservoir host, and then it must

    (A) find a means of transmission   **(D)** find a reservoir host

    (B) find a means of entrance   **(E)** none of the above

    (C) have a susceptible host

    (A) is correct. A pathogen must find a means of transmission after exiting its reservoir host. This is how the organism spreads. It does this by either direct transmission, which is contact with an infected person (as with cough or sneeze droplets from an infected person), or contact with the infected person's bodily fluids (as in HIV).

    (B) After a means of transmission has been found, the pathogen must find a means of entrance (mouth, nose, eyes, intestines, urinary tract, or an open wound).

    (C) Once the pathogen has gained entrance, it must have a susceptible host (one that can support growth and reproduction).

    (D) With the right environment, the pathogen can reach infectious levels. When this occurs, the susceptible host becomes a reservoir agent.

8. In order for a pathogen to reproduce and grow within the host, it must

    (A) find a means of transmission   **(D)** find a reservoir host

    (B) find a means of entrance   **(E)** none of the above

    (C) find a susceptible host

    (C) is correct. In order for a pathogen to reproduce and grow within a host, it must find a susceptible host.

9. Human immunodeficiency virus (HIV) is transmitted by

    (A) indirect transmission   **(D)** droplets produced by sneezing

    (B) contact with droplets   **(E)** none of the above

    (C) direct contact

    (C) is correct. HIV is transmitted by direct contact with an infected person or infected bodily fluids.

10. During the inflammatory response, white blood cells overpower and consume the pathogenic microorganisms in a process called

(A) suppuration

(B) septicemia

(C) specific defense

(D) phagocytosis

(E) nonspecific defense

(D) is correct. Phagocytosis is the process in which white blood cells (phagocytes) overpower and consume pathogenic microorganisms.

(A) Suppuration is the process of pus formation. Another term for suppuration is pyopoiesis.

(B) Septicemia is the spread of infection to the bloodstream.

(C) Specific defense is a term used to describe immunity. Immunity is a means of protection from disease due to the production of antibodies. Antibodies are specific predators, that is, antibody A can only kill antigen B. It cannot kill other antigens; therefore, it is specific in its nature of defense.

(E) Nonspecific defense mechanisms can protect the body from many different kinds of antigens. Some examples of nonspecific defense mechanisms are skin, mucous membranes, hair, saliva, tears, stomach acid, and the lymphatic system.

11. The skin can protect the body from many different types of disease by simply not allowing a pathogen to enter the body. What type of defense is this?

(A) antigen

(B) antibody

(C) nonspecific defense

(D) specific defense

(E) inflammation

(C) is correct. Nonspecific defense can protect the body from many different types of disease by not allowing a pathogen to enter the body.

12. The entrance of a disease-producing organism into a cell or organism is referred to as a/an

(A) disease

(B) infection

(C) pathogen

(D) microorganism

(E) infestation

(B) is correct. The entrance of a disease-producing organism into a cell or organism is an infection. It may or may not alter the normal structure, function, or metabolism of a cell or organism.

(A) A disease occurs when any sustained harmful alteration of the normal structure, function, or metabolism of a cell or organism comes about.

(C) A pathogen is a disease-producing organism.

(D) A microorganism is a tiny living organism that is not visible to the naked eye.

(E) An infestation is the presence of parasites in the environment.

13. Which is a disease-producing microbe?

(A) asepsis

(B) infestation

(C) pathogen

(D) germicide

(E) antiseptic

(C) is correct. A pathogen is a disease-producing microbe or microorganism.

(A) Asepsis is a condition free of germs or infection.

(B) Infestation refers to the presence of parasites.

(D) A germicide is a chemical used to kill pathogenic microorganisms, but it is too harsh to be used on people.

(E) An antiseptic is a substance that prevents the growth of microorganisms without necessarily killing them and is generally safe to use on people.

14. A substance that can kill many organisms but is not effective on spores is

(A) an antiseptic

(B) a disinfectant

(C) a germicide

(D) formaldehyde

(E) a bactericide

(B) is correct. A disinfectant is not effective on spores and, in most cases, is not used on people. The exceptions are alcohol and betadine, which are classified as both antiseptic and/or disinfectant. An antiseptic does not single out and kill bacteria, as a bactericide does, or pathogens, as a germicide does.

(A) An antiseptic is a substance that prevents the growth of microorganisms without necessarily killing them and is generally safe to use on people.

(C) A germicide is a chemical used to kill pathogenic microorganisms, but it is too harsh to be used on people.

(D) Formaldehyde is used as a disinfectant, fixative, or preservative.

(E) A bactericide is destructive to bacteria and too harsh to be used on people.

15. A substance that prevents the growth of microorganisms without necessarily killing them and is generally safe for use on people is

(A) a bactericide

(B) a germicide

(C) disinfectant

(D) an antiseptic

(E) formaldehyde

(C) is correct.

16. A mixture of 1:10 bleach and water is a substance that can kill microorganisms but not spores and is not used on people. It can be classified as

(A) a bactericide

(B) a germicide

(C) a disinfectant

(D) an antiseptic

(E) formaldehyde

(C) is correct. A solution of 1:10 bleach and water is a disinfectant.

17. What is a form that is resistant to heat, drying, and chemicals, but that can be killed by steam under pressure (as in autoclaving)?

(A) virus

(B) spore

(C) HIV

(D) TB

(E) ARC

(B) is correct. A spore is the dormant form assumed by some bacteria that acts as a protective environment for the bacteria. Under the right conditions, the spore may revert back to an active form of bacteria.

(A) A virus is not resistant to heat, drying, or chemicals. It is, however, resistant to antibiotics. It is a very small parasitic microorganism that can only duplicate if within a living cell of an organism.

(C) Human immunodeficiency virus (HIV) is the virus that causes acquired immune deficiency syndrome (AIDS).

(D) Tuberculosis (TB) is caused by a bacteria that is not resistant to heat, drying, or chemicals.

(E) AIDS-related complex (ARC) is a less serious condition than AIDS. It occurs when the HIV has seriously damaged the immune system but before the final stage of an HIV infection (AIDS).

18. What type of bacteria usually forms grape-like clusters of pus-producing organisms (as seen in boils, wound infections, impetigo, and osteomyelitis)?

(A) staphylococci

(D) bacilli

(B) streptococci

(E) spirilla

(C) diplococci

(A) is correct. Staphylococci is a type of bacteria that forms grape-like clusters of pus-producing organisms. They stain gram-positive, which appears purple or blue in color.

(B) Streptococci form chains of round cells, as seen in strep throat, rheumatic heart disease, scarlet fever, or glomerulonephritis. They stain gram-negative, which appears reddish/pink in color.

(C) Diplococci form in pairs in chains of round cells, such as seen in gonorrhea, pneumonia, and meningitis. They stain gram-negative.

(D) Bacilli are rod-shaped bacteria, as seen in tuberculosis (TB), tetanus, diphtheria, and gas gangrene. These are all examples of gram-positive bacilli (Escherichia coli or E. coli).

(E) Spirilla are spiral-shaped bacteria, as seen in syphilis and cholera. They usually stain gram-negative.

19. This type of bacteria form pairs and stain gram negative. It is seen in gonorrhea and pneumonia.

(A) streptococci

(D) bacilli

(B) staphylococci

(E) spirilla

(C) diplococci

(C) is correct.

20. Which of the following are examples of diseases caused by fungi?

(A) amebic dysentery, malaria, trichomonas, and giardiasis

(B) Rocky Mountain spotted fever, typhus, rickettsial pox, trench fever, and Brill's disease

(C) thrush, athlete's foot, jock itch, ringworm, and candidiasis

(D) tetanus, diphtheria, whooping cough, UTI, syphilis, pneumonia, strep throat, boils, and meningitis

(E) herpes I and II, HIV, common cold, influenza, hepatitis A and B, MMR, polio, and warts

(C) is correct. Thrush, athlete's foot, jock itch, ringworm, and candidiasis are all caused by a fungus.

(A) Amebic dysentery, malaria, trichomonas, and giardiasis are examples of diseases caused by single-celled organisms called protozoa.

(B) Rocky Mountain spotted fever, typhus, rickettsial pox, trench fever, and Brill's disease are examples of rickettsiae diseases, which are transmitted by insects.

(D) Tetanus, diphtheria, whooping cough, UTI, syphilis, pneumonia, strep throat, boils, and meningitis are examples of diseases caused by bacteria, which are unicellular and can be treated with antibiotics. Note that both pneumonia and meningitis can be caused by either bacteria or virus.

(E) Herpes I and II, HIV, common cold, influenza, hepatitis A and B, MRR (mumps, measles, rubella), polio, and warts are examples of diseases caused by viruses, which are the smallest microorganisms and are not susceptible to antibiotics.

21. Which of the following conditions is NOT favorable for the growth of bacteria?

(A) moisture

(D) oxygen

(B) temperature of 98.6°F

(E) dampness

(C) direct sunlight

(C) is correct. Direct sunlight can kill bacterial growth. (A), (B), (D), and (E) are all examples of conditions that are favorable for the growth of bacteria (aerobic bacteria require oxygen, and anaerobic bacteria thrive without oxygen).

22. What type of immunity would one have if given tetanus immune serum globulin (TIG)?

    (A) passive acquired natural immunity (PANI)

    (B) passive acquired artificial immunity (PAAI)

    (C) active acquired natural immunity (AANI)

    (D) active acquired artificial immunity (AAAI)

    (E) all of the above

    (B) is correct. TIG (tetanus immune serum globulin) and TAT or TA (tetanus antitoxin) are examples of temporary protection against tetanus and are acquired through the process of passive acquired artificial immunity (PAAI).

    (A) PANI is naturally acquired from someone else's antibodies, such as from mother to fetus through the placenta or through breast milk.

    (C) AANI occurs by having the disease, which results in production of antibodies and "memory cells" that respond when the antigen reappears again.

    (D) AAAI is acquired by the administration of a vaccine, which actively stimulates production of one's own antibodies and "memory cells" to prevent that disease from occurring.

23. The first tier of the Centers for Disease Control (CDC) 1994 isolation guidelines focuses on

    (A) standard precautions (SPs)   (D) contact precautions (CPs)

    (B) airborne precautions (APs)   (E) transmission-based precautions

    (C) droplet precautions (DPs)

    (A) is correct. These precautions are used when caring for all patients, regardless of the patient's diagnosis or whether or not the patient has a known infectious disease. Major features of universal precautions are stated under Tier I.

    (B) Airborne precautions (APs) are part of Tier II, which focuses on patients who either are suspected of carrying an infectious disease or are already infected. It requires extra precautions in addition to the standard precautions and is known as transmission-based precautions. APs are used to reduce the transmission of diseases like TB, measles, or chickenpox. Precautions include isolation if hospitalized, mask and protective gown worn by health care workers, washing hands before gloving and after removing gloves, transporting patients with a mask, and limiting transportation.

    (C) Droplet precautions (DPs) are part of Tier II. Droplet precautions (DPs) are used to reduce the transmission of diseases such as meningitis, pneumonia, sepsis, diphtheria, pertussis, streptococcal pneumonia, scarlet fever, mumps, and rubella. Precautions include isolation if hospitalized, washing hands before gloving and after removing gloves, gloves and gowns being worn if coming into contact with bodily fluids or blood of the patient, wearing a mask if within 3 feet of the patient, and limiting transport of patients. All reusable equipment should be cleaned and disinfected.

    (D) Contact precautions (CPs) are part of Tier II. These precautions are used for patients known to be infected with a microorganism that is not easily treated with antibiotics or that is easily transmitted to others. Examples of these diseases are intestinal infections; respiratory, skin, or wound infections; diphtheria; herpes simplex virus; impetigo; hepatitis A; scabies; pediculosis; and herpes zoster. Precautions include isolation if hospitalized, gloves and gown worn when in contact with the patient, and mask and eyewear worn when there is potential for exposure to infectious body materials and fluids. When possible, patient care equipment should not be used on other patients.

    (E) Transmission-based precautions is the descriptive title given to the second tier (Tier II) of the CDC guidelines.

24. Caring for patients who have meningitis or pneumonia requires what type of precautions?

(A) standard precautions   (D) contact precautions

(B) airborne precautions   (E) transmission-based precautions

(C) droplet precautions

(C) is correct. Droplet precautions are required when caring for patients with meningitis or pneumonia.

25. Universal precautions (Ups) under the Occupational Safety and Health Administration (OSHA) are

(A) guidelines   (D) law

(B) suggestions   (E) bills

(C) recommendations

(D) is correct. Ups are the law and must be observed by employers of health care personnel.

26. Which of the following is appropriate when hand washing?

(A) use hot water and hold hands upward

(B) use cool water and hold hands downward

(C) use cold water and hold hands upward

(D) use tepid or lukewarm water and hold hands downward

(E) use hot water under pressure and hold hands outward

(C) is correct.

27. The destruction of organisms after they leave the body is called

(A) incubation   (D) surgical asepsis

(B) phagocytosis   (E) opportunistic infections

(C) medical asepsis

(C) is correct. Medical asepsis is the destruction of organisms after they leave the body.

(A) Incubation refers to a period of time during which a disease develops after the person is exposed.

(B) Phagocytosis is the process of engulfing, digesting, and destroying pathogens.

(D) Surgical asepsis is a technique practiced to maintain a sterile environment.

(E) Opportunistic infections, such as pneumonia, occur in a body when there is a reduced immune system (for example, as seen in AIDS).

28. Sterilization time requirements in the autoclave for surgical instruments that are double-thickness wrapped are

(A) 10 minutes   (D) 30 minutes

(B) 15 minutes   (E) 1 hour

(C) 20 minutes

(D) is correct.

29. The symptoms of HBV are

(A) slow onset of symptoms, fever, loss of appetite, jaundice, nausea, vomiting, malaise, dark urine, and whitish stools

(B) rapid onset of symptoms, fever, chills, diarrhea with clay-colored stools, orange-brown urine, anorexia, enlarged liver, and jaundice

(C) T-cell count less than 200, unexplained weight loss, swelling or hardening of lymph nodes, discolored or purplish growths and spots on the skin and inside the mouth, and an altered state of consciousness

(D) A and C

(E) B and C

(B) is correct. HBV (hepatitis B or serum hepatitis) generally has a rapid onset of symptoms with an incubation period of 60 to 90 days.

(A) Hepatitis A (acute infective hepatitis) has a very slow onset of symptoms with an incubation period of 14 to 50 days.

(C) The symptoms of AIDS include a T-cell count of less than 200, unexplained weight loss, swelling or hardening of lymph nodes, discolored or purplish growths and spots on the skin and inside the mouth, and an altered state of consciousness.

▶ CHAPTER 7, PART TWO: PHARMACOLOGY AND MEDICATION ADMINISTRATION

1. The prevention of disease is

(A) contraindicated   (D) prophylaxis

(B) habituation   (E) toxicity

(C) idiosyncrasy

(D) is correct.

(A) Contraindicated is a condition in which a specific drug should not be used.

(B) Habituation is the development of an emotional dependence on a drug, due to repeated use.

(C) Idiosyncrasy is an unusual or abnormal response to a drug or food by an individual.

(E) Toxicity is the extent or degree to which a substance is poisonous.

2. A condition in which the use of a drug should NOT be used is

(A) contraindicated   (D) prophylaxis

(B) habituation   (E) toxicity

(C) idiosyncrasy

(A) is correct. Pregnancy, high blood pressure, kidney disease, and other diseases may prevent an individual from being allowed to use certain drugs.

(B) Habituation is the development of an emotional dependence on a drug, due to repeated use.

(C) Idiosyncrasy is an unusual or abnormal response to a drug or food.

(D) Prophylaxis is the prevention of disease.

(E) Toxicity is the extent or degree to which a substance is poisonous.

3. A response to a drug other than the effect desired is

   (A) addiction   **(D)** placebo

   (B) side effects   **(E)** habituation

   (C) toxicity

   (B)   is correct.

   (A)   Addiction is an acquired physical and psychological dependence on a drug.

   (C)   Toxicity is the extent or degree to which a substance is poisonous.

   (D)   Placebo is an inactive, harmless substance used to satisfy a patient's desire for medication.

   (E)   Habituation is the development of an emotional dependence on a drug, due to repeated use.

4. A drug tolerance is

   (A) an acquired physical and psychological dependence on a drug

   (B) the ability of a drug to be effective against a wide range of microorganisms

   (C) to weaken the strength of a substance by the addition of something else

   (D) the development of an emotional dependence on a drug, due to repeated use

   (E) a decrease in susceptibility to a drug after the continued use of the drug

   (E)   is correct.

5. The official federal agency with responsibility for the regulation of food, drugs, cosmetics, and medical devices is the

   (A) BNDD   **(D)** USP-NF

   (B) FDA   **(E)** DEA

   (C) PDR

   (B)   is correct.

   (A)   BNDD is the Bureau of Narcotics and Dangerous Drugs, which enforces drug control.

   (C)   PDR is the Physician's Desk Reference, a book used as a quick reference on drugs.

   (D)   USP-NF is the United States Pharmacopeia-National Formulary, a drug book listing all the official drugs that are authorized for use in the United States.

   (E)   DEA is the Drug Enforcement Agency, which controls the use of narcotics.

6. The proprietary name of a drug is also known as the

   (A) trade name   **(D)** A & B

   (B) brand name   **(E)** A & C

   (C) generic name

   (D)   is correct. The trade name or brand name is the commercial name that is patented by the pharmaceutical company that manufactures the drug.

   (C)   The generic name is the common name by which a drug or product is known (for example, aspirin).

7. An OTC drug is
   (A) a drug that can only be ordered by a physician
   (B) accessible without a prescription
   (C) controlled due to a potential for addiction
   (D) labeled: Caution: Federal law prohibits dispensing without a prescription
   (E) a drug that must be administered directly by a physician

   (B)   is correct.

8. Which schedule for controlled substances has a high potential for addiction and abuse?
   (A) Schedule I   **(D)** Schedule IV
   (B) Schedule II   **(E)** Schedule V
   (C) Schedule III

   (B)   is correct.
   (A)   Schedule I has the highest potential for addiction and abuse.
   (C)   Schedule III has a moderate to low potential for addiction.
   (D)   Schedule IV has a lower potential for addiction and abuse than Schedule III.
   (E)   Schedule V has the lowest potential for addiction and abuse.

9. The drug classification that relieves pain without the loss of consciousness is
   (A) adrenergic   **(D)** antibiotic
   (B) analgesic   **(E)** antiseptic
   (C) anesthetic

   (B)   is correct.
   (A)   Adrenergic increases the rate and strength of the heart muscle.
   (C)   Anesthetic produces a lack of feeling, which may be of local or general effect.
   (D)   Antibiotic destroys or prohibits the growth of microorganisms.
   (E)   Antiseptic prevents the growth of microorganisms.

10. The drug classification that controls nausea and vomiting is
   (A) antacid   **(D)** antipruritics
   (B) antidote   **(E)** antipyretic
   (C) anti-emetic

   (C)   is correct.
   (A)   Antacid neutralizes acid in the stomach.
   (B)   Antidote counteracts the effects of poisons.
   (D)   Antipruritic relieves itching.
   (E)   Antipyretic reduces fever.

11. The drug classification that controls itching is

   (A) antacid   **(D)** antipruritic
   (B) antidote   **(E)** antipyretic
   (C) anti-emetic

   (D) is correct.

12. The drug classification that lowers blood sugar is

   (A) antihistamine   **(D)** hemostatic
   (B) antihypertensive   **(E)** hypoglycemic
   (C) diuretic

   (E) is correct.
   (A) Antihistamine counteracts histamine and controls allergic reactions.
   (B) Antihypertensive controls high blood pressure.
   (C) Diuretic increases the excretion of urine, which promotes the loss of water and salt from the body.
   (D) Hemostatic controls bleeding.

13. The drug classification that controls or relieves coughing is

   (A) antibiotic   **(D)** decongestant
   (B) antitussive   **(E)** expectorant
   (C) bronchodilator

   (B) is correct.
   (A) Antibiotic destroys or prohibits the growth of microorganisms.
   (C) Bronchodilator dilates or opens the bronchi to improve breathing.
   (D) Decongestant reduces nasal congestion and swelling.
   (E) Expectorant assists in the removal of secretions from the bronchopulmonary membranes.

14. Anesthetics

   (A) increase peripheral circulation and decrease blood pressure and vasodilation
   (B) produce relaxation without causing sleep
   (C) produce sleep
   (D) produce a lack of feeling, which may be of local or general effect
   (E) are used to reduce mental anxiety and tensions

   (D) is correct.
   (A) Adrenergic blocking agents increase peripheral circulation and decrease blood pressure and vasodilation.
   (B) Sedatives produce relaxation without causing sleep.
   (C) Hypnotics produce sleep.
   (E) Tranquilizers are used to reduce mental anxiety and tensions.

15. Mydriatics

    (A) dilate the pupils   **(D)** stimulate bowel movements

    (B) strengthen the heart muscle   **(E)** are given to promote resistance to infectious diseases

    (C) control bleeding

    (A) is correct.

    (B) Cardiogenics strengthen the heart muscle.

    (C) Hemostatics control bleeding.

    (D) Purgatives stimulate bowel movements.

    (E) Vaccines are given to promote resistance to infectious diseases.

16. Acetaminophen is the generic name for

    (A) aspirin   **(D)** Demerol

    (B) Advil   **(E)** Valium

    (C) Tylenol

    (C) is correct.

    (A) Acetylsalicylic acid is aspirin.

    (B) Ibuprofen is Advil.

    (D) Meperidine is Demerol.

    (E) Diazepam is Valium.

17. Darvon is classified as a/an

    (A) analgesic   **(D)** anesthetic

    (B) anti-anxiety   **(E)** antipyretic

    (C) antibiotic

    (A) is correct. Darvon, an analgesic, relieves pain.

    (B) An anti-anxiety drug relieves or reduces anxiety.

    (C) An antibiotic destroys or prohibits the growth of microorganisms.

    (D) An anesthetic drug produces a lack of feeling.

    (E) An antipyretic drug reduces fever.

18. Xanax is classified as a/an

    (A) antibiotic   **(D)** stimulant

    (B) anti-anxiety   **(E)** tranquilizer

    (C) psychedelic

    (E) is correct. Xanax is used as a tranquilizer to reduce mental tensions.

    (A) An antibiotic destroys or prohibits the growth of microorganisms.

    (B) An anti-anxiety drug relieves or reduces anxiety and muscle tension.

    (C) A psychedelic drug can produce visual hallucinations.

    (D) A stimulant acts to speed up the heart and respiratory system.

19. Lanoxin is classified as a/an

    (A) antibiotic   **(D)** antitussive

    (B) diuretic   **(E)** laxative

    (C) cardiogenic

    (C) is correct. Lanoxin, a cardiogenic, strengthens the heart.

    (A) An antibiotic destroys or prohibits the growth of microorganisms.

    (B) A diuretic drug increases the excretion of urine.

    (D) An antitussive drug controls or relieves coughing.

    (E) A laxative is used to promote normal bowel function.

20. Premarin is classified as a/an

    (A) antibiotic   **(D)** antihypertensive

    (B) decongestant   **(E)** estrogen

    (C) expectorant

    (E) is correct. Premarin is a replacement for estrogen.

    (A) An antibiotic destroys or prohibits the growth of microorganisms.

    (B) A decongestant reduces nasal congestion and swelling.

    (C) An expectorant assists in the removal of secretions from pulmonary membranes.

    (D) An antihypertensive drug prevents or controls high blood pressure.

21. Tenormin is classified as a/an

    (A) antibiotic   **(D)** diuretic

    (B) beta-blocker   **(E)** antidiabetic

    (C) antihistamine

    (B) is correct. Tenormin is a beta-blocker that reduces blood pressure, which works for the good of the heart.

22. Dyazide is classified as a/an

    (A) antibiotic   **(D)** diuretic

    (B) antihypertensive   **(E)** emetic

    (C) antihistamine

    (D) is correct. Dyazide, a diuretic, causes an increased production of urine.

23. Dilantin is classified as a/an

    (A) emetic   **(D)** analgesic

    (B) bronchodilator   **(E)** anticonvulsant

    (C) diuretic

    (E) is correct. Dilantin, an anticonvulsant, helps to reduce or control seizure activity in the epileptic.

    (A) An emetic induces vomiting.

    (B) A bronchodilator opens or dilates the bronchi.

    (C) A diuretic increases the excretion of urine.

    (D) An analgesic relieves pain.

24. Micronase is classified as a/an

 (A) antibiotic

 (B) decongestant

 (C) oral hypoglycemic agent

 (D) antihypertensive

 (E) antacid

 (C) is correct. Micronase, an oral hypoglycemic, works to reduce blood sugar and is given orally.

25. Coumadin is classified as a/an

 (A) anticoagulant

 (B) antibiotic

 (C) expectorant

 (D) antihypertensive

 (E) antitussive

 (A) is correct. Coumadin, an anticoagulant, delays or prevents blood from clotting. Patients taking Coumadin must have their blood monitored frequently to make sure that the blood isn't too thick or too thin. Aspirin is contraindicated when using Coumadin since aspirin is a blood thinner in itself.

26. Prozac is classified as a/an

 (A) tranquilizer

 (B) sedative

 (C) hypnotic

 (D) anesthetic

 (E) antidepressant

 (E) is correct. Prozac, an antidepressant, elevates the mood of a depressed individual.

27. Theo-Dur is classified as a

 (A) bronchodilator

 (B) beta-blocker

 (C) tranquilizer

 (D) diuretic

 (E) vasoconstrictor

 (A) is correct. Theo-Dur, a bronchodilator, opens the bronchi to make breathing easier.

28. Vasotec is classified as a/an

 (A) antidiarrheal

 (B) antihypertensive

 (C) vasodilator

 (D) vasoconstrictor

 (E) vitamin

 (B) is correct. Vasotec, an antihypertensive, lowers blood pressure.

29. Synthroid is classified as a/an

 (A) antibiotic

 (B) cardiogenic

 (C) analgesic

 (D) hormone

 (E) anti-inflammatory

 (D) is correct. Synthroid is used either to replace the hormone lacking in hypothyroidism or if the thyroid has been removed surgically.

30. Motrin is classified as a/an

(A) analgesic   (D) decongestant

(B) anti-inflammatory   (E) anti-emetic

(C) antacid

(B) is correct. Motrin, an anti-inflammatory, is prescribed for inflammatory conditions of the musculoskeletal system.

31. An injection under the skin and fat layers is

(A) intradermal   (D) intravenous

(B) subcutaneous   (E) intracavity

(C) intramuscular

(B) is correct. A subcutaneous injection is administered under the skin and fat layers.

(A) An intradermal injection is administered within the top layer of the skin.

(C) An intramuscular injection is given into a muscle.

(D) An intravenous injection is administered into a vein.

32. An injection into the veins is

(A) intradermal   (D) intravenous

(B) subcutaneous   (E) intracavity

(C) intramuscular

(D) is correct. Medical assistants are not permitted to administer intravenous medications.

33. The method commonly used in skin testing for allergies and tuberculosis is

(A) intradermal   (D) intravenous

(B) subcutaneous   (E) intracavity

(C) intramuscular

(A) is correct. The intradermal method is a very shallow injection, just within the top layer of skin.

34. Rx is Latin for

(A) take thou   (D) name

(B) mark   (E) prescription

(C) taken by mouth

(A) is correct. Rx is taken from the Latin term recipe, which means "take thou."

35. Which one is NOT a part of a prescription?

(A) patient's name and address   (D) instructions for taking drug

(B) name of drug   (E) the FDA number

(C) method of taking drug

(E) is correct. The DEA number is usually listed on a prescription in the event the drug is a narcotic. FDA is the Food and Drug Administration, a federal agency that regulates food, drugs, cosmetics, and medical devices.

36. Which is NOT one of the "six rights" of medication administration?

 (A) right patient   **(D)** right dosage

 (B) right medication   **(E)** right route

 (C) right physician

 (C) is correct. The "six rights" are right patient, right medication, right dosage, right route, right time, and right documentation.

37. Bid is an abbreviation for

 (A) once a day   **(D)** four times a day

 (B) twice a day   **(E)** every day

 (C) three times a day

 (B) is correct. Bid means to give the medication twice a day.

38. OD is an abbreviation for

 (A) overdose   **(D)** once daily

 (B) right ear   **(E)** right eye

 (C) after meals

 (E) is correct. OD is right eye, OS is left eye, and OU is both eyes.

39. PRN is an abbreviation for

 (A) stat   **(D)** after meals

 (B) before meals   **(E)** evening

 (C) as needed

 (C) is correct. PRN means that the medication is only given when the patient needs it.

40. The abbreviation for "hours of sleep" is

 (A) PO   **(D)** hs

 (B) H   **(E)** s

 (C) ss

 (D) is correct. hs means hours of sleep.

 (A) PO means after meals.

 (B) H means hour.

 (C) ss means one-half.

 (E) s means without.

41. Which weight or measure is NOT in the metric system?

 (A) mL   **(D)** L

 (B) cc   **(E)** gr

 (C) gm

 (E) is correct. The grain (gr) is an apothecary measurement.

42. To change grams to milligrams, the decimal point is moved how many spaces?

    (A) 2 spaces to the left   (D) 2 spaces to the right
    (B) 3 spaces to the left   (E) none of the above
    (C) 3 spaces to the right

    (C) is correct. To convert grams to milligrams, multiply by 1,000, or move the decimal three places to the right. Example: 15 grams = 15,000 milligrams.

43. To change grams to kilograms, the decimal point is moved how many spaces?

    (A) 2 spaces to the left   (D) 2 spaces to the right
    (B) 3 spaces to the left   (E) none of the above
    (C) 3 spaces to the right

    (B) is correct. To change grams to kilograms, divide grams by 1,000, or move the decimal point 3 spaces to the left. Example: 150 grams = 0.15 kilogram.

44. The equivalent metric measurement of the apothecary measurement of 1 dram is

    (A) 15 mL   (D) 4 mL
    (B) 30 cc   (E) 1 ounce
    (C) 1 m

    (D) is correct. 1dr (dram) = 4 mL (milliliter).

45. The equivalent metric measurement of the apothecary measurement of 1 fl. oz. is

    (A) 5 mL   (D) 30 mL
    (B) 10 mL   (E) 50 mL
    (C) 15 mL

    (D) is correct. 1 fl. oz. (fluid ounce) = 30 mL (milliliter).

46. The equivalent metric measurement of the apothecary measurement of 1 oz. is

    (A) 5 cc   (D) 30 cc
    (B) 10 cc   (E) 50 cc
    (C) 15 cc

    (D) is correct. 1 cc (cubic centimeter) = 1 mL (milliliter). Therefore 1 ounce (oz.) is equal to 30 cc or 30 mL.

47. The common household measurement of 1 T is equal to how many milliliters?

    (A) 1 mL   (D) 15 mL
    (B) 5 mL   (E) 30 mL
    (C) 10 mL

    (D) is correct. 1 T (tablespoon) = 15 mL (milliliter).

48. The common household measurement of 1 t is equal to how many milliliters?

(A) 1 mL   (D) 15 mL

(B) 5 mL   (E) 30 mL

(C) 10 mL

(B) is correct. 1 t (teaspoon) = 5 mL (milliliter).

49. The common household measurement of 15 gtts is equal to the apothecary measurement of

(A) 1 m   (D) 15 m

(B) 5 m   (E) 30 m

(C) 10 m

(D) is correct. 1 gtt (drop) = 1 m (minim). Therefore 15 drops = 15 minims.

50. The household measurement of 1 t is equal to the apothecary measurement

(A) 1 fl. dr   (D) 4 fl. dr

(B) 2 fl. dr   (E) 5 fl. dr

(C) 3 fl. dr

(A) is correct. 1 t (teaspoon) = 1 fl. dr (fluid dram).

51. Which pediatric dosage calculation is based on the child's age (if over 1 year)?

(A) Clark's rule   (D) West's nomogram

(B) Fried's law   (E) none of the above

(C) Young's rule

(C) is correct. To use Young's rule, divide the child's age in years by the same number plus 12. Multiply this number by the adult dose to determine the correct pediatric dose.

52. Which pediatric dosage calculation is based on the child's weight?

(A) Clark's rule   (D) West's nomogram

(B) Fried's law   (E) none of the above

(C) Young's rule

(A) is correct. Clark's rule divides the weight of the child by 150 pounds and multiplies this number by the adult dose to arrive at the pediatric dosage.

53. To take medication by injection is to take medication

(A) orally   (D) by inhalation

(B) sublingually   (E) parenterally

(C) topically

(E) is correct. Parenteral medication is administered by injection.

(A) Orally is by mouth.

(B) Sublingually is under the tongue.

(C) Topically is applied on the outside of the body on the skin.

(D) By inhalation is by breathing in the medication.

54. When administering oral or sublingual medication
    (A) assemble all equipment using aseptic technique
    (B) use the "three befores" and select the correct medication
    (C) pour the medication into the bottle cap instead of the hand
    (D) A and C
    (E) A, B, and C

    (E) is correct.

55. Which one of the following is NOT a parenteral route to administer medication?
    (A) intradermal   **(D)** elixir
    (B) intramuscular   **(E)** Z-track
    (C) subcutaneous

    (D) is correct. Elixir is given orally.

56. The 3/8-inch needle length is used in a/an
    (A) intradermal injection   **(D)** intravenous injection
    (B) subcutaneous injection   **(E)** Z-track injection
    (C) intramuscular injection

    (A) is correct.
    (B) Subcutaneous injection uses a ½-inch or ⅝-inch needle.
    (C) Intramuscular injection uses a 1- to 3-inch needle.
    (D) Intravenous injections are not given by medical assistants.
    (E) Z-track is a deep intramuscular injection and ranges from 1½ to 3 inches.

57. The most common gauge(s) for subcutaneous injections is/are
    (A) 27–28   **(D)** 27
    (B) 25–26   **(E)** 23
    (C) 20–23

    (B) is correct.

58. Infants' immunizations are usually injected into the
    (A) deltoid muscle   **(D)** bicep muscle
    (B) gluteus medius muscle   **(E)** tricep muscle
    (C) vastus lateralis muscle

    (C) is correct. The vastus lateralis muscle is used in infants because their gluteus medius muscle is not well developed yet.

59. The angle at which subcutaneous injections are administered is
    (A) 10–15 degrees   **(D)** 45 degrees
    (B) 25 degrees   **(E)** 90 degrees
    (C) 30 degrees

    (D) is correct. Subcutaneous injections are administered at a 45-degree angle, except for insulin and heparin, which are given at a 90-degree angle.

60. Immunizations scheduled for a child 4 to 5 months of age are
    (A) HBV 1, DPT 1, oral polio 1
    (B) DPT 2, oral polio 2, HIB 2
    (C) DPT 1, oral polio 1, HBV 2, HIB 1
    (D) DPT 1, oral polio 2, HBV 2
    (E) DPT 2, oral polio 2, MMR

    (B) is correct.

61. Immunizations scheduled for a child 1 year of age are
    (A) TB test, rubeola   (D) DPT 3, MMR
    (B) DPT 3, HBV 3   (E) MMR, TB test
    (C) DPT booster, oral polio booster

    (E) is correct. Immunizations for a 1-year-old child are mumps, measles, and rubella (MMR), and a TB test.

62. Gauge 20–23, length 1–3 inches is the needle size for
    (A) intradermal injections   (D) insulin injections
    (B) subcutaneous injections   (E) tuberculin skin tests
    (C) intramuscular injections

    (C) is correct.
    (A) Intradermal injections use 27–28, ⅜-inch needles.
    (B) Subcutaneous injections use 25–26, ½- or ⅝-inch needles.
    (D) Insulin injections are given subcutaneously.
    (E) Tuberculin skin tests are done intradermally.

63. The intradermal injection is administered at what degree of angle?
    (A) 5-degree angle   (D) 45-degree angle
    (B) 15-degree angle   (E) 90-degree angle
    (C) 20-degree angle

    (B) is correct.

64. Intradermal injections are given for
    (A) influenza prevention   (D) tuberculin skin testing
    (B) iron-replacement therapy   (E) pain management
    (C) insulin therapy

    (D) is correct. The Mantoux tuberculin test is administered intradermally.

65. Which site is used in administering intradermal injections?
    (A) lateral thigh   (D) upper arm
    (B) deltoid   (E) forearm
    (C) stomach

    (E) is correct. The inner center aspect of the forearm, as well as the upper chest and upper back, is an intradermal injection site.

66. When administering an intradermal injection, a visible sign of proper technique is a

(A) slight allergic reaction

(B) small wheal

(C) needlestick mark

(D) small cyst

(E) discoloration of the site

(B) is correct. Intradermal injections enter only the top level of skin where the substance injected leaves a wheal or bubble on the skin.

67. Which site can be used for subcutaneous injections?

(A) deltoid

(B) forearm

(C) upper chest

(D) buttocks

(E) abdomen

(E) is correct. Subcutaneous injections are administered in the abdomen, upper outer arm, anterior thigh, and subscapular portion of the back.

68. Which site can be used for intramuscular injections?

(A) upper chest

(B) abdomen

(C) vastus lateralis

(D) forearm

(E) subscapular portion of back

(C) is correct. Intramuscular injections can be given in the deltoid, vastus lateralis, and the gluteus medius muscles.

69. The muscle site most commonly used for administering tetanus boosters in adults is

(A) quadriceps

(B) vastus lateralis

(C) deltoid

(D) gluteus medius

(E) biceps

(C) is correct.

70. The muscle site that is considered the safest for an intramuscular injection is

(A) vastus lateralis

(B) deltoid

(C) gluteus medius

(D) quadriceps

(E) gluteus maximus

(A) is correct. The vastus lateralis muscle has fewer major blood vessels located in it and is considered safest.

71. When administering intramuscular injections in the dorsogluteal muscle, there must be care not to damage the

(A) femur

(B) spinal cord

(C) sciatic nerve

(D) iliac crest

(E) pelvic girdle

(C) is correct. To avoid the sciatic nerve, draw an imaginary line from the greater trochanter of the femur to the posterior superior iliac spine, and inject above and lateral to the imaginary line.

72. The agency that issues universal precautions pertaining to the handling of body fluids is the

(A) DEA

(B) OSHA

(C) FDA

(D) AAMA

(E) AMA

(B) is correct. OSHA is the Occupational Safety and Health Administration.

(A) DEA is the Drug Enforcement Agency.

(C) FDA is the Food and Drug Administration.

(D) AAMA is the American Association of Medical Assistants.

(E) AMA is the American Medical Association.

73. Epinephrine for allergic reactions is administered

(A) SC (subcutaneous)

(B) IM (intramuscular)

(C) IV (intravenous)

(D) Z-track (deep intramuscular)

(E) ID (intradermal)

(A) is correct.

74. A small sealed glass tube that contains medication is called a/an

(A) single-dose vial

(B) multidose vial

(C) ampule

(D) prefilled cartridge

(E) none of the above

(C) is correct.

75. To remove all of the medication from the neck of an ampule

(A) gently shake the ampule

(B) gently roll the ampule

(C) tip the ampule upside down

(D) gently tap the neck of the ampule on the counter

(E) snap your thumb and middle finger gently against the tip of the ampule

(E) is correct. Tapping the ampule in this manner rids the neck of the medication. Do not use your bare fingers to break the neck of the ampule to remove the medication.

76. A formula that is frequently used in dosage calculations is

(A) D/Q × H

(B) D/H × Q

(C) H/Q × D

(D) Q/D × H

(E) Q/H × D

(B) is correct. D/H × Q means desired strength divided by the strength on hand, multiplied by the quantity per cc of the on-hand strength. This equals the quantity to be given for the desired strength.

77. The physician has ordered 50 mg of Demerol to be administered. Demerol on hand is 25 mg/cc. How much should be given?

   (A) 0.5 cc   (D) 2 cc
   (B) 1 cc   (E) 2.5 cc
   (C) 1.5 cc

   (D) is correct. 50 mg divided by 25 mg multiplied by 1 cc equals 2 cc. 50/25 = 2 × 1 cc = 2 cc

78. The physician has ordered 5 mg of Compazine to be administered. Compazine on hand is 10 mg/cc. How much should be given?

   (A) 0.5 cc   (D) 2.5 cc
   (B) 1 cc   (E) 3 cc
   (C) 2 cc

   (A) is correct. 5 mg divided by 10 mg multiplied by 1 cc equals 0.5 cc. 5/10 = 0.5 × 1 cc = 0.5 cc

79. The physician has ordered 1,000 mg of Keflin to be administered. Keflin on hand is 1 g/2 cc. How much should be given?

   (A) 0.5 cc   (D) 2.5 cc
   (B) 1 cc   (E) 3 cc
   (C) 2 cc

   (C) is correct. 1,000 mg equals 1 g multiplied by 2 cc equals 2 cc. 1,000 mg = 1 g; 1/1 = 1 × 2 cc = 2 cc

80. The physician has ordered 250 mg of penicillin to be administered. Penicillin on hand is 0.25 g/5 cc. How much should be given?

   (A) 1 cc   (D) 4 cc
   (B) 2 cc   (E) 5 cc
   (C) 3 cc

   (E) is correct. 250 mg divided by 250 mg multiplied by 5 cc equals 5 cc. 0.25 g = 250 mg; 250/250 = 1 × 5 cc = 5 cc

▶ CHAPTER 7, PART THREE: ASSISTING WITH MINOR SURGERY

1. Outpatient surgery is generally limited to that which lasts less than

   (A) 15 minutes   (D) 90 minutes
   (B) 30 minutes   (E) 120 minutes
   (C) 60 minutes

   (C) is correct. Outpatient surgery usually lasts less than 60 minutes. Longer procedures are performed in a surgical center or hospital.

2. Outpatient surgery can be

   (A) an emergency procedure   (D) performed in a surgicenter
   (B) optional surgery   (E) all of the above
   (C) elective surgery

(E) is correct.

(A) Emergency surgery is required to immediately save a life, such as in the case of hemorrhage, or to prevent further injury or infection.

(B) Optional surgery may not be medically necessary, but the patient wishes to have it performed (for example, cosmetic surgery or a vasectomy).

(C) Elective surgery is considered medically necessary, but it can be performed when the patient wishes.

(D) A surgicenter is a medical facility that performs ambulatory surgery.

3. Any invasive procedure in which the body is entered requires

(A) oral permission

(B) the skin to be sterilized

(C) written permission

(D) written and oral permission

(E) a board-certified surgeon

(C) is correct.

4. Another name for surgical asepsis is

(A) sterile asepsis

(B) medical asepsis

(C) sterile technique

(D) surgical sterilization

(E) none of the above

(C) is correct. Sterile technique is the same as surgical asepsis.

5. Because the purpose of the surgical scrub clothes is to protect the patient from exposure to pathogens, the scrubs should

(A) be changed between each patient

(B) be white only

(C) be washed separately

(D) not be worn home by the medical assistant

(E) all of the above

(D) is correct. The medical assistant should not wear surgical scrubs home.

6. The surgical hand-washing procedure is performed

(A) for 10 minutes using a clean hand brush

(B) for 10 minutes using a sterile hand brush

(C) by scrubbing for 2 minutes after removing all rings and jewelry

(D) using a germicidal soap

(E) with a brush and disinfectant

(D) is correct. A germicidal soap is used for the surgical hand-washing procedure. Each hand and wrist is scrubbed with a sterile brush for 5 minutes, moving toward the elbows. After rinsing, the hands are given a second lather of germicidal soap and scrubbed for 3 minutes.

7. A germicidal soap dispenser is preferable to bar soap when doing a surgical scrub primarily because

   (A) it produces more lather

   (B) it can be sterilized

   (C) bar soap is frequently a compatible medium for the growth of bacteria

   (D) it is less messy

   (E) all of the above

   (C) is correct. A germicidal soap dispenser does not provide a medium for bacterial growth.

8. When performing a surgical scrub, it is best that the water temperature be

   (A) hot for the first scrub, warm for the second   **(D)** warm for the first scrub, hot for the second

   (B) tolerably hot   **(E)** none of the above

   (C) warm

   (C) is correct. The water temperature should be comfortably warm when performing a surgical scrub.

9. When applying sterile gloves

   (A) apply the gloves before setting up the equipment

   (B) pick up the first glove under the cuff and pull over the other hand slowly

   (C) hold the gloves over the sink while applying them since the sink is considered "clean"

   (D) leave the cuffs turned down after applying since the cuff will catch any spilled fluids

   (E) place the fingers of the gloved hand under the cuff of the second glove, and then apply

   (E) is correct. Place the fingers of the gloved hand under the cuff of the second sterile glove, and then apply the second glove. The first sterile glove is applied by using the thumb of the left hand to pick up the first glove by grasping the folded inside edge of the cuff. This glove is pulled onto the right hand using only the thumb and fingers of the left hand. The fingers must not touch the rest of the sterile glove.

10. The rationale for turning surgical gloves inside out while removing them is to

   (A) maintain the sterility of the gloves

   (B) seal in blood and bodily fluids

   (C) make them easier to remove

   (D) identify them more readily as used and contaminated

   (E) none of the above

   (B) is correct. Turning the gloves inside out during the removal stage seals in the blood and bodily fluids.

11. What is the correct method for shaving a surgical patient during the skin prep?

   (A) dry shave going against the grain

   (B) wet shave going against the grain

   (C) wet shave going with the grain

   (D) wet shave before preparing the patient's skin

   (E) dry shave after preparing the patient's skin

   (C) is correct. A wet shave going with the grain of the hair is the correct method for shaving a surgical patient during the skin prep.

12. A sterile assistant who passes instruments, among other duties, is called a/an

(A) surgical assistant

(B) scrub assistant

(C) second "hand"

(D) operating room assistant

(E) circulating assistant

(B) is correct. The scrub assistant has "scrubbed" or performed a surgical hand-washing scrub and wears sterile gown, mask, and gloves. This person passes instruments during the surgical procedure. The person in charge of handing instruments is called a "surgical technologist/technician."

13. Another name for a local anesthetic is

(A) conduction

(B) general

(C) intravenous

(D) hypnotic

(E) none of the above

(A) is correct. A local anesthetic is also known as a conduction type of anesthesia.

(B) A general anesthetic is one in which the patient loses consciousness.

(C) An intravenous (IV) is often used to administer a general anesthetic such as sodium pentothal.

(D) A hypnotic anesthetic produces sleep when administered in large doses. This is a type of general anesthetic.

14. An example of a local infiltration anesthetic is lidocaine hydrochloride, which is more commonly known as

(A) benzocaine

(B) Novocain

(C) Solarcaine

(D) Xylocaine

(E) none of the above

(D) is correct. Xylocaine is the local anesthetic lidocaine hydrochloride.

15. An example of a small-gauge suture used for the skin is

(A) stainless steel 0

(B) stainless steel 5-0

(C) chromic gut 2-0

(D) plain gut 3-0

(E) nylon 2-0

(B) is correct. Stainless steel 5-0 is an example of a small-gauge suture used for the skin.

16. Of the different types of absorbable sutures, which is absorbed the fastest?

(A) plain cat gut

(B) surgical cat gut

(C) chromic cat gut

(D) black silk

(E) none of the above

(A) is correct. Plain cat gut is absorbed the fastest. It is used in areas where there is rapid healing, such as highly vascular areas of the lips and tongue.

(B) Surgical cat gut is used on tissues in which there is fast healing, such as the vaginal area.

(C) Chromic cat gut has a slower absorption rate and can be used to hold tissue together longer, such as for muscle repair.

(D) Black silk is nonabsorbable suture material.

17. Absorbable suture materials are used
    (A) in areas in which they do not have to be removed
    (B) when absorption will occur within 5 to 20 days
    (C) for internal organs such as the bladder and intestines
    (D) for ligating and tying off of blood vessels
    (E) all of the above

    (E) is correct.

18. An all-purpose suture, which is considered one of the most dependable types, is
    (A) nylon   (D) steel
    (B) silk   (E) cotton
    (C) polyester

    (B) is correct. Silk, while the most expensive, is also considered the most dependable suture material. Black silk is the most commonly used nonabsorbable suture material.

19. The size, which is gauge or diameter of suture material,
    (A) increases in size with the number of zeros
    (B) decreases in size with the number of zeros
    (C) indicates the amount of scarring that will be present
    (D) A and C only
    (E) B and C only

    (E) is correct. The size decreases with the number of zeros. For example, 6-0 (000000) is the smallest and 0 is the thickest. Very fine suture, such as 5-0 and 6-0, leaves little scarring.

20. The smallest suture material is
    (A) 0   (D) 5-0
    (B) 2-0   (E) 6-0
    (C) 4-0

    (E) is correct. 6-0 is the smallest suture gauge.

21. A swaged needle is one in which
    (A) no needle is required
    (B) the needle and suture are combined in one length
    (C) the needle has a large cutting portion
    (D) the surgeon is allowed to go in and out of tissue in a confined space
    (E) none of the above

    (B) is correct. A swaged needle is one in which the needle and suture are combined in one length.

22. Facial sutures, in order to prevent scarring, may be removed after only

(A) 12 to 24 hours
(B) 24 to 48 hours
(C) 48 to 72 hours

(D) 3 to 5 days
(E) they are not removed at all

(B) is correct. Facial sutures may be removed after 24 to 48 hours.

23. If instructed to cut suture material once the wound has been closed, cut both ends

(A) ¼ to ½ of an inch above the knot
(B) ⅛ to ¼ of an inch above the knot
(C) ½ to ¾ of an inch above the knot
(D) ¾ to 1 inch above the knot
(E) none of the above

(B) is correct. The suture should be cut ⅛ to ¼ of an inch above the knot.

24. An instrument used by an obstetrician to measure an expectant mother's pelvis is the

(A) vaginal speculum
(B) dilator
(C) curette

(D) pelvimeter
(E) none of the above

(D) is correct. A pelvimeter is used to measure the expectant mother's pelvis to determine the size and growth of the baby.

(A) A vaginal speculum is used to visualize the vagina and cervix.

(B) A dilator is used to expand the diameter of a vessel or an opening.

(C) A curette is a spoon-shaped scraping instrument.

25. The portion of the hemostat located near the handle, which protects it from slipping once it is closed, is the

(A) tooth
(B) clamp
(C) ratchet

(D) serrated tip
(E) lock

(C) is correct. The ratchet is the portion of the hemostat located near the handle, which protects it from slipping once it is closed.

26. Hemostats include

(A) mosquito forceps
(B) Pennington forceps
(C) curved forceps

(D) sponge forceps
(E) all of the above

(E) is correct.

27. A hemostat with clawlike teeth at the tip to grasp and hold tissue is called a
  (A) thumb forceps   **(D)** needle holder
  (B) tissue forceps   **(E)** splinter forceps
  (C) sterilizer or transfer forceps

  (B) is correct. A tissue forceps has clawlike teeth to grasp and hold tissue.
  (A) Thumb forceps are tweezer-like forceps that are used to grasp sterile objects, such as dressings and tissue.
  (C) Sterilizer or transfer forceps have a long handle and are used to remove materials and objects from sterilizers and containers.
  (D) Needle holders are forceps that are used to grasp the needle during a suturing.
  (E) Splinter forceps are a type of thumb forceps that have a fine pointed tip to grasp foreign objects imbedded in the skin.

28. A sharply pointed instrument that fits inside a sheath or cannula to act as a guide for the cannula as it moves into an organ, body cavity, or vessel is a/an
  (A) probe   **(D)** sound
  (B) obturator   **(E)** laryngoscope
  (C) trocar

  (C) is correct. A trocar is a sharply pointed instrument that fits inside a sheath or cannula to act as a guide for the cannula as it moves into an organ, body cavity, or vessel.
  (A) A probe is a slender instrument that is used to enter and explore body cavities.
  (B) An obturator is an instrument that fits inside a speculum or scope and assists in guiding the speculum or scope into a vessel, organ, or canal.
  (D) A sound is a long slender probe.
  (E) A laryngoscope is an instrument, containing a light, that is used to examine the larynx.

29. An endoscope is a hollow, cylindrical instrument containing a light source. An endoscope that is used to examine the urinary bladder is called a/an
  (A) otoscope   **(D)** cystoscope
  (B) anoscope   **(E)** sigmoidoscope
  (C) proctoscope

  (D) is correct. A cystoscope is used to examine the urinary bladder.
  (A) An otoscope is used to examine the external and middle ear.
  (B) An anoscope is used to examine the superficial rectum (anus).
  (C) A proctoscope is used to examine the rectum.
  (E) A sigmoidoscope is used to visualize the sigmoid colon.

30. A typical surgical setup consists of
  (A) scalpel, blades, trocar, probe, scope
  (B) scalpel, blades, hemostat, probe, scope
  (C) scalpel, blades, hemostat, scissors, suture, scope
  (D) scalpel, blades, hemostat, scissors, suture
  (E) scalpel, blades, scissors, suture, speculum

(D) is correct. The typical surgical setup consists of a scalpel and several blades, hemostat(s), scissors, and suture. Other instruments are added as determined by the nature of the procedure.

31. Scalpel blades come in various sizes, depending on the

(A) manufacturer

(B) surgeon's preference

(C) type of tissue and incision

(D) size of the surgeon's hand

(E) whether the patient is an adult or a child

(C) is correct. The most important criteria for selecting the correct scalpel and blade are the type of tissue being operated upon and the type of incision being made.

32. Orthopedic instruments include

(A) drill set   (D) forceps

(B) wire cutters   (E) all of the above

(C) bone clamp

(E) is correct.

33. Surgical scissors used to cut tissue and sutures may be

(A) curved or straight   (D) sharp-blunt

(B) sharp-sharp   (E) all of the above

(C) blunt-blunt

(E) is correct.

34. Bandage scissors have

(A) a sharp-sharp edge

(B) a hook near the tip to facilitate moving under and cutting

(C) a knobby tip to facilitate moving under the bandage

(D) long handles

(E) blades with edges that do not touch

(C) is correct. Bandage scissors have a knobby tip to facilitate placing the edge under a bandage without injuring or cutting the patient's skin.

35. What is the name of the small table used to hold instruments during a surgical procedure?

(A) surgical table   (D) Mayo stand

(B) Lister stand   (E) none of the above

(C) sterile stand

(D) is correct. A Mayo stand is the small table used to hold instruments during a surgical procedure.

36. When transferring sterile solutions to a sterile field
   (A) discard the liquid remaining in the bottle
   (B) place the cap on a surface with outside edges of the cap facing up
   (C) place the cap on a surface with the inside edges of the cap facing up
   (D) place the cap on the Mayo stand
   (E) pour the liquid by stabilizing the bottle on the edge of the basin

   (C) is correct. To avoid contamination of the inside ring of the cap, it is placed on another surface, such as a table, with the inside of the cap facing up.

37. The area that is considered contaminated on a draped Mayo stand is
   (A) within a 1-inch border   **(D)** outside a 2-inch border
   (B) outside a 1-inch border   **(E)** the entire drape is sterile
   (C) within a 2-inch border

   (B) is correct. The area outside a 1-inch border on the draped Mayo stand is considered contaminated since it is in contact with the nonsterile work surface.

38. Which of the following should NOT touch a sterile field?
   (A) sterile instrument container   **(D)** used instruments
   (B) 4 × 4s   **(E)** transfer forceps
   (C) gloved hands

   (D) is correct. Used instruments are contaminated and should not touch a sterile work surface. All the other items listed are considered sterile, including the tips of the transfer forceps.

39. The air immediately above a sterile field is considered
   (A) unsterile
   (B) part of the sterile field
   (C) contaminated by droplets in the air
   (D) part of the perimeter of the sterile field
   (E) none of the above

   (B) is correct. The air immediately above the sterile field is considered part of the sterile field. This means that no ungloved hand or unsterile container should be placed over the sterile field.

40. You have an open sore on your hand. What procedure should you follow when preparing to assist the surgeon?
   (A) try to be excused from assisting with the procedure until the sore is completely healed
   (B) if you are not excused from assisting with the procedure, cover the sore with a dressing or bandage and then correctly apply gloves
   (C) if you are not excused from the procedure, apply two sets of sterile gloves
   (D) all of the above are correct
   (E) none of the above is correct

   (D) is correct depending on office policy.

41. When a patient is awakening from a surgical procedure, which of the following complaints needs to be IMMEDIATELY conveyed to the surgeon?

(A) nausea and vomiting   **(D)** all of the above

(B) pain   **(E)** none of the above

(C) bleeding

(C) is correct. While all of the complaints need to be conveyed to the surgeon, the most immediate need for action is in the case of bleeding.

42. When patients are scheduled to have outpatient surgery, the medical assistant would tell them

(A) that another person should accompany them

(B) what food and drink they may take before coming in for the procedure

(C) that there will be minimal pain

(D) that the surgeon has performed this procedure many times, and there is no danger to having the procedure

(E) A and B only

(E) is correct. Patients should be told about needing someone to accompany them and what food and drink are permissible, but the MA should not make promises about the amount of pain or the outcome of the procedure.

43. The father of a 6-year-old tonsillectomy and adenoidectomy (T & A) postoperative patient has just purchased orange juice through a vending machine and given it to the patient. The father was instructed to give only ice chips to the boy as needed. What does the medical assistant do?

(A) tell the father he may not stay with his son

(B) inform the surgeon

(C) explain that orange juice can cause nausea and vomiting

(D) remain with the boy

(E) B, C, and D only

(E) is correct.

44. What should be done when trying to obtain a written, surgical informed consent form from a patient who is an immigrant and does not speak or understand English?

(A) contact a relative who can interpret for the patient

(B) use hand signs and pantomime to explain the procedure to the patient

(C) explain the procedure in English since the obligation is to explain the procedure, not to interpret it for the patient

(D) inform the surgeon

(E) A and D only

(E) is correct. If the patient does not understand the surgical consent form, it is not considered to be an informed consent and is, therefore, illegal.

45. Cryosurgery is surgery done with

(A) heat

(B) freezing temperatures

(C) sufficient anesthesia to cause no pain

(D) chemicals designed to kill cancer cells

(E) laser beams

(B) is correct. Cryosurgery is performed with freezing temperatures.

46. Small electrocautery units used to perform minor cautery procedures are called

(A) hyfrecators

(B) hemostats

(C) trocars

(D) lasers

(E) cryosurgical units

(A) is correct. A hyfrecator is a small electrocautery unit.

(B) Hemostats are applied to blood vessels to hold vessels until they can be sutured.

(C) A trocar is used to withdraw fluids from cavities.

(D) A laser is an intense beam of light used in a variety of surgical procedures, including the removal of tumors.

(E) Cryosurgerical units use extreme cold to control bleeding and treat lesions.

47. A wound in which the outer layers of skin are rubbed away due to scraping is a/an

(A) incision

(B) laceration

(C) puncture

(D) abrasion

(E) none of the above

(D) is correct. An abrasion is a wound in which the outer layers of skin are rubbed away.

(A) An incision is a smooth cut resulting from a surgical scalpel or sharp material, such as razor or glass. This may result in excessive bleeding if deep and scarring.

(B) A laceration is a wound in which the edges are torn in an irregular shape. This can cause profuse bleeding and scarring.

(C) A puncture wound is made by a sharp pointed instrument, such as a bullet, needle, nail, or splinter. External bleeding is usually small, but infection may occur due to penetration with a contaminated object.

48. A patient with a wound should be asked when he or she last received a tetanus shot, and the physician should be notified if it has been more than

(A) 1 year

(B) 3 years

(C) 5 years

(D) 8 years

(E) 10 years

(E) is correct. A tetanus shot is good for 10 years.

49. An EMB consists of

(A) using a curette or suction tool to remove uterine tissue

(B) the tying and cutting of the vas deferens

(C) an incision and drainage (I & D)

(D) an examination of the vagina and cervix, performed using a lighted instrument

(E) none of the above

(A)   is correct. An endometrial biopsy (EMB) consists of using a curette or suction tool to remove uterine tissue for testing.

(B)   A vasectomy consists of tying and cutting the vas deferens. This is considered a permanent form of birth control for the male.

(C)   An incision and drainage (I & D) is performed to relieve the buildup of purulent (pus) material as a result of infection.

(D)   A colposcopy is an examination of the vagina and cervix, performed using a lighted instrument called a colposcope.

Section Four
APPENDICES

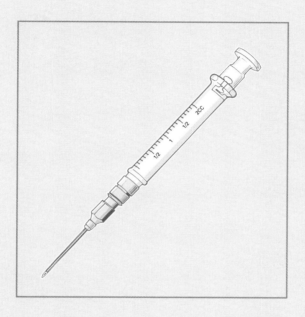

Appendix A

SYLLABUS AND CALENDARS

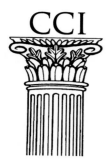

CORINTHIAN COLLEGES, INC.
Medical Assisting Program
MODULE B—CLINICAL ASSISTING AND PHARMACOLOGY
Syllabus and Topic Outline

Prerequisite: None

Date:

Time:

Module Length: 20 days

Instructor:

Module Description:

Module B stresses the importance of asepsis and sterile technique in today's health care environment. Students learn about basic bacteriology and its relationship to infection and disease control. Students identify the purpose and expectations of the Occupational Health and Safety Administration (OSHA) and the Clinical Laboratory Improvement Amendments (CLIA) regarding disease transmission in the medical facility. Students become familiar with the principles and various methods of administering medication. Basic pharmacology, therapeutic drugs, their uses, inventory, and classification and effects on the body are included. Students participate in positioning and draping of patients for various examinations and prepare for and assist with minor office surgical procedures. Students gain an understanding of basic anatomy and physiology of the muscular system, common diseases and disorders, and medical terminology related to this system. Students study essential medical terminology, build on their keyboarding and word processing skills, and become familiar with the self-directed job search process by identifying their personal career objective, create a neat, accurate, well-organized cover letter, resume, and job application.

Module B is comprised of three sections:

Semester Credits		**Quarter Credits**	
Theory	41 hours/ 2.73 credit units	Theory	40 hours/ 4 credit units
Clinical/Lab	30 hours/ 1 credit unit	Clinical/Lab	30 hours/ 1.5 credit units
Computers	10 hours/ .33 credit units	Computers	10 hours/ .5 credit units
Total:	81 hours / 4 credit units	Total:	80 hours / 6 credit units

Student must receive a grade of 70% or above to pass this module.

Module B Textbook:

Medical Assisting: Module B—Clinical Assisting and Pharmacology; Corinthian Colleges, Inc., 2004

Reference Material:

Insurance Handbook for the Medical Office; 8th edition; Marilyn T. Fordney, W.B. Saunders, 2002.
Student Workbook for the Insurance Handbook for the Medical Office; 8th edition; Marilyn T. Fordney, W.B. Saunders, 2002.
Medical Transcribing: Techniques and Procedures; 5th edition; Diehl and Fordney, W.B. Saunders, 2003.
Microsoft Word 2000; Nita Rutkosky, EMC Paradigm Publishers, 2000.

Additional Reference material: Medical management software, Video series, Medical dictionary and Physicians Desk Reference

Instructional Methods:

Instructors for Module B will utilize lectures, classroom discussions, hands-on experiences, laboratory exercises, role playing, presentations, demonstrations, research and student assignments (depending on section requirements) to facilitate students' achievement of course objectives.

Grading:

The Clinical/Laboratory section grade will be determined as follows:

Hands-on practice and experiences	50%
Tests/quizzes	50%

The grade distribution for Module B is as follows:

Theory	30%
Clinical/Laboratory	40%
Computer/Keyboarding	30%
Total Module B Grade	100%

Attendance:

Students are expected to attend every class session. Make up work will be allowed only with instructor's approval. Refer to catalog for explanation of attendance policy.

Date of last Revision: June 2004

Objectives and Topic Outline:

Upon successful completion of this course the student will be able to:

1. Identify and define terms related to basic medical terminology, including prefixes, suffixes, word parts, abbreviations and symbols. Define and spell the glossary terms for each chapter.
2. Briefly describe the purpose and function of the muscular system.
3. Describe the structure of the skeletal, smooth and cardiac muscles and define the function of each.
4. Name the major skeletal muscles of the body.
5. Briefly explain the types of muscle movement.
6. Identify common disorders and diseases of the muscular system.
7. List and explain common diagnostic tests performed on muscles.
8. Identify common microorganisms and the structure of each.
9. Explain the difference between direct and indirect disease transmission.
10. Describe the chain of infection.
11. Explain some of the body's natural defense mechanisms to prevent the spread of infection.
12. Identify common factors that influence the growth of microorganisms.
13. Identify recommended universal and standard precautions in regard to human tissue, blood and body fluids.
14. Identify the expectations and the purpose of the Occupational Health and Safety Administration (OSHA) and the Clinical Laboratory Improvement Amendments (CLIA) regarding disease transmission in the medical facility.
15. Describe the difference between medical asepsis (clean technique) and surgical asepsis (sterile technique).
16. Explain the difference between sanitization, disinfection and sterilization.
17. Explain the function of the autoclave and demonstrate proper procedure for preparing and wrapping instruments to be autoclaved.
18. Identify the preventative measures taken in the medical facility to ensure the personal safety and well being of staff and patients.
19. Explain the importance of and demonstrate proper handwashing technique.
20. Identify guidelines for laboratory safety.
21. Describe the surgical process for scheduling, preoperative and postoperative preparation for the patient having a minor surgery.
22. Briefly describe common surgical procedures performed in the medical office.
23. Describe the medical assistant's role in the surgical process and assisting with surgery.
24. Demonstrate a minor surgery tray set-up and preparation of the treatment room prior to surgery.
25. Describe how to assemble equipment and supplies needed for a minor office surgery.
26. Demonstrate surgical aseptic technique for preparing the patients skin for minor surgery.
27. Demonstrate proper technique for putting on sterile gloves.
28. List and describe instruments for: cutting, dissecting, grasping, clamping, probing and dilating.

29. Demonstrate how to assist a physician with suturing.
30. Demonstrate how to remove sutures as directed by a physician.
31. Briefly identify the uses and sources of drugs in regards to pharmacology.
32. Demonstrate how to put medications, used in the medical office, in its proper classification.
33. Identify the drugs that are under federal regulation according to category, or Schedules I through V.
34. Utilize the Physicians' Desk Reference (PDR) for information regarding prescriptions and nonprescription medications.
35. Identify and describe the various methods of administering medication.
36. Explain the importance of and demonstrate the "Six Rights" prior to administering medication.
37. Demonstrate how to write a prescription as ordered by the physician.
38. Explain the proper procedure for phoning a prescription in to the pharmacy.
39. Identify necessary information required for the patients' medical record when administering medication and demonstrate how to record that information properly.
40. Define common abbreviations used for medications and administering medications.
41. Demonstrate how to maintain and inventory the medications that are kept locked in a physician's office, and the laboratory supplies
42. Identify medical, legal, and ethical concerns regarding medications.
43. Identify considerations regarding drug action in the body.
44. Demonstrate and apply knowledge of the apothecary and metric systems.
45. Demonstrate and apply knowledge of various drug calculation formulas, including pediatric dosage formulas.
46. Correctly identify the parts of a syringe and needle.
47. Demonstrate how to recap a needle properly using the OSHA approved scoop method.
48. Demonstrate how to prepare a patient for an injection.
49. Demonstrate the correct method for discarding a used needle and syringe.
50. Demonstrate how to administer intradermal, intramuscular, and subcutaneous injections properly.
51. List and explain the immunization schedule for normal infants, children, and adults.
52. Briefly discuss the legal and ethical concerns regarding administering medication.
53. Identify a personal career objective and describe the necessary basic universal skills and workplace competencies necessary to be successful on the job.
54. Identify the necessary components of a successful job search.
55. Prepare a neat, accurate, and well-organized resume and job application.
56. Identify three contacts that can assist you as a reference or with a letter of recommendation.
57. Explain the purpose of and prepare a neat well-written cover letter to accompany a resume.
58. Identify the necessary tools to create a career portfolio.
59. Demonstrate increasing speed and accuracy on the computer keyboard, medical transcription, and acceptable progress through the identified text(s).
60. Demonstrate knowledge and skill in medical terminology and anatomy & physiology by utilizing software to enhance learning and assist in research material for essay assignments.
61. Demonstrate progressive skill acquisition related to word processing, computerized medical office application, and processing of insurance claim forms with acceptable progress through the identified text(s).

Topic Outline

I.   Terminology associated with Clinical Assisting and Pharmacology
   A. Three types of word parts
      1. Prefixes
      2. Suffixes
      3. Root terms
   B. Prefixes
      1. Numbers
      2. Colors
      3. Opposites
      4. Negative
      5. Size/Comparison
      6. Position
   C. Suffixes
      1. Condition
      2. Surgical
      3. Diagnostic
      4. Clinical
      5. Miscellaneous
   D. Root Terms
   E. Anatomical Terms
   F. Medical Abbreviations
   G. The Medical Record
   H. Prescription and Delivery
   I. Using the Medical Dictionary (MedWords)
   J. Anatomy & Physiology of Muscular System (Ch. 6 – MedWorks)

II. Muscular System
   A. Three types of muscle tissue and purpose
      1. Skeletal
      2. Smooth
         a. Peristalsis
      3. Cardiac
   B. Functions of muscles
   C. Structure of skeletal muscles
      1. Grouped in bundles
         a. myofibrils
         b. filaments
         c. sarcomeres
   D. Nerve cell and muscle link
      1. Muscle activity directed by the brain
         a. motor neuron
         b. neuromuscular junction
         c. muscle contraction
      2. Sarcomeres
   E. The work of muscles
      1. How muscles perform work
      2. "Muscle team"
      3. Partially contracted at all times
      4. Isometric
      5. Isotonic
      6. Atrophy
      7. Contracture
      8. Glycogen
         a. Uses

    b. Changes
    c. Body heat
    d. Fatigued
  F. Muscle Attachment / Structure and Function
    1. Tendons
    2. Ligaments
    3. Fascia
      a. Origin
      b. Insertion
  G. Sheaths / Purpose
  H. Bursae / Structure and Function
  I. Sphincter / Structure and Function
III. Major Skeletal Muscles
  A. Muscles of the head, face and neck
  B. Muscles of the trunk
  C. Muscles of the upper extremities
  D. Muscles of the lower extremities
IV. Types of Movement
V. Disorders and Diseases
  A. Strain
  B. Cramp or spasm
  C. Bursitis
  D. Tendonitis
  E. Fibromyalgia
  F. Muscular Dystrophy
  G. Torticollis
VI. Diagnostic Tests
  A. X-rays
  B. Electromyography (EMG)
  C. Electroneurography
  D. Blood Tests
  E. Muscle Biopsy
VII. Infection Control / Asepsis
  A. Microbiology
  B. Microorganisms
    a. Pathogenic
    b. Nonpathogenic
  C. Infection
VIII. Common Microorganisms
  A. Bacteria
  B. Virus
  C. Protozoa
  D. Fungi
  E. Animal Parasites
  F. Rickettsiae and Chlamydiae
IX. Transmission of Disease
  A. Epidemiology
  B. Communicable disease
  C. Communicable period
  D. Incubation time
  E. Direct transmission
  F. Indirect transmission
X. Chain of Infection
  A. Reservoir Host

        B. Means of exit
        C. Means of transmission
        D. Means of entry
        E. Susceptible host
   XI. Body's Natural Defenses Against Infection
        A. Coughing and sneezing
        B. Cilia
        C. Skin
        D. Tears and sweat
        E. Acid environment in urinary bladder and vagina
        F. Hydrochloric acid in stomach
        G. Immune response
   XII. Factors that Influence the Growth of Microorganisms
        A. Nutrition
        B. Oxygen
            1. Aerobes
            2. Anaerobes
        C. Light
        D. Moisture
        E. Temperature
        F. PH
   XIII. Universal (Standard) Precautions
        A. Assumption
        B. Preventative Measures
   XIV. Regulatory Agencies
        A. OSHA
        B. CLIA
        C. Center for Disease Control
   XV. Sanitazation, Disinfection, and Sterilization
        A. General Information
            1. Asepsis
            2. Medical asepsis (Clean technique)
            3. Surgical asepsis (Sterile technique)
        B. Sanitazation
        C. Disinfection
        D. Sterilization
            1. Autoclave (function)
        E. Dry Heat Methods
            1. Incineration
            2. Dry Heat Oven
   XVI. Proper Procedure for Wrapping Instruments for the Autoclave
   XVII. Preventative Measures for Safety in Medical Office
        A. Medical Assistants Role in Infection Control
        B. Professional Cleaning Services
        C. Latex Gloves
        D. Handwashing
        E. Guidelines to Prevent the Spread of Disease
        F. Prevent Accidents
        G. Guidelines for Laboratory Safety
   XVIII. Understanding the Surgical Process
        A. Scheduling
        B. Common minor office surgeries
        C. Day before surgery
            1. Prepare instruments and supplies

          2. Patient preparation
      D. Before surgery (preoperative)
          1. Consent form
          2. Prepare room
          3. Assemble equipment and supplies
      E. During surgery
          1. Prepare patient
          2. Prepare skin
          3. Assisting with surgery
      F. After surgery (postoperative)

XIX. Common Instruments used in Minor Office Surgery
      A. Cutting
      B. Dissecting
      C. Grasping
      D. Clamping
      E. Probing
      F. Dilating

XX. Assisting with Suturing and Suture Removal

XXI. Pharmacology-study of Drugs
      A. Uses
      B. Sources
      C. Classification
          1. Chemical name
          2. Generic name
          3. Brand or trade name
      D. Schedule of Controlled Substances
          1. Schedule I
          2. Schedule II
          3. Schedule III
          4. Schedule IV
          5. Schedule V
      E. Physician's Desk Reference (PDR)
      F. Routes and Methods of Drug Administration
          A. Six Rights
          B. Methods of Administration
             1. Oral
             2. Sublingual
             3. Buccal
             4. Inhalation
             5. Topical
             6. Transdermal patch
             7. Vaginal
             8. Injections

XXII. Writing Prescriptions
      A. Prescription content
      B. Phoning in prescriptions to pharmacy
      C. Recording medications
      D. Standard abbreviations

XXIII. Legal and ethical concerns regarding medications

XXIV. Frequently Administered Drugs

XXV. Factors that Affect how the body responds to drugs.

XXXVI. Dosage Calculations
      A. Basic math
      B. Apothecary system

C. Metric system

D. Calculation formulas

E. Calculation formulas for pediatrics

    1. Clark's Rule

    2. Fried's Rule

    3. Young's Rule

XXVII. Injections

XXVIII. Parts of a syringe and needle

A. Syringe

    1. Barrel

    2. Flange

    3. Plunger

    4. Tip

B. Needle

    1. Hub

    2. Hilt

    3. Shaft

    4. Bevel

    5. Lumen

    6. Point

XXIX. Injection Technique

A. OSHA approved scoop method for recapping needle

B. Patient preparation

C. Disposal of needles and syringe (Biohazard containers)

D. Intradermal (ID) Injection

E. Subcutaneous (SC) Injection

F. Intramuscular (IM) Injection

G. Intravenous (IV) Injection

XXX. Immunizations

A. Immunization Schedules

XXXI. Maintain and inventory of locked medication

XXXII. Maintain and inventory of laboratory supplies

XXXIII. Legal and Ethical concerns regarding medications.

XXXIV. Career Development / Job Search Success

A. Personal Career Objective

    1. Universal Work skills

        a. Positive attitude

        b. How is your attitude?

    2. Workplace competencies

    3. Qualities employers want

B. Components of a successful job search

    1. Well-written Resume

    2. References or letters of recommendation

    3. Finding job openings

    4. Well-written cover letter

    5. Career Portfolio

    6. Employment application

    7. Interviewing

    8. Assessing job offers

    9. Declining / accepting job offers

C. Conducting a Successful Job Search

    1. Developing a personalized job search

    2. Writing your resume

        a. content

          b. order

          c. requirements

       3. Completing employment applications

          a. purpose

          b. directions

          c. discriminatory information

       4. Obtaining References

          a. Positive feedback

          b. Letters of recommendation

       5. Writing your cover letter

          a. Purpose

          b. Order of content

XXXV.   Technical Communication and Professional Development

     A. Medical Terminology

     B. Anatomy & Physiology

     C. Keyboarding

     D. Word Processing

     E. Medical Operations Software

     F. Medical Insurance

     G. Medical Transcribing

     H. Disease short essays

Day and Evening Schedule

Module B
Clinical Assisting / Pharmacology
Lecture Calendar

One (1) hour per day

(One (1) hour per day)

	Day 1 / Day 2 / Day 3	Day 4	Day 5
Unit I Day 1	**Lecture:** A & P of the Muscular System Chapter 1 & 2	**Lecture:** Career Development	**Unit I Theory test** Chapter 1 & 2 **Unit I S/T test**
Unit 2 Day 6	**Lecture:** Infection Control: Asepsis Chapter 3 **Lab Lecture:** Infection Control: Asepsis cont'd	**Lecture:** Assisting with Minor Surgery Chapter 4 **Lab Lecture:** Assisting with Minor Surgery cont'd	**Unit II Theory test** Chapter 3, 4 **Unit II S/T test**
Unit 3 Day 11	**Lecture:** Pharmacology Chapter 5	**Lecture:** Pharmacology Chapter 5	**Unit III Theory test** Chapter 5 **Unit III S/T test**
Unit 4 Day 16	**Lecture:** Administering Medications Chapter 6	**Lecture:** Administering Medications Chapter 6	**Theory Final Exam** Chapter 1-6

Notes on full day-by-day layout:

- Unit I: Day 1, Day 2, Day 3 — Lecture: A & P of the Muscular System Chapter 1 & 2; Day 4 — Lecture: Career Development; Day 5 — Unit I Theory test Chapter 1 & 2, Unit I S/T test
- Unit 2: Day 6, Day 7 — Lecture: Infection Control: Asepsis Chapter 3, Lab Lecture: Infection Control: Asepsis cont'd; Day 8, Day 9 — Lecture: Assisting with Minor Surgery Chapter 4, Lab Lecture: Assisting with Minor Surgery cont'd; Day 10 — Unit II Theory test Chapter 3, 4, Unit II S/T test
- Unit 3: Day 11, Day 12, Day 13, Day 14 — Lecture: Pharmacology Chapter 5; Day 15 — Unit III Theory test Chapter 5, Unit III S/T test
- Unit 4: Day 16, Day 17, Day 18, Day 19 — Lecture: Administering Medications Chapter 6; Day 20 — Theory Final Exam Chapter 1-6

MEDICAL ASSISTING - MODULE B
Standard Lab / Clinical Calendar

Two (2) hours per day

Day and Evening Schedule

	Day 1	Day 2	Day 3	Day 4	Day 5
	Demo VS	Demo injections	Demo Venipuncture	Demo Coding	Demo PDR
1	practice core	practice core	practice core	practice core	practice core
2	practice core	practice core	practice core	practice core	practice core
3	practice core	practice core	practice core	practice core	practice core
4	practice core	practice core	practice core	practice core	practice core

	Day 6	Day 7	Day 8	Day 9	Day 10
	Demo Autoclave	Demo Glove & Tray	Demo Skin Prep	Demo Suture Removal	Demo Ampule
1	check-off core	practice scrub & glove	practice tray set-up	suture removal	practice ampule
2	practice autoclave	check-off core	practice scrub & glove	suture removal	practice tray set-up
3	practice autoclave	practice tray set-up	check-off core	suture removal	practice scrub & glove
4	practice autoclave	practice tray set-up	practice scrub & glove	suture removal	check-off core

	Day 11	Day 12	Day 13	Day 14	Day 15
1	practice skin prep	check-off	practice autoclave	practice meds/ampule	practice tray set-up
2	practice autoclave	practice CPX	check-off	practice skin prep	practice meds/ampule
3	practice meds/ampule	practice meds/ampule	practice skin prep	check-off	practice autoclave
4	practice meds/ampule	practice skin prep	practice CPX	practice autoclave	check-off

	Day 16	Day 17	Day 18	Day 19	Day 20
	Demo Med exercises				
1	med exercises	open practice	open practice	open practice	check-offs
2	med exercises	open practice	open practice	open practice	check-offs
3	med exercises	open practice	open practice	open practice	check-offs
4	med exercises	open practice	open practice	open practice	check-offs

MODULE CHECK-OFFS:

Surgical Tray	Medication Exercises	Intradermal Injections
Instrument Prep & Autoclave	Ampule Withdrawal	Subcutaneous Injections
Skin Preparation	Charting	Deltoid Injections
Scrub & Glove	Professionalism	Glute/Z-Track Injections
Suture Removal	CPT/ICD-9 Coding	
Oral Medication Admin.	PDR Exercises	
	Vital Signs I & II	
	Venipuncture	

Group 1

Group 2

Group 3

Group 4

Appendix B

PROCEDURE COMPETENCY CHECKLISTS AND ASSIGNMENTS

Student Name (Print)   Instructor's Name (Print)   Date

MODULE B
STUDENT ASSIGNMENTS AND PROCEDURE LOCATION LIST

It is recommended that students read the assigned chapters thoroughly every week. Be sure to include the items labeled in the chapters: Med Tips located in the chapter, and On The Job, Legal and Ethical Issues, and the Study Outline and Chapter Review that are located *at the end of the chapters.*

To assist you in preparing for the Certification Exam to become a Certified Medical Assistant when your program is complete, we have provided review questions to study at the end of each chapter and at the end of your textbook.

Your instructor will assign 25 vocabulary words from the chapters you are reading for the week to study for your weekly Spelling & Terminology Exam.

In addition to your regular assignments, every module you will be expected to complete ICD-9 (Page 305), CPT Coding (Page 307), and PDR (Page 309) exercises that you have in your text. It is recommended that you begin these exercises as soon as the module begins to ensure that they are complete by the end of the module. If you have never done these exercises before, your instructor will go over them with you.

WEEK 1 ASSIGNMENTS:

Read:

Chapter 1 & 2—Medical Terminology and A & P of the Muscular System

The Career Development reading assignment is located in the appendix of your student handbook. This reading assignment must to be completed prior to your scheduled career development lecture that will be conducted this week.

Assignment:

Complete the following assignments that are due according to your instructor's direction:

Chapter 1, Pages 27-35

Chapter 2, Pages 57-63

WEEK 2 ASSIGNMENT:

Read:

Chapter 3—Infection Control: Asepsis, Assisting with Minor Surgery & Physical Exams

Assignment:

Complete the following assignments that are due according to your instructor's direction:

Chapter 3, Pages 99-109

Chapter 4, Pages 152-163

WEEK 3 ASSIGNMENT:

Read:

Chapter 5—Pharmacology

Assignment:

Complete the Mathematical Review and Dosage Calculations (pages 313-323) according to your instructor's direction. ✓

Chapter 5, Pages 186-197

WEEK 4 ASSIGNMENT:

Read:

Chapter 6—Administering Medications

Assignment:

Complete the Inventory for Locked Medication (Page 310) and Lab Supplies (Page 311) according to your instructor's direction.

Chapter 6, Pages 237-247 ✓

PROCEDURE LOCATION LIST

Procedure:	Located in textbook on:
Hand washing	Pages 81 & 82
Gloving	Page 85
Surgical Tray Set-ups	Pages 135-138, 150-151, 328
Instruments & Autoclaving	Pages 86, 123-131 and 88, 91-92
Surgical Skin Preparation	Page 143
Surgical Scrub & Glove	Pages 114-115 & 117
Assisting with Suturing	Page 138
Removal of Sutures	Page 147
Administering Oral Medication	Pages 181-182, 210, 212
Ampule Withdrawal	Pages 218-219
Vital Signs	Located in the appendix of your Student Handbook
Intradermal Injection	Pages 232-233
Subcutaneous or Intramuscular Injection	Pages 227-228
Z-Track Injection	Page 230

MATHEMATICS REVIEW FOR DOSAGE CALCULATIONS
MODULE B

SECTION 1—WHOLE NUMBERS

ADDITION: In order to add whole numbers; align the last digit of each number in a vertical column. Add the digits in the last column on the right first. If the total is more than 9, you must **carry** the extra digit. Continue adding vertical columns from right to left.

<u>EXAMPLE</u>

$1,237 + 592 = ?$

$$
\begin{array}{r}
1 \\
1,237 \\
+592 \\
\hline
1,829
\end{array}
$$

Do the following practice problems without a calculator:

1) $108 + 45 + 8$
2) $856 + 4,710$

SUBTRACTION: In order to subtract whole numbers, align the last digit of each number in a vertical column. Subtract the digits in the last column on the right first. If the bottom digit is larger than the top digit, it is necessary to **borrow** from the next digit on the left. Continue from right to left until complete.

<u>EXAMPLE:</u>

$1,295 - 426 = ?$

$$
\begin{array}{r}
^{0\,12\,8\,15} \\
\cancel{1,295} \\
-426 \\
\hline
869
\end{array}
$$

Do the following practice problems without a calculator:

3) $1,727 - 48$
4) $808 - 199$
5) $347 - 277$

MULTIPLICATION: Is a shortcut for repeated addition. For example $5 \times 4 = 5 + 5 + 5 + 5$.

<u>EXAMPLE</u>

$37 \times 24 = ?$
- Multiply 7 by 4. $7 \times 4 = 28$. Write the 8, carry the 2
- Multiply 3 by 4. $3 \times 4 = 12$. Add the carried 2. Write 14

Now you drop down to the next line and shift your answer to the left. You may want to enter a zero as a placeholder.
- Multiply 7 by 2. Write the 4 under the 4 and carry the 1.
- Multiply 3 by 2. $3 \times 2 = 6$. Add the carried 1 to get 7
- Add the two lines to get the resulting answer of 888

$$
\begin{array}{r}
^{1}_{2} \\
37 \\
\times 24 \\
\hline
148 \\
740 \\
\hline
888
\end{array}
$$

Do the following practice problems without a calculator.

6) 612×37
7) 46×32

DIVISION: When figuring out problems by hand, long division is usually the best method. The problem gets separated into smaller, easier parts to arrive at the final answer.

<u>EXAMPLE</u>

$232 \div 8 = ?$

Since there are no 8's in 2, divide 8 into 23. We estimate there are 2 8's in 23. the 2 is placed over the 23. Multiply the 2 by the divisor 8, place the product under the 23. Subtract 16 from 23. Bring down the next digit. Repeat the steps. There is no remainder. The quotient is 29.

$$
\begin{array}{r}
29 \\
8{\overline{\smash{)}232}} \\
\underline{16} \\
72 \\
\underline{72} \\
0
\end{array}
$$

Do the following problems without a calculator.

8) $1,358 \div 23$
9) $1,331 \div 11$
10) $10,000 \div 10$

SECTION 2 - FRACTIONS

FRACTIONS: A fraction is written with the numerator (top) over the denominator (bottom). A fraction symbolizes a part of a whole. The fraction also indicates division. Thus:

$$\frac{2}{3} = 2 \div 3 = \sqrt[3]{2}$$ In this case 2 is the numerator and 3 is the denominator.

A) Simplifying Fractions: Sometimes fractions can be made simpler.

$$\frac{4}{4} = 1 \quad \frac{10}{10} = 1$$

B) Reducing Fractions:

$$\frac{8}{12} = \frac{8}{12} \div \frac{4}{4} = \frac{2}{3}$$

C) Improper Fractions: It is helpful to convert any mixed numbers to improper fractions before attacking the problem. Multiply the denominator (bottom) by the whole number, then add the numerator(top) to the result. Place this sum over the original denominator. (3 x 3 = 9, 9 + 2 = 11)

$$3 + \frac{2}{3} = 3\frac{2}{3} = \frac{11}{3}$$

D) Multiplication of Fractions: To multiply two or more fractions together, multiply the numerators, then multiply the denominators.

$$\frac{2}{3} \times \frac{5}{9} = \frac{10}{27} \qquad \frac{1}{2} \times \frac{3}{4} = \frac{3}{8}$$

Do the following practice problems without a calculator.

11) $\dfrac{5}{8} \times \dfrac{3}{4}$

12) $\dfrac{5}{8} \times \dfrac{5}{9}$

E) Division of Fractions: Division problems involving fractions are rewritten as multiplication problems reversing the numerator (top) and denominator (bottom). Always reverse the second fraction only.

$$\frac{1}{2} \div \frac{2}{3} = \frac{1}{2} \times \frac{3}{2} = \frac{3}{4}$$

Do the following practice problems without a calculator

13) $\frac{8}{21} \div \frac{8}{9}$

14) $\frac{12}{17} \div 6$

F) Addition and subtraction of fractions: If the fraction has the same denominator (bottom): Add or subtract the numerators (top). Write the result over the *common* denominator. Reduce, if necessary.

$$\frac{2}{13} + \frac{7}{13} = \frac{9}{13} \qquad \frac{8}{15} - \frac{4}{15} = \frac{4}{15}$$

If the fractions have different denominators, an extra step is required. You must first multiply both the top and the bottom of each fraction by the bottom of the other fraction.

For example:

$$\frac{1}{5} + \frac{9}{13} = \frac{1}{5} \times \frac{13}{13} \quad + \quad \frac{9}{13} \times \frac{5}{5}$$

$$= \frac{13}{65} \quad + \quad \frac{45}{65}$$

$$= \frac{58}{65}$$

Do the following practice problems without a calculator:

15) $\frac{3}{7} + \frac{2}{5}$

16) $\frac{4}{5} - \frac{1}{3}$

17) $\frac{8}{21} + \frac{8}{9}$

18) $\frac{6}{8} - \frac{1}{8}$

19) $\frac{5}{8} + \frac{7}{9} + \frac{11}{12}$

SECTION 3—DECIMAL NUMBERS

A) ADDITION AND SUBTRACTION OF DECIMAL NUMERS:

To add or subtract decimal numbers, rewrite the problem vertically making sure to line up the decimal points. Add or subtract and bring down the decimal point in line with the other decimal points.

$$1.2 + 0.04 + 22 = ?$$

$$\begin{array}{r} 1.2 \\ 0.04 \\ +22.00 \\ \hline 23.24 \end{array}$$

B) MULTIPLICATION OF DECIMAL NUMBERS:

1. Arrange the numbers vertically, preferably with the number containing the most digits on top.
2. Multiply the numbers as if they were whole numbers, disregarding temporarily the decimal points.
3. Count the number of places to the right of the decimal point in each number and add together.
4. Starting to the right of the last digit in the answer, count as many places to the left as you totaled in step 3. Sometimes, zeros need to be added in the answer to account for the decimal places.

$$18.07 \times 2.9 = ?$$

$$\begin{array}{r} 18.07 \\ \times 2.9 \\ \hline 16263 \\ 36140 \\ \hline 52.403 \end{array}$$

C) DIVISION OF DECIMAL NUMBERS:

1. Change the divisor to a whole number by moving the decimal point to the right of the last digit.
2. Move the decimal point under the division sign to the right the same number of places.
3. Bring up the decimal point.
4. Divide

$$234.56 \div .04 = ? \qquad .04\overline{)234.56} \ = 4.\overline{)23456.}^{\,5864}$$

Do the following practice problems without a calculator

20) 0.335 ÷ 5
21) 12.7 x 1.2
22) 90 x 4.91
23) 0.439 x 349
24) (0.5 + 0.7) ÷ 0.24
25) 88.013 + 85 + 8.213
26) 4.24 + 1.7

SECTION 4—PERCENTAGES

The word *percent* means *out of 100*. Thus, $45\% = \dfrac{45}{100} = 0.45$

Decimal numbers can be expressed as a percent number, and percent numbers can be expressed as a decimal number.

1. Percent to decimal number
    a. move the decimal point two places to the left
    b. drop the percent sign $23\% = 0.23$
2. Decimal to percent number
    a. move the decimal two places to the right.
    b. Add the percent sign. $0.025 = 2.5\%$

Most word problems involving percent ask to find one of three numbers.

1. The missing percent (What percent of 15 is 3?)
2. A percent of a number (70% of 49 is what?)
3. The number of which a percent is taken (32% of what number is 60?)

Note that in these problems "of" means "x" and "is" means "equals".

In case number 2 (70 % of 49 is what?) convert the percent to a decimal number and solve.

$$70\% \times 49 = ? \qquad 0.70 \times 49 = 34.3$$

In case number 1 & 3, notice that the unknown is on the left side of the equals sign. In both cases simply divide the number on the right side of the equals sign by the number on the left side of the equals sign.

$$1. \text{ What percent} \times 15 = 3 = \quad 3 \div 15 = 15\overline{)3.0}^{0.2} = 0.20 = 20\%$$

$$3. \, 32\% \times \text{ what} = 60 \qquad 60 \div 32\% = 60 \div 0.32 = 0.32\overline{)60} = 32\overline{)6000.0}^{187.5}$$

Do the following practice problems without a calculator.

27) 12% of 25 is what?
28) 93 is 110% of what
29) Six co-workers got together for dinner after work one evening. The bill totaled $79.50. If the bill was divided evenly among the six, how much did each pay?
30) Dave bought two plant stands regularly priced at $44.95 each for $ 26.95 each. How much did he save in all?
31) A clothing store buys a suit for $185 and uses a 45% markup rate. What is the selling price.
32) The mad dasher can walk to school in 5/6 of an hour. He can jog the same distance in 3/4 of an hour. How much longer does it take him to walk to school than to jog?

MEDICATION LEARNING EXERCISE

STUDENT _____

INSTRUCTOR _____

MOD & UNIT _____

DATE _____

1. Locate the Drug Name in PINK section (Alphabetical Index by Brand Name) of the PDR (Physicians Desk Reference). This will give the page number of the WHITE section to complete the exercise.

2. Give indications. Some lists will be extensive, select a few uses.

3. Drug Classification will be given under indications or action (i.e., antibiotic, diuretic).

4. Contraindications: Conditions when the drug would not be used.

5. Dosage—Give the usual dose. Also list the forms of the drug (i.e., tablets, suppositories).

6. Side Effects or Adverse Reactions: Conditions that may arise as a result of taking the drug. (i.e., nausea, vomiting)

NAME OF DRUG CATEGORY (GENERIC/TRADE)	INDICATION (USE)	CONTRAINDICATIONS (PRECAUTIONS/WARNINGS)	FORM, DOSAGE AND INSTRUCTIONS	SIDE EFFECTS

NAME OF DRUG	INDICATION (USE)	CONTRAINDICATIONS (PRECAUTIONS/WARNINGS)	FORM, DOSAGE AND INSTRUCTIONS	SIDE EFFECTS

NAME OF DRUG	INDICATION (USE)	CONTRAINDICATIONS (PRECAUTIONS/WARNINGS)	FORM, DOSAGE AND INSTRUCTIONS	SIDE EFFECTS

NAME OF DRUG	INDICATION (USE)	CONTRAINDICATIONS (PRECAUTIONS/WARNINGS)	FORM, DOSAGE AND INSTRUCTIONS	SIDE EFFECTS

NAME OF DRUG	INDICATION (USE)	CONTRAINDICATIONS (PRECAUTIONS/WARNINGS)	FORM, DOSAGE AND INSTRUCTIONS	SIDE EFFECTS

CORE PROCEDURE COMPETENCY REQUIREMENTS
MODULE B

Document each patient in proper charting format

VITAL SIGNS I & II

Date/Time	Patient	T	P	R	B/P	MA Signature
1.						
2.						
3.						
4.						
5.						

INJECTIONS

Date/Time	Patient	Location	Reaction	MA Signature

Deltoid

1. _____
2. _____
3. _____

Subcutaneous

1. _____
2. _____
3. _____

Intradermal

1. _____
2. _____
3. _____

Gluteal/Z-track

1. _____
2. _____
3. _____

VENIPUNCTURE

MA Signature

1. _____

2. _____

3. _____

4. _____

PROCEDURE COMPETENCY REQUIREMENTS
MODULE B

Document each patient in proper charting format

Date/Time   Patient   MA Signature

INSTRUMENT PREPARATION & AUTOCLAVE

1. _____

2. _____

3. _____

4. _____

5. _____

SURGICAL SKIN PREPARATION

1. _____

2. _____

3. _____

SURGICAL SCRUB & GLOVE

1. _____

2. _____

3. _____

SURGICAL TRAY SET UP

I & D Tray

1. _____

2. _____

3. _____

Laceration repair tray

1. _____

2. _____

3. _____

Suture removal tray

1. _____

2. _____

3. _____

ADMINISTER ORAL MEDICATION

MA Signature

1. _____

2. _____

WITHDRAW MEDICATION FROM AN AMPULE

1. _____

2. _____

——— Appendix C

REFERENCE TO COMMON ALLERGIES, INFECTIONS, DISORDERS, PROCEDURES, AND TESTS

TABLE 1   Common Types of Allergies

Allergy	Description
Allergic rhinitis	Inflammation of the nasal mucosa which results in nasal congestion, rhinorrhea (runny nose), sneezing and itching of the nose. Seasonal allergic rhinitis, such as seen in hay fever, occurs only during certain seasons of the year. Children suffering from this type of allergy may rub their nose in an upward movement, called the "allergic salute."
Asthma	A condition seen most frequently in early childhood in which wheezing, coughing, and dyspnea are the major symptoms. Asthmatic attacks may be caused by allergens inhaled from the air, food, and drugs. The patient's airway is affected by a constriction of the bronchial passages. Treatment is medication and control of the causative factors.
Contact dermatitis	Inflammation and irritation of the skin due to contact with an irritating substance, such as soap, perfume, cosmetics, plastic, dyes, and plants such as poison ivy. Symptoms include itching, redness, and skin lesions with blistering and oozing. Treatment consists of topical and systemic medications and removal of the causative item.
Eczema	A superficial dermatitis accompanied by papules, vesicles, and crusting. This condition can be acute or chronic.
Urticaria	A skin eruption of pale reddish wheals (circular elevations of the skin) with severe itching. It is usually associated with a food allergy, stress, or drug reactions. Also called hives.

TABLE 2   Common Skin Lesions

Type of Lesion	Description
Cyst	A fluid-filled sac or pouch under the skin.
Fissure	Crack-like lesion or groove in the skin.
Macule	Small, flat discolored area that is flush with the skin surface. An example would be a freckle and the flat rash of roseola.
Nodule	Solid, raised group of cells.
Papule	Small, solid, circular raised spot on the surface of the skin.
Polyp	Small tumor with a pedicle or stem attachment. They are commonly found in vascular organs such as the nose, uterus, and rectum.
Pustule	Raised spot on the skin containing pus.
Vesicle	Small, fluid-filled raised spot on the skin; blister.
Wheal	Small, round, raised area on the skin that may be accompanied by itching.

TABLE 3   Common Skin Infections

Infection	Description
Boil	Acute inflammation of the subcutaneous layer of skin, or hair follicle. Also called a furuncle. Treatment consists of the application of moist heat until the boil comes to a "head" or softens. An incision and drainage (I&D) may be performed to allow the purulent material to drain. Antibiotics may be prescribed.
Carbuncle	Inflammation and infection of the skin and hair follicle that may result from several untreated boils. They are most commonly found on the neck, upper back, or head. Treatment is similar to that for a single boil. Systemic antibiotics may be prescribed. A gauze bandage is applied when drainage is present.
Furuncle	Staphylococcal skin abscess with redness, pain and swelling. Also called a boil.
Herpes simplex	Infectious disease caused by the herpes simplex virus 1 and characterized by thin vesicles that tend to recur in the same area such as the lips or conjunctiva. Treatment consists of the drug acyclovir either locally or orally.
Herpes zoster	A painful, infectious viral disease which attacks the nerve endings. It is also called shingles and is caused by the same virus as chickenpox. Treatment consists of analgesics to relieve pain, and antiviral medications, such as acyclovir. In severe cases a nerve block may be necessary to relieve pain.
Impetigo	A highly contagious inflammatory skin disease with pustules that become crusted and rupture. Treatment consists of thorough cleansing using separate towels and wash cloths for the patient. These should be washed daily. Topical medications may be prescribed.
Scabies	Contagious skin disease caused by an egg-laying mite that causes intense itching. The lesions appear as small, red papules and vesicles between the fingers, toes, genitalia, and beneath the breasts. Treatment consists of a methrin cream from the neck down. All clothing and bedding need careful laundering.
Sebaceous cyst	Cyst filled with sebum (oil) from a sebaceous gland. This can grow to a large size and may need to be excised.

(continued)

TABLE 3   *(continued)*

Infection	Description
Tinea	A fungal skin disease resulting in itching, scaling lesions. Tinea pedis is also called athlete's foot. Diagnosis of tinea is made with the use of a Wood's light which are ultraviolet rays used to detect fluorescent materials in the skin and hair of patients with tinea. Topical treatment consists of fungicidal agents, such as griseofulvin.
Verruca	A benign neoplasm (tumor), which has a rough surface that is removed by chemicals and /or laser therapy, and is caused by a virus. Also called warts.

TABLE 4   Neoplasms

Benign (non-cancerous) Neoplasms	Description
Dermatofibroma	A fibrous tumor of the skin. It is painless, round, firm, red, and generally found on the extremities.
Hemangioma	Benign tumor of dilated vessels.
Keloid	The formation of a scar after an injury or surgery, which results in a raised, thickened, red area.
Keratosis	Overgrowth and thickening of cells in the epithelium located in the epidermis of the skin.
Leukoplakia	A change in the mucous membrane that results in thick, white patches on the mucous membrane of the tongue and cheek. It is considered precancerous and is associated with smoking.
Lipoma	Fatty tumor that generally does not **metastasize** (spread).
Nevus	A pigmented (colored) congenital skin blemish. It is usually benign but may become cancerous. Also called a birthmark or mole.

Malignant (cancerous) Neoplasms	Description
Basal cell carcinoma	An epithelial tumor of the basal cell layer of the epidermis. A frequent type of skin cancer that rarely metastasizes.
Kaposi's sarcoma	A form of skin cancer frequently seen in acquired immune deficiency syndrome (AIDS) patients. It consists of brownish-purple papules that spread from the skin and metastasize to internal organs.
Malignant melanoma	A dangerous form of skin cancer caused by an overgrowth of melanin in the skin. It may metastasize.
Squamous cell carcinoma	Epidermal cancer that may go into deeper tissue but does not generally metastasize.

TABLE 5   Diagnostic Procedures and Tests Relating to the Integumentary System

Procedure/Test	Description
Adipectomy	Surgical removal of fat.
Biopsy	Removal of a piece of tissue by syringe and needle, knife, punch, or brush to examine under a microscope as an aid in diagnosis.
Cauterization	The destruction of tissue with a caustic chemical, electric current, freezing, or hot iron.
Chemobrasion	Abrasion of the skin using chemicals. Also called a chemical peel.
Cryosurgery	The use of extreme cold to freeze and destroy tissue.
Curettage	The removal of superficial skin lesions with a curette or scraper.
Debridement	The removal of foreign material or dead tissue from a wound.
Dermabrasion	Abrasion or rubbing using wire brushes or sandpaper.
Dermatoplasty	The transplantation of skin. Also called skin grafting. May be used to treat large birthmarks (hemangiomas) and burns.
Electrocautery	To destroy tissue with an electric current.
Exfoliative cytology	Scraping cells from tissue and then examining them under a microscope.
Frozen section	Taking a thin piece of tissue from a frozen specimen for rapid examination under a microscope. This is often performed during a surgical procedure to detect the presence of cancer in a diseased organ.
Fungal scrapings (FS)	Scrapings taken with a curette or scraper of tissue from lesions are placed on a growth medium and examined under a microscope to identify fungal growth.
Incision and drainage (I & D)	Making an incision to create an opening for the drainage of material such as pus.
Laser therapy	Removal of skin lesions and birthmarks using a laser that emits intense heat and power at close range. The laser converts frequencies of light into one small beam.
Lipectomy	The surgical removal of fat.
Marsupialization	Creating a pouch to promote drainage by surgically opening a closed area, such as a cyst.
Needle biopsy	Using a sterile needle to remove tissue for examination under a microscope.
Plication	Taking tucks surgically in a structure to shorten it.
Rhytidectomy	Surgical removal of excess skin to eliminate wrinkles. Commonly referred to as a face lift.
Skin grafts	The transfer of skin from a normal area to cover another site. Used to treat burn victims and after some surgical procedures.
Sweat test	Test performed on sweat to see the level of chloride. There is an increase in skin chloride in some diseases, such as cystic fibrosis.

TABLE 6   Disorders of the Cardiovascular System

Disorder	Description
Anemia	A reduction in the number of circulating red blood cells per cubic millimeter of blood. It is not a disease but a symptom of disease.
Aneurysm	An abnormal dilation of a blood vessel, usually an artery, due to a congenital weakness or defect in the wall of the vessel.
Angina pectoris	Condition in which there is severe pain with a sensation of constriction around the heart. It is caused by a deficiency of oxygen to the heart muscle.
Angioma	Tumor, usually benign, consisting of blood vessels.
Angiospasm	Spasm or contraction of blood vessels.
Aortic aneurysm	Localized, abnormal dilation of the aorta, causing pressure on the trachea, esophagus, veins, or nerves. This is due to a weakness in the wall of the blood vessel.
Aortic insufficiency	A failure of the aortic valve to close completely which results in leaking and inefficient heart action.
Aortic stenosis	Condition caused by a narrowing of the aorta.
Arrhythmia	An irregularity in the heartbeat or action.
Arterial embolism	Blood clot moving within an artery. This can occur as a result of arteriosclerosis.
Arteriosclerosis	Thickening, hardening, and loss of elasticity of the walls of arteries.
Atherosclerosis	This is the most common form of arteriosclerosis. It is caused by the formation of yellowish plaques of cholesterol building up on the inner walls of the arteries.
Bradycardia	An abnormally slow heart rate (under 60 beats per minute).
Congenital heart disease	Heart defects that are present at birth, such as patent ductus arteriosus, in which the opening between the pulmonary artery and the aorta fails to close at birth. This condition requires surgery.
Congestive heart failure	Pathological condition of the heart in which there is a reduced outflow of blood from the left side of the heart. This results in weakness, breathlessness, and edema.
Coronary artery disease	A narrowing of the coronary arteries that is sufficient enough to prevent adequate blood supply to the myocardium.
Coronary thrombosis	Blood clot in a coronary vessel of the heart causing the vessel to close completely or partially.
Embolus	Obstruction of a blood vessel by a blood clot that moves from another area.
Endocarditis	Inflammation of the membrane lining the heart. May be due to microorganisms or to an abnormal immunological response.
Fibrillation	Abnormal quivering or contractions of heart fibers. When this occurs within the fibers of the ventricle of the heart, arrest and death can occur. Emergency equipment to defibrillate, or convert the heart to a normal beat, will be necessary.
Hypertensive heart disease	Heart disease as a result of persistently high blood pressure which damages the blood vessels and ultimately the heart.
Hypotension	A decrease in blood pressure. This can occur in shock, infection, anemia, cancer, or as death approaches.
Infarct	Area of tissue within an organ or part that undergoes necrosis (death) following the cessation of the blood supply.
Ischemia	A localized and temporary deficiency of blood supply due to an obstruction to the circulation.
Mitral stenosis	Narrowing of the opening (orifice) of the mitral valve which causes an obstruction in the flow of blood from the atrium to the ventricle on the left side of the heart.
Mitral valve prolapse (MVP)	Common and serious condition in which the cusp of the mitral valve drops back (prolapses) into the left atrium during systole.
Murmur	A soft blowing or rasping sound heard upon auscultation of the heart.
Myocardial infarction	Condition caused by the partial or complete occlusion or closing of one or more of the coronary arteries. Symptoms include a squeezing pain or heavy pressure in the middle of the chest. A delay in treatment could result in death. This is also referred to as MI or heart attack.
Myocarditis	An inflammation of the myocardial lining of the heart resulting in extremely weak and rapid beat, and irregular pulse.
Patent ductus arteriosus	Congenital presence of a connection between the pulmonary artery and the aorta that remains after birth. This condition is normal in the fetus.
Pericarditis	Inflammatory process or disease of the pericardium.
Phlebitis	Inflammation of a vein.
Reynaud's phenomenon	Intermittent attacks of pallor or cyanosis of the fingers and toes associated with the cold or emotional distress. There may also be numbness, pain, and burning during the attacks. It may be caused by decreased circulation due to smoking.
Rheumatic heart disease	Valvular heart disease as a result of having had rheumatic fever.
Tetralogy of Fallot	Combination of four symptoms (tetralogy), resulting in pulmonary stenosis, a septal defect, abnormal blood supply to the aorta, and the hypertrophy of the right ventricle. A congenital defect that is present at birth and needs immediate surgery to correct.
Thrombophlebitis	Inflammation and clotting of blood within a vein.
Thrombus	A blood clot.
Varicose veins	Swollen and distended veins, usually in the legs, resulting from pressure, such as occurs during a pregnancy.

TABLE 7   Diagnostic Procedures and Tests Relating to the Cardiovascular System

Procedure/Test	Description
Aneurysmectomy	The surgical removal of the sac of an aneurysm, which is an abnormal dilatation of a blood vessel.
Angiography	X-rays taken after the injection of an opaque material into a blood vessel. Can be performed on the aorta as an aortic angiogram, on the heart as an angiocardiogram, and on the brain as a cerebral angiogram.
Angioplasty	A surgical procedure of altering the structure of a vessel by dilating the vessel using a balloon inside the vessel.
Arterial blood gases	Measurement of the amount of oxygen (O_2), carbon dioxide (CO_2), and nitrogen in the blood. Also gives a pH reading of the blood. Blood gases are performed in emergency situations and provide valuable evaluation of cardiac failure, hemorrhage, and kidney failure.
Artery graft	A piece of blood vessel that is transplanted from a part of the body to the aorta to repair a defect.
Artificial pacemaker	Electrical device that substitutes for the natural pacemaker of the heart. It controls the beating of the heart by a series of rhythmic electrical impulses. An external pacemaker has the electrodes on the outside of the body. An internal pacemaker will have the electrodes surgically implanted within the chest wall.
Cardiac catheterization	Passage of a thin tube (catheter) through an arm vein and the blood vessels leading into the heart. It is done to detect abnormalities, to collect cardiac blood samples, and to determine the pressure within the cardiac area.
Cardiac enzymes	Complex proteins that are capable of inducing chemical changes within the body. Cardiac enzymes are taken by blood sample to determine the amount of heart disease or damage.
Cardiac magnetic resonance imaging (MRI)	A noninvasive procedure in which images of the heart and blood vessels are captured for examination to determine effects.
Cardiolysis	A surgical procedure to separate adhesions which involves a resection of the ribs and sternum over the pericardium.
Cardiorrhaphy	Surgical suturing of the heart.
Cardioversion	Converting a cardiac arrhythmia (irregular heart action) to a normal sinus rhythm using a cardioverter to give countershocks to the heart.
Commissurotomy	Surgical incision to change the size of an opening. For example in mitral commissurotomy, a stenosis or narrowing is corrected by cutting away at the adhesions around the mitral opening (orifice).
Coronary artery bypass surgery	Open-heart surgery in which a shunt is created to permit blood to travel around the constriction in coronary blood vessel(s).
Doppler ultrasonography	Measurement of sound-wave echoes as they bounce off tissues and organs to produce an image. Can assist in determining heart and blood vessel damage. Also called echocardiogram.
Electrocardiogram	Record of the electrical activity of the heart. Useful in the diagnosis of abnormal cardiac rhythm and heart muscle (myocardium) damage. This procedure is explained fully in Chapter 29.
Electrolytes	Measurement of blood sodium (Na), potassium (K), and chlorides (Cl).
Embolectomy	Surgical removal of an embolus or clot from a blood vessel.
Heart transplantation	Replacement of a diseased or malfunctioning heart with a donor's heart.
Holter monitor	Portable ECG monitor worn by the patient for a period of a few hours to a few days to assess the heart and pulse activity as the person goes through the activities of daily living. Used to assess a patient who experiences chest pain and unusual heart activity during exercise and normal activities when a cardiogram is inconclusive.
Lipoproteins	Measurement of blood to determine serum cholesterol and triglycerides.
Open-heart surgery	Surgery that involves the heart, coronary arteries, or the heart valves. The heart is actually entered by the surgeon.
Percutaneous balloon valvuloplasty	Insertion through the skin of a balloon catheter across a narrowed or stenotic heart valve. When the balloon is inflated, the narrowing or constriction is decreased.
Percutaneous transluminal coronary angioplasty (PTCA)	Method for treating localized coronary artery narrowing. A balloon catheter is inserted through the skin into the coronary artery and inflated to dilate the narrow blood vessel.
Phleborrhaphy	Suturing of a vein.
Prothrombin time	Measurement of the time it takes for a sample of blood to coagulate.
Stress testing	Method for evaluating cardiovascular fitness. The patient is placed on a treadmill or bicycle and then subjected to steadily increasing levels of work. An EKG and oxygen levels are taken while the patient exercises. The test is stopped if abnormalities occur on the EKG.
Treadmill test	Also called a stress test.
Valve replacement	Surgical procedure to excise a diseased heart valve and replace with an artificial valve.
Venography	X-ray of the veins by tracing the venous flow. Also called phlebography.

TABLE 8   Disorders of the Endocrine System

Disorder	Description
Acidosis	Excessive acidity of bodily fluids due to the accumulation of acids, as in diabetic acidosis.
Acromegaly	Chronic disease of middle-aged persons which results in an elongation and enlargement of the bones of the head and extremities. There can also be mood changes.
Addison's disease	A disease resulting from a deficiency in adrenocortical hormones. There may be an increased pigmentation of the skin, generalized weakness, and weight loss.
Adenoma	A neoplasm or tumor of a gland.
Cretinism	Congenital condition due to a lack of thyroid, which may result in arrested physical and mental development.
Cushing's syndrome	Set of symptoms which result from hypersecretion of the adrenal cortex. This may be the result of a tumor of the adrenal glands. The syndrome may present symptoms of weakness, edema, excess hair growth, skin discoloration, and osteoporosis.
Diabetes insipidus (DI)	Disorder caused by the inadequate secretion of the antidiuretic hormone ADH by the posterior lobe of the pituitary gland. There may be polyuria and polydipsia.
Diabetes mellitus (DM)	Chronic disorder of carbohydrate metabolism which results in hyperglycemia and glycosuria. Type I diabetes mellitus (IDDM) involves insulin dependency, which requires that the patient take daily injections of insulin. Type II (NIDDM) patients may not be insulin dependent.
Diabetic retinopathy	Secondary complication of diabetes mellitus (DM) which affects the blood vessels of the retina, resulting in visual changes and even blindness.
Dwarfism	Condition of being abnormally small. It may be the result of a hereditary condition or an endocrine dysfunction.
Gigantism	Excessive development of long bones of the body due to overproduction of the growth hormone by the pituitary gland.
Goiter	Enlargement of the thyroid gland.
Graves' disease	Disease that results from an over activity of the thyroid gland and can result in a crisis situation. Also called hyperthyroidism.
Hashimoto's disease	A chronic form of thyroiditis.
Hirsutism	Condition of having an excessive amount of hair on the body. This term is used to describe females who have the adult male pattern of hair growth. Can be the result of a hormonal imbalance.
Hypercalcemia	Condition of having an excessive amount of calcium in the blood.
Hyperglycemia	Having an excessive amount of glucose (sugar) in the blood.
Hyperkalemia	Condition of having an excessive amount of potassium in the blood.
Hyperthyroidism	Condition that results from over activity of the thyroid gland. Also called Graves' disease.
Hypothyroidism	Result of a deficiency in secretion by the thyroid gland. This results in a lowered basal metabolism rate with obesity, dry skin, slow pulse, low blood pressure, sluggishness, and goiter. Treatment is replacement with synthetic thyroid hormone.
Ketoacidosis	Acidosis due to an excess of ketone bodies (waste products) which can result in death for the diabetic patient if not reversed.
Myasthenia gravis	Condition in which there is great muscular weakness and progressive fatigue. There may be difficulty in chewing and swallowing and drooping eyelids. If a thymoma is causing the problem, it can be treated with removal of the thymus gland.
Myxedema	Condition resulting from a hypofunction of the thyroid gland. Symptoms can include anemia, slow speech, enlarged tongue and facial features, edematous skin, drowsiness, and mental apathy.
Thyrotoxicosis	Condition that results from overproduction of the thyroid gland. Symptoms include a rapid heart action, tremors, enlarged thyroid gland, exophthalmos, and weight loss.
von Rechlinghausen's disease	Excessive production of parathyroid hormone, which results in degeneration of the bones.

TABLE 9   Procedures and Tests Relating to the Endocrine System

Procedure/Test	Description
Basal metabolic rate (BMR)	Somewhat outdated test to measure the energy used when the body is in a state of rest.
Blood serum test	Blood test to measure the level of substances such as calcium, electrolytes, testosterone, insulin, and glucose. Used to assist in determining the function of various endocrine glands.
Fasting blood sugar	Blood test to measure the amount of sugar circulating throughout the body after a 12-hour fast.
Glucose tolerance test (GTT)	Test to determine the blood sugar level. A measured dose of glucose is given to a patient either orally or intravenously. Blood samples are then drawn at certain intervals to determine the ability of the patient to utilize glucose. Used for diabetic patients to determine their insulin response to glucose.
Parathyroidectomy	Excision of one or more of the parathyroid glands. This is performed to halt the progress of hyperparathyroidism.
Protein bound iodine (PBI) test	Blood test to measure the concentration of thyroxin (T4) circulating in the bloodstream. The iodine becomes bound to the protein in the blood and can be measured. This test is useful in establishing thyroid function.
Radioactive iodine uptake (RAIU) test	Test in which radioactive iodine is taken orally (PO) or intravenously (IV) and the amount that is eventually taken into the thyroid gland (the uptake) is measured to assist in determining thyroid function.
Radioimmunoassay (RIA) test	Test used to measure the levels of hormones in the plasma of the blood.
Serum glucose test	Blood test performed to assist in determining insulin levels and useful for adjusting medication dosage. Surgical removal of the thymus gland.
Thymectomy	Ultrasound examination of the thyroid which can assist in distinguishing a thyroid nodule from a cyst.
Thyroid echogram	Surgical removal of the thyroid gland. The patient is then placed on replacement hormone (thyroid) therapy.

(continued)

TABLE 9   *(continued)*

Procedure/Test	Description
Thyroidectomy	Blood tests used to measure the levels of T3, T4, and TSH in the bloodstream to assist in determining thyroid function.
Thyroid function tests	Surgical removal (excision) of the thyroid and parathyroid glands.
Thyroparathyroidectomy	Test in which a radioactive element is administered which localizes in the thyroid gland. The gland can then be
Thyroid scan	visualized with a scanning device to detect pathology such as tumors.
Total calcium	Blood test to measure the total amount of calcium to assist in detecting parathyroid and bone disorders.
Two-hour postprandial glucose tolerance test	Blood test to assist in evaluating glucose metabolism. The patient eats a high-carbohydrate diet and fasts overnight before the test. A blood sample is then taken two hours after a meal.

TABLE 10   Disorders and Pathology of the Digestive System

Disorder/Pathology	Description
Anorexia	Loss of appetite that can accompany other conditions such as a gastrointestinal (GI) upset.
Ascites	Collection or accumulation of fluid in the peritoneal cavity.
Bulimia	Eating disorder that is characterized by recurrent binge eating and then purging of the food with laxatives and vomiting.
Cholecystitis	Inflammation of the gallbladder.
Cholelithiasis	Formation or presence of stones or calculi in the gallbladder or common bile duct.
Cirrhosis	Chronic disease of the liver.
Cleft lip	Congenital condition in which the upper lip fails to come together. This is often seen along with cleft palate and is corrected with surgery.
Cleft palate	Congenital condition in which the roof of the mouth has a split or fissure. It is corrected with surgery.
Constipation	Experiencing difficulty in defecation or infrequent defecation.
Crohn's disease	Form of chronic inflammatory bowel disease affecting the ileum and/or colon. Also called regional ileitis.
Diverticulitis	Inflammation of a diverticulum or sac in the intestinal tract, especially in the colon.
Diarrhea	Passing of frequent, watery bowel movements. Usually accompanies gastrointestinal (GI) disorders.
Dyspepsia	Indigestion.
Emesis	Vomiting usually with some force.
Enteritis	Inflammation of only the small intestine.
Esophageal stricture	Narrowing of the esophagus which makes the flow of foods and fluids difficult.
Fissure	Cracklike split in the rectum or anal canal or roof of mouth.
Fistula	Abnormal tubelike passage from one body cavity to another.
Gastritis	Inflammation of the stomach which can result in pain, tenderness, nausea, and vomiting.
Gastroenteritis	Inflammation of the stomach and small intestine.
Halitosis	Bad or offensive breath, which is often a sign of disease.
Hepatitis	Inflammation of the liver.
Ileitis	Inflammation of the ileum of the small intestine.
Inflammatory bowel syndrome	Ulceration of the mucous membranes of the colon of unknown origin. Also known as ulcerative colitis.
Inguinal hernia	Hernia or outpouching of intestines into the inguinal region of the body. May require surgical correction.
Intussusception	Result of the intestine slipping or telescoping into another section of intestine just below it. More common in children.
Irritable bowel syndrome	Disturbance in the functions of the intestine from unknown causes. Symptoms generally include abdominal discomfort and an alteration in bowel activity.
Malabsorption syndrome	Inadequate absorption of nutrients from the intestinal tract. May be caused by a variety of diseases and disorders, such as infections and pancreatic deficiency.
Peptic ulcer	Ulcer occurring in the lower portion of the esophagus, stomach, and duodenum thought to be caused by the acid of gastric juices. Some peptic ulcers are now successfully treated with antibiotics.
Pilonidal cyst	Cyst in the sacrococcygeal region due to tissue being trapped below the skin.
Polyphagia	To eat excessively.
Polyps	Small tumors that contain a pedicle or footlike attachment in the mucous membranes of the large intestine (colon).
Reflux esophagitis	Acid from the stomach backs up into the esophagus causing inflammation and pain. Also called GERD (gastroesophageal reflux disease).
Regurgitation	Return of fluids and solids from the stomach into the mouth. Similar to emesis but without the force.
Ulcerative colitis	Ulceration of the mucous membranes of the colon of unknown source. Also known as inflammatory bowel disease.
Volvulus	Condition in which the bowel twists upon itself and causes an obstruction. Painful and requires immediate surgery.

TABLE 11   Procedures and Tests Relating to the Digestive System

Procedure/Test	Description
Abdominal ultrasonography	Using ultrasound equipment for producing sound waves to create an image of the abdominal organs.
Air contrast barium enema	Using both barium and air to visualize the colon on x-ray.
Anastomosis	Creating a passageway or opening between two organs or vessels.
Appendectomy	Surgical removal of the appendix.
Barium enema (Lower GI)	Radiographic examination of the small intestine, large intestine, or colon in which an enema containing barium is administered to the patient while the x-ray pictures are taken.
Barium swallow (Upper GI)	A barium mixture swallowed while x-ray pictures are taken of the esophagus, stomach, and duodenum used to visualize the upper gastrointestinal tract. Also called esophagram.
Colectomy	Surgical removal of the entire colon.
Cholecystectomy	Surgical excision of the gallbladder. Removal of the gallbladder through the laparoscope is a newer procedure with fewer complications than the more invasive abdominal surgery. The laparoscope requires a small incision into the abdominal cavity.
Cholecystogram	Dye given orally to the patient is absorbed and enters the gallbladder. An x-ray is then taken.
Choledocholithotomy	Removal of a gallstone through an incision into the bile duct.
Choledocholithotripsy	Crushing of a gallstone in the common bile duct. Commonly called lithotripsy.
Colonoscopy	A flexible fiberscope passed through the anus, rectum, and colon is used to examine the upper portion of the colon. Polyps and small growths can be removed during the procedure.
Colostomy	Surgical creation of an opening of some portion of the colon through the abdominal wall to the outside surface.
Diverticulectomy	Surgical removal of a diverticulum.
Endoscopic retrograde cholangiopancreatography (ERCP)	Using an endoscope to x-ray the bile and pancreatic ducts.
Esophagoscopy	The esophagus is visualized by passing an instrument down the esophagus. A tissue sample for biopsy may be taken.
Esophagram (barium swallow)	As barium is swallowed the solution is observed traveling from the mouth into the stomach over a television monitor.
Esophagogastrostomy	Surgical creation of an opening between the esophagus and the stomach. Also called Upper GI.
Esophagostomy	Surgical creation of an opening into the esophagus.
Exploratory laparotomy	Abdominal operation for the purpose of examining the abdominal organs and tissues for signs of disease or other abnormalities.
Fistulectomy	Excision of a fistula.
Gastrectomy	Surgical removal of a part of or whole stomach.
Gastrointestinal endoscopy	A flexible instrument or scope is passed either through the mouth or anus to facilitate visualization of the gastrointestinal (GI) tract.
Glossectomy	Complete or partial removal of the tongue.
Hemorrhoidectomy	Surgical excision of hemorrhoids from the anorectal area.
Hepatic lobectomy	Surgical removal of a lobe of the liver.
Ileostomy	Surgical creation of a passage through the abdominal wall into the ileum. The fecal material (stool) drains into a bag worn on the abdomen.
Intravenous cholangiogram	A dye is administered intravenously to the patient that allows for visualization of the bile vessels.
Intravenous cholecystography	A dye is administered intravenously to the patient that allows for visualization of the gallbladder.
Jejunostomy	Surgical creation of a permanent opening into the jejunum.
Lithotripsy	Crushing of a stone located within the gallbladder.
Liver biopsy	Excision of a small piece of liver tissue for microscopic examination. This is generally used to determine if cancer is present.
Liver scan	A radioactive substance is administered to the patient by an intravenous (IV) route. This substance enters the liver cells, and this organ can then be visualized. This is used to detect tumors, abscesses, and other hepatomegaly.

TABLE 12   Disorders and Pathology of the Lymphatic System

Disorder/Pathology	Description
Acquired immune deficiency syndrome (AIDS)	A disease that involves a defect in the cell-mediated immunity system. A syndrome of opportunistic infections occur in the final stages of infection with the human immunodeficiency virus (HIV). This virus attacks T4 lymphocytes and destroys them, which reduces the person's ability to fight infection.
AIDS-related complex (ARC)	A complex of symptoms which appears in the early stages of AIDS. This is a positive test for the virus but only mild symptoms of weight loss, fatigue, skin rash, and anorexia.
Elephantiasis	Inflammation, obstruction, and destruction of the lymph vessels which results in enlarged tissues due to edema.
Epstein-Barr virus	Virus which is believed to be the cause of infectious mononucleosis.
Hodgkin's disease	Lymphatic system disease that can result in solid tumors in any lymphoid tissue.
Lymphadenitis	Inflammation of the lymph glands. Referred to as swollen glands.
Lymphangioma	A benign mass of lymphatic vessels.
Lyphoma	Malignant tumor of the lymph nodes and tissue.
Lymphosarcoma	Malignant disease of the lymphatic tissue.
Mononucleosis	Acute infectious disease with a large number of atypical lymphocytes. Caused by the Epstein-Barr virus. There may be abnormal liver function and spleen enlargement.
Multiple sclerosis	Autoimmune disorder of the central nervous system in which the myelin sheath of nerves is attacked.
Non-Hodgkin's lymphoma	Malignant, solid tumors of lymphoid tissue.
Peritonsillar abscess	Infection of the tissues between the tonsils and the pharynx. Also called quinsy sore throat.
Sarcoidoisis	Inflammatory disease of the lymph system in which lesions may appear in the liver, skin, lungs, lymph nodes, spleen, eyes, and small bones of the hands and feet.
Splenomegaly	Enlargement of the spleen.
Systemic lupus erythematosis (SLE)	A chronic autoimmune disorder of connective tissue that causes injury to the skin, joints, kidneys, mucous membranes, and nervous system.
Thymoma	Malignant tumor of the thymus gland.

TABLE 13   Procedures and Tests Relating to the Lymphatic System

Procedure/Test	Description
Bone marrow aspiration	Removing a sample of bone marrow by syringe for microscopic examination. Useful for diagnosing such diseases as leukemia. For example, a proliferation (massive increase) of white blood cells could confirm the diagnosis of leukemia.
ELISA	Enzyme immunoassay test used to test blood for an antibody to the AIDS virus. A positive test means that the person has been exposed to the virus. There may be a false-positive reading and then the Western blot test would be used to verify the results.
Lymphadenectomy	Excision of a lymph node. This is usually done to test for a malignancy.
Lymphangiogram	X-ray taken of the lymph vessels after the injection of dye into the foot. The lymph flow through the chest is traced.
Splenopexy	The artificial fixation of a movable spleen.
Tonsillectomy	The surgical removable of the tonsils. Usually the adenoids are removed at the same time. This procedure is known as a T & A.
Western Blot	The test that is used as backup to the ELISA blood test to detect the presence of the antibody to HIV (AIDS virus) in the blood.

TABLE 14   Disorders of the Musculoskeletal System

Disorder	Description
Arthritis	Inflammation of the bone joints.
Bunion	Enlargement of the joint at the base of the great toe caused by inflammation of the bursa of the great toe.
Bursitis	Inflammation of the bursa, the connective tissue surrounding a joint.
Carpal tunnel syndrome	Pain caused by compression of the nerve as it passes between the bones and tendons of the wrist.
Gout	Inflammation of the joints caused by excessive uric acid.
Kyphosis	Abnormal increase in the outward curvature of the thoracic spine. Also known as hunchback or humpback.
Lordosis	Abnormal increase in the forward curvature of the lumbar spine. Also known as swayback.
Muscular dystrophy	Inherited disease causing a progressive muscle weakness and atrophy.
Myasthenia gravis	An autoimmune disorder causing loss of muscle strength and paralysis.
Osteoarthritis	Noninflammatory type of arthritis resulting in degeneration of the bones and joints, especially those bearing weight.
Osteomalacia	Softening of the bones caused by a deficiency of phosphorus or calcium. It is thought that in children the cause is insufficient sunlight and vitamin D.
Osteomyelitis	Inflammation of the bone and bone marrow due to infection; can be difficult to treat.
Osteoporosis	Decrease in bone mass that results in a thinning and weakening of the bone with resulting fractures. The bones become more porous, especially in the spine and pelvis.
Paget's disease	A fairly common metabolic disease of the bone from unknown causes. It usually attacks middle-aged and elderly people and is characterized by bone destruction and deformity.

(continued)

TABLE 14   *Continued*

Disorder	Description
Polymyositis	A disease causing muscle inflammation and weakness from an unknown cause.
Rheumatoid arthritis	Chronic form of arthritis with inflammation of the joints, swelling, stiffness, pain, and changes in the cartilage that can result in crippling deformities.
Rickets	Deficiency in calcium and vitamin D in early childhood which results in bone deformities, especially bowed legs.
Ruptured intervertebral disk	Herniation or outpouching of a disk between two vertebrae—also called a slipped or herniated disk.
Scoliosis	Abnormal lateral curvature of the spine.
Spinal stenosis	Narrowing of the spinal canal causing pressure on the cord and nerves.
Supernumerary bone	An extra bone, generally a finger or toe, found in newborns.
Talipes	Congenital deformity of the foot. This is also referred to as a clubfoot.
Tumors: *Benign*	
• Epidermoid cyst	Cysts located in the skull and phalanges of the fingers.
• Ganglion cyst	Cyst found at the end of long bones.
• Giant cell tumor	Benign tumor that appears at the epiphysis but does not interfere with joint movement. It may become malignant or return after removal.
• Osteoblastoma	A benign lesion or tumor which is generally found on the spine, where it may result in paralysis.
• Osteochondroma	Tumor composed of both cartilage and bony substance.
• Osteoid osteoma	Painful tumor usually found in the lower extremities.
Malignant	
• Ewing's sarcoma	Malignant growth found in the shaft of the long bones that spreads through the periosteum. Removal is treatment of choice, as this tumor will metastasize or spread to other organs.
• Fibrosarcoma	Tumor that contains connective tissue that occurs in bone marrow. It is found most frequently in the femur, humerus, and jaw bone.
• Myeloma	Malignant neoplasm originating in plasma cells in the bone.
Whiplash	Injury to the bones in the cervical spine as a result of a sudden movement forward and backward of the head and neck. Can occur as a result of a rear-end auto collision.

TABLE 15   Procedures and Diagnostic Tests Relating to the Musculoskeletal System

Procedure/Test	Description
Amputation	Partial or complete removal of a limb for a variety of reasons, including tumors, gangrene, intractable pain, crushing injury, or uncontrollable infection.
Anterior cruciate ligament (ACL) reconstruction	Replacing a torn ACL with a graft by means of arthroscopy.
Arthrocentesis	Removal of synovial fluid with a needle from a joint space, such as in the knee, for examination.
Arthrodesis	Surgical reconstruction of a joint.
Arthrography	Visualization of a joint by a radiographic study after injection of a contrast medium into a joint space.
Arthroplasty	Surgical reconstruction of a joint.
Arthroscopic surgery	Use of an arthroscope, a lighted instrument with camera/video capabilities, to facilitate performing surgery on a joint.
Arthrotomy	Surgically cutting into a joint.
Bone graft	Piece of bone taken from the patient that is used to take the place of a removed bone or a bony defect at another site, or to be wedged between bones for fusion of a joint.
Bone scan	Use of scanning equipment to visualize bones. It is especially useful in observing progress of treatment for osteomyelitis and cancer metastases to the bone.
Bunionectomy	Removal of the bursa at the joint of the great toe.
Carpal tunnel release	Surgical cutting of the ligament in the wrist to relieve nerve pressure caused by repetitive motion, for example typing (carpal tunnel disease).
Computerized axial tomography (CAT)	Computer-assisted x-ray used to detect tumors and fractures. Also referred to as CT-scan.
Electromyography	Study and record of the strength of muscle contractions as a result of electrical stimulation. Used in the diagnosis of muscle disorders and to distinguish nerve disorders from muscle disorders,.
Fasciectomy	Surgical removal of the fascia, which is the fibrous membrane covering and supporting muscles.
Laminectomy	Removal of the vertebral posterior arch to correct severe back problems caused by compression of the lamina.
Magnetic resonance imaging (MRI)	Medical imaging that uses radio-frequency radiation as its source of energy. It does not require the injection of contrast medium or exposure to ionizing radiation. The technique is useful for visualizing large blood vessels, the heart, brain, and soft tissues.

(continued)

TABLE 15 *Continued*

Procedure/Test	Description
Menisectomy	Removal of the knee cartilage (meniscus).
Muscle biopsy	Removal of muscle tissue for pathological examination.
Myelography	Study of the spinal column after injecting opaque contrast material.
Photon absorptiometry	Measurement of bone density using an instrument for the purpose of detecting osteoporosis.
Reduction	Correcting a fracture by realigning the bone fragments. A closed reduction of the fracture is the manipulation of the bone into alignment and the application of a cast or splint to immobilize the part during the healing process. Open reduction is the surgical incision at the site of the fracture to perform the bone re-alignment. This is necessary when there are bone fragments to be removed.
Spinal fusion	Surgical immobilization of adjacent vertebrae. This may be done for several reasons, including correction of a herniated disk.
Total hip replacement	Surgical reconstruction of a hip by implanting a prosthetic or artificial joint.

TABLE 16 Disorders and Diseases of the Nervous System

Disorder/Disease	Description
Amnesia	Loss of memory in which people forget their identity as a result of head injury or a disorder, such as epilepsy, senility, and alcoholism. This can be either temporary or permanent.
Amyotrophic lateral sclerosis (ALS)	Disease with muscular weakness and atrophy due to degeneration of motor neurons of the spinal cord. Also called Lou Gehrig's disease, after the New York Yankees' baseball player who died from the disease.
Aneurysm	Localized abnormal dilatation of a blood vessel, usually an artery; the result of a congenital defect or weakness in the wall of the vessel.
Anorexia nervosa	Loss of appetite, which generally occurs in females between the ages of 12 and 21, due to a fear of obesity. The patient believes that she is fat even when thin. Psychiatric treatment may be necessary if the patient refuses to eat, since death can occur.
Aphasia	Loss of ability to speak.
Asthenia	Lack or loss of strength, causing extreme weakness.
Astrocytoma	Tumor of the brain or spinal cord that is composed of astrocytes.
Ataxia	Lack of muscle coordination as a result of a disorder or disease.
Autism	Form of mental introversion in which the patient, usually a child, shows no interest in anything or anyone except himself or herself.
Bell's palsy	One-sided facial paralysis caused by herpes simplex virus. The person cannot control salivation, tearing of the eyes, or expression but will usually recover.
Brain tumor	Intracranial mass, either benign or malignant. A benign tumor of the brain can be fatal since it will grow and cause pressure on normal brain tissue. The most malignant form of brain tumor in children is the glioma.
Cerebral palsy	Nonprogressive paralysis resulting from a defect or trauma at the time of birth.
Cerebrovascular accident (CVA)	Hemorrhagic lesion in the brain which can result in paralysis and the inability to speak.
Chorea	Involuntary nervous disorder that results in muscular twitching of the limbs or facial muscles.
Coma	Abnormal deep sleep or stupor resulting from an illness or injury.
Concussion	Injury to the brain that results from an illness or injury.
Convulsion (seizure)	Sudden severe involuntary muscle contractions and relaxations. These have a variety of causes, such as head injury, epilepsy, fever, and toxic conditions.
Encephalitis	Inflammation of the brain due to disease factors, such as rabies, influenza, measles, or smallpox.
Embolism	Obstruction of a blood vessel by a blood clot or foreign substance, such as air and/or fat.
Epidural hematoma	Mass of blood in the space outside the dura mater of the brain and spinal cord.
Epilepsy	A recurrent disorder of the brain in which convulsive seizures and loss of consciousness occurs.
• Grand mal	Severe seizures in which loss of consciousness and muscular contractions occur.
• Petit mal	Form of epilepsy in which there is an alteration in the level of consciousness but an absence of seizures or convulsions.
• Jacksonian	A localized form of epilepsy with spasms confined to one part or one group of muscles.
Glioma	Sarcoma of neurological origin.
Hematoma	Swelling or mass of blood confined to a specific area, such as in the brain.
Herniated nucleus pulposa	Protrusion of the nucleus pulposa of the intervertebral disk into the spinal canal. This is also called a herniated disk.
Huntington's chorea	Disease of the central nervous system that results in progressive dementia with bizarre involuntary movements of parts of the body.
Hydrocephalus	Accumulation of cerebrospinal fluid within the ventricles of the brain, causing pressure on the brain and for the head to be enlarged. It is treated by creating an artificial shunt for the fluid to leave the brain.
Meningioma	Slow-growing tumor in the meninges of the brain.
Meningitis	Inflammation of the membranes of the spinal cord and brain that is caused by a microorganism.

(continued)

TABLE 16 *(continued)*

Disorder/Disease	Description
Meningocele	Congenital hernia in which the meninges, or membranes, protrude through an opening in the spinal column or brain.
Multiple sclerosis	Degenerative, demyelination, inflammatory disease of the central nervous system in which there is extreme weakness and numbness.
Narcolepsy	Chronic disorder in which there is an extreme uncontrollable desire to sleep.
Neuritis	Inflammation of a nerve or nerves, causing pain.
Neuroblastoma	Malignant metastatic hemorrhagic tumor that originates in the sympathetic nervous system, especially in the adrenal medulla. Occurs mainly in infants and children.
Palsy	Temporary or permanent loss of the ability to control movement.
Paralysis	A temporary or permanent loss of the ability to control movement.
• Paraplegia	Paralysis of the lower portion of the body and both legs.
• Hemiplegia	Paralysis of only one side of the body. This is the same as hemiparesis.
• Quadriplegia	Paralysis of all four limbs. This is the same as tetraplegia.
Parkinson's disease	Chronic progressive disorder of the nervous system with fine tremors, muscular weakness, rigidity, and a shuffling gait.
Pica	An eating disorder in which there is a craving for material that is not food, such as clay, grass, wood, dirt, paper, soap, and plaster.
Reye's syndrome	A combination of symptoms that generally occurs in children under 15 years of age one week after they have had viral infection. It begins with a rash, vomiting, and confusion and may lead to coma, seizures, or respiratory arrest.
Shingles	Eruption of vesicles on the trunk of the body along a nerve path. Can be painful and generally occurs on only one side of the body. It is caused by the herpes zoster.
Spina bifida	Congenital defect in the walls of the spinal canal in which the laminae of the vertebra do not meet or close. May cause membranes and/or the spinal cord to herniate through the opening. This condition can also result in other defects such as hydrocephalus (fluid on the brain).
Subdural hematoma	Mass of blood forming beneath the dura mater of the brain.
Syncope	Fainting.
Tic douloureaux	Painful condition in which the trigeminal nerve is affected by pressure or degeneration. The pain is of a severe stabbing nature and radiates from the jaw and along the face.
Transient ischemic attack (TIA)	Temporary interference with blood supply to the brain, causing neurological symptoms, such as dizziness, numbness, and hemiparesis. May lead eventually to a full-blown stroke (CVA).

TABLE 17   Procedures and Tests Relating to the Nervous System

Procedure/Test	Description
Babinski's sign	Reflex test developed by John Babinski, a French neurologist, to determine lesions and abnormalities in the nervous system. The Babinski reflex is present, for a positive Babinski, if the great toe extends instead of flexes when the lateral sole of the foot is stroked. The normal response to this stimulation would be a flexion, or upward movement of the toe.
Brain scan	Injection of radioactive isotopes into the circulation to determine the function and abnormality of the brain.
Carotid endarterectomy	A surgical procedure for removing an obstruction within the carotid artery. It was developed to prevent strokes but is found to be useful only in severe stenosis with TIA.
Cerebral angiogram	X-ray of the blood vessels of the brain after the injection of radiopaque dye.
Cerebrospinal fluid shunts	Surgical creation of an artificial opening to allow for the passage of fluid. Used in the treatment of hydrocephalus.
Cordectomy	Removal of part of the spinal cord.
Craniotomy	Surgical incision into the brain through the cranium.
Cryosurgery	Use of extreme cold to produce areas of destruction in the brain. Used to control bleeding and treat brain tumors.
Echoencephalogram	Recording of the ultrasonic echoes of the brain. Useful in determining abnormal patterns of shifting in the brain.
Electromyogram	Written recording of the contraction of muscles as a result of receiving electrical stimulation.
Laminectomy	Removal of a vertebral posterior arch.
Lumbar puncture	Puncture with a needle into the lumbar area (usually the fourth intervertebral space) to withdraw fluid for examination and for the injection of anesthesia.
Nerve block	A method of regional anesthetic to stop the passage of sensory stimulation along a nerve path.
Pneumoencephalography	X-ray examination of the brain following withdrawal of cerebrospinal fluid and injection of air or gas via spinal puncture.
Positron emission tomography (PET)	Use of positive radionuclides to reconstruct brain sections. Measurement can be taken of oxygen and glucose uptake, cerebral blood flow, and blood volume.
Romberg's sign	Test developed to establish neurological function in which the person is asked to close their eyes and place their feet together. This test for body balance is positive if the patient sways when the eyes are closed.
Spinal puncture	Puncture with a needle into the spinal cavity to withdraw spinal fluid for microscopic analysis. Anesthetic is also administered by this route. This is also called a spinal tap.
Sympathectomy	Excision of a portion of the sympathetic nervous system. Could include a nerve or ganglion.
Transcutaneous electrical nerve stimulation (TENS)	Application of a mild electrical stimulation to skin electrodes placed over a painful area, causing interference with the transmission of the painful stimuli. Can be used in pain management to interfere with the normal pain mechanism.
Trephination	Process of cutting out a piece of bone in the skull to gain entry into the brain to relieve pressure.
Vagotomy	Surgical incision into the vagus nerve. Medication can be administered into the nerve to prevent its function.

TABLE 18   Common Disorders of the Eye

Disorder	Description
Achromatopsia	The condition of color blindness. This is more common in males.
Astigmatism	An eye disorder in which light rays are focused unevenly on the retina, resulting in a distorted image due to the abnormal curvature of the cornea.
Blepharitis	Inflammatory condition of the eyelash follicles and glands of the eyelids which results in swelling, redness, and crusts of dried mucus on the lids. This can be the result of allergy or infection.
Blepharochalasis	In this condition, the upper eyelid increases in size due to loss of elasticity, which is followed by swelling and recurrent edema of the lids. The skin may droop over the edges of the eyes when the eyes are open.
Cataract	Diminished vision resulting from the lens of the eye becoming opaque or cloudy. Treatment is usually surgical removal of the cataract.
Chalazion	A small, hard tumor or mass, similar to a sebaceous cyst, developing on the eyelid. This may require incision and drainage (I & D).
Conjunctivitis	An inflammation of the conjunctiva which is also called pinkeye.
Diabetic retinopathy	Small hemorrhages and edema that develop as a result of diabetes mellitus. Laser surgery and vitrectomy may be necessary for treatment.
Ectropion	Refers to an enversion (outward turning) of the eyelid, exposing the conjunctiva.
Entropion	Inversion (inward turning) of the eyelid.
Esotropia	Inward turning of the eye. An example of strabismus (muscle weakness of the eye).
Exophthalmus	Abnormal protrusion of the eyeball. Can be due to hyperthyroidism.
Esotropia	Outward turning of the eye. Also an example of strabismus (muscle weakness of the eye).
Glaucoma	Increase in intraocular pressure, which, if untreated, may result in atrophy (wasting away) of the optic nerve and blindness. Glaucoma is treated with medication and surgery. There is an increased risk of developing glaucoma in persons over 60 years of age, in people of African ancestry, after sustaining a serious eye injury, and in anyone with a family history of diabetes or glaucoma. Figure 22-8 [ID23-19] illustrates a glaucoma test.
Hemianopia	Loss of vision in half of the visual field. A stroke patient may suffer from this condition.
Hordeolum	Refers to a sty which is a small purulent inflammatory infection of a sebaceous gland of the eye. This is treated with hot compresses and, if necessary, surgical incision.
Hyperopia	With this condition a person can see things in the distance but has trouble reading material at close vision. It is also known as farsightedness.
Keratitis	Inflammation of the cornea.
Macular degeneration	Degeneration or deterioration of the macular area of the retina of the eye. It may be treated with laser surgery to destroy the blood vessels beneath the macula.
Myopia	With this condition a person can see things close up but distance vision is blurred. It is also known as nearsightedness.
Nystagmus	Jerky-appearing involuntary eye movement.
Presbyopia	Visual change due to aging, resulting in difficulty in focusing for near vision (such as reading).
Retinal detachment	A disorder that occurs when the two layers of the retina become separated or detached. The treatment is surgery.
Retinitis pigmentosa	Progressive disease of the eye which results in the retina becoming hard (sclerosed), pigmented, and atrophying (wasting away). There is no known cure for this condition.
Strabismus	An eye muscle weakness resulting in the eyes looking in different directions at the same time. (The eyes may be divergent or convergent). May be corrected with glasses, and/or surgery. Also called lazy eye, crossed eyes, or squint.
Trachoma	A chronic infectious disease of the conjunctiva and cornea caused by bacteria. This occurs more commonly in people living in hot, dry climates. Untreated, it may lead to blindness when the scarring invades the cornea. Trachoma can be treated with antibiotics.

TABLE 19   Procedures and Diagnostic Tests Relating to the Eye

Disorder	Description
Fluorescein angiography	The process of injecting a dye (fluorescein) to observe the movement of blood for detecting lesions in the macular area of the retina. This is used to determine if there is a detachment of the retina.
Gonioscopy	Use of an instrument called a gonioscope to examine the anterior chamber of the eye to determine ocular motility and rotation.
Keratometry	Measurement of the cornea using an instrument called a keratometer.
Laser Surgery	Surgical procedure performed with a laser handpiece that transfers light into intense, small beams capable of destroying or fixing tissue in place.
Slit lamp microscope	The instrument used in ophthalmology for examining the posterior surface of the cornea.
Tonometry	Measurement of the intraocular pressure of the eye using a tonometer to check for the condition of glaucoma. After a topical anesthetic is applied, the physician places the tonometer lightly upon the eyeball and a pressure measurement is taken. An air-puff tonometer similarly records the cornea's resistance to pressure, but uses more expensive equipment. This is generally part of a normal eye examination for adults.
Visual acuity	Measurements of the sharpness of a patient's vision. Usually a Snellen chart is used for this test and the patient identifies letters from a distance of 20 feet.
Vitrectomy	A surgical procedure for replacing the contents of the vitreous chamber of the eye.

TABLE 20   Common Disorders of the Ear

Disorder	Description
Acoustic neuroma	Benign tumor of the eighth cranial nerve sheath which can cause symptoms from pressure being exerted on tissues.
Anacusis	Total loss of hearing. Also called deafness.
Cerumen block	Ear wax causing a blockage in the external canal of the ear.
Conductive hearing loss	Loss of hearing as a result of the blocking of sound transmission in the middle ear or outer ear.
Meniere's disease	An abnormal condition within the labyrinth of the inner ear that can lead to a progressive hearing loss. The symptoms are dizziness or vertigo, hearing loss, and tinnitus (ringing in the ears).
Otitis media	Commonly referred to as a middle ear infection. This is seen frequently in children and is often preceded by an upper respiratory infection.
Otosclerosis	Progressive hearing loss caused by immobility of the stapes bone.
Presbycusis	Loss of hearing that can accompany the aging process.

TABLE 21   Procedures and Diagnostic Tests Relating to the Ear

Procedure/Test	Description
Audiogram	A chart that shows the faintest sounds a patient can hear during audiometry testing.
Audiometric test	A test of hearing ability by determining the lowest and highest intensity and frequencies that a person can distinguish. The patient may sit in a soundproof booth and receive sounds through earphones as the technician decreases and changes the volume or tones.
Falling test	A test used to observe balance and equilibrium. The patient is observed on one foot, then with one foot in front of the other, and then walking forward with eyes open. The same test is conducted with the patient's eyes closed. Swaying and falling with the eyes closed can indicate an ear and equilibrium malfunction.
Mastoid antrotomy	Surgical opening made in the cavity within the mastoid process to alleviate pressure from infection and allow for drainage.
Mastoid x-ray	X-ray taken of the mastoid bone to determine the presence of an infection, which can be an extension of a middle ear infection.
Myringoplasty	Surgical reconstruction of the eardrum.
Myringotomy	Surgical puncture of the eardrum with removal of fluid and pus from the middle ear, to eliminate a persistent ear infection and excessive pressure on the tympanic membrane. A tube is placed in the tympanic membrane to allow for drainage of the middle ear cavity.
Otoplasty	Corrective surgery to change the size of the external ear or pinna. The surgery can either enlarge or decrease the size of the pinna.
Otoscopy	The use of a lighted instrument (otoscope) to examine the external auditory canal and the middle ear.
Rinne and Weber tuning-fork tests	The physician holds a tuning fork, an instrument that produces a constant pitch when it is struck, against or near the bones on the side of the head. These tests assess both nerve and bone conduction of sound.
Sensorineural hearing loss	A type of hearing loss in which the sound is conducted normally through the external and middle ear but there is a defect in the inner ear or with the auditory nerve (eighth cranial nerve), resulting in the inability to hear.
Stapedectomy	Removal of the stapes bone to treat otosclerosis (hardening of the bone). A prosthesis or artificial stapes is implanted.
Tympanometry	Measurement of the movement of the tympanic membrane. Can indicate the presence of pressure in the middle ear.
Tympanoplasty	Another term for the surgical reconstruction of the eardrum. Also called myringoplasty.

TABLE 22   Common Disorders and Pathology of the Reproductive System

Disorder/Pathology	Description
Abruptio placenta	An emergency condition in which the placenta tears away from the uterine wall before the 20th week of pregnancy. This requires immediate delivery of the baby.
Amenorrhea	An absence of menstruation, which can be the result of many factors, including pregnancy, menopause, and dieting.
Breech presentation	Position of the fetus within the uterus in which the buttocks or feet are presented first for delivery rather than the head.
Carcinoma in situ	Malignant tumor that has not extended beyond the original site.
Cervical cancer	A malignant growth in the cervix of the uterus. This is an especially difficult type of cancer to treat, and causes 5 percent of the cancer deaths in women. PAP tests have helped to detect early cervical cancer.
Cervical polyps	Fibrous or mucous tumor or growth found in the cervix of the uterus. These are removed surgically if there is a danger that they will become malignant.
Cervicitis	Inflammation of the cervix of the uterus.
Choriocarcinoma	A rare type of cancer of the uterus which may occur following a normal pregnancy or abortion.
Condyloma	A wartlike growth on the external genitalia. *(continued)*

TABLE 22   *(continued)*

Disorder/Pathology	Description
Cystocele	Hernia or outpouching of the bladder that protrudes into the vagina. This may cause urinary frequency and urgency.
Dysmenorrhea	Painful cramping that is associated with menstruation.
Eclampsia	Convulsive seizures and coma occurring between the 20th week of pregnancy and the first week of postpartum.
Ectopic	A fetus that becomes abnormally implanted outside the uterine cavity. This is a condition requiring immediate surgery.
Endometrial cancer	Cancer of the endometrial lining of the uterus.
Fibroid tumor	Benign tumor or growth that contains fiberlike tissue. Uterine fibroid tumors are the most common tumors in women.
Mastitis	Inflammation of the breast, which is common during lactation but can occur at any age.
Menorrhagia	Excessive bleeding during the menstrual period. Can be either in the total number of days or the amount of blood or both.
Ovarian carcinoma	Cancer of the ovary.
Ovarian cyst	Sac that develops within the ovary.
Pelvic inflammatory disease (PID)	Any inflammation of the female reproductive organs, generally bacterial in nature.
Placenta previa	When the placenta has become attached to the lower portion of the uterus and, in turn, blocks the birth canal.
Preeclampsia	Toxemia of pregnancy which if untreated can result in true eclampsia. Symptoms include hypertension, headaches, albumin in the urine, and edema.
Premature birth	Delivery in which the infant (neonate) is born before the thirty-seventh week of gestation (pregnancy).
Premenstrual syndrome (PMS)	Symptoms that develop just prior to the onset of a menstrual period, which can include irritability, headache, tender breasts, and anxiety.
Prolapsed uterus	A fallen uterus that can cause the cervix to protrude through the vaginal opening. It is generally caused by weakened muscles from vaginal delivery or as a result of pelvic tumors pressing down.
Rh factor	A condition developing in the baby when the mother's blood type is Rh-negative and the father's is Rh-positive. The baby's red blood cells can be destroyed as a result of this condition. Treatment is early diagnosis and blood transfusion.
Salpingitis	Inflammation of the fallopian tube or tubes.
Spontaneous abortion	Loss of a fetus without any artificial aid. Also called a miscarriage.
Stillbirth	Birth in which the fetus dies before or at the time of delivery.
Toxic shock syndrome	Rare and sometimes fatal staphylococcus infection that generally occurs in menstruating women.
Tubal pregnancy	Implantation of a fetus within the fallopian tube instead of the uterus. This requires immediate surgery.
Vaginitis	Inflammation of the vagina, generally caused by a microorganism.

TABLE 23   Procedures and Diagnostic Tests Relating to the Female Reproductive System

Procedure/Test	Description
Abortion	The termination of a pregnancy before the fetus reaches a viable point in development.
Amniocentesis	Puncturing of the amniotic sac using a needle and syringe for the purpose of withdrawing amniotic fluid for testing. Can assist in determining fetal maturity, development, and genetic disorders.
Cauterization	The destruction of tissue using an electric current, a caustic product, a hot iron, or freezing.
Cervical biopsy	Taking a sample of tissue from the cervix to test for the presence of cancer cells.
Cesarean section (C-section)	Surgical delivery of a baby through an incision into the abdominal and uterine walls.
Colposcopy	Visual examination of the cervix and vagina.
Conization	Surgical removal of a core of cervical tissue or a partial removal of the cervix.
Cryosurgery	Exposing tissues to extreme cold in order to destroy tissues. This procedure is used in treating malignant tumors, to control pain and bleeding.
Culdoscopy	Examination of the female pelvic cavity using an endoscope.
Dilation and curettage (D&C)	Surgical procedure in which the opening of the cervix is dilated and the uterus is scraped or suctioned of its lining or tissue. A D & C is performed after a spontaneous abortion and to stop excessive bleeding from other causes.
Doppler ultrasound	Using an instrument placed externally over the uterus to detect the presence of fibroid tumors to outline the shape of the fetus.
Endometrial biopsy	Taking a sample of tissue from the lining of the uterus to test for abnormalities.
Episiotomy	Surgical incision of the perineum to facilitate the delivery process. Can prevent an irregular tearing of tissue during birth.
Fetal monitoring	Using electronic equipment placed on the mother's abdomen to monitor the baby's heart rate and strength of uterine contractions during labor.
Hymenectomy	Surgical removal of the hymen.
Hysterectomy	Surgical removal of the uterus.
Hysterosalpingography	Taking an x-ray after injecting radiopaque material into the uterus and oviducts.
Hysteroscopy	Inspection of the uterus using a special endoscope instrument.
Intrauterine device (IUD)	A device inserted into the uterus by a physician for the purpose of contraception.

(continued)

TABLE 23 *(continued)*

Procedure/Test	Description
Kegel exercises	Exercises named after A.H. Kegel, an American gynecologist, who developed them to strengthen female pelvic muscles. The exercises are useful in treating incontinence and as an aid in childbirth.
Laparoscopy	Examination of the peritoneal cavity using an instrument called a laparoscope. The instrument is passed through a small incision made by the surgeon into the peritoneal cavity.
Laparotomy	Making a surgical opening into the abdomen.
Oophorectomy	Surgical removal of an ovary.
Panhysterectomy	Excision of the entire uterus, including the cervix.
Panhysterosalpingo-oophorectomy	Surgical removal of the entire uterus, cervix, ovaries, and fallopian tubes. Also called a total hysterectomy.
PAP (Papanicolaou) smear	Test for the early detection of cancer of the cervix named after the developer of the test, George Papanicolaou, a Greek physician. A scraping of cells is removed from the cervix for examination under a microscope.
Pelvic examination	The physical examination of the vagina and adjacent organs performed by a physician by placing the fingers of one hand into the vagina. A visual examination is performed using a speculum.
Pelvimetry	Measurement of the pelvis to assist in determining if the birth canal will allow the passage of the fetus for a vaginal delivery.
Pelvic ultrasonography	The use of ultrasound waves to produce an image or photograph of organ or fetus.
Pregnancy test	A chemical test on urine that can determine pregnancy during the first few weeks. This can be performed in the physician's office or with an at-home test.
Salpingo-oophorectomy	Surgical removal of the fallopian tube and ovary.
Tubal ligation	Surgical tying off of the fallopian tube to prevent conception from taking place. This results in the sterilization of the female.

TABLE 24   Disorders of the Male Reproductive System

Disorder	Description
Anorchism	A congenital absence of one or both testes.
Aspermia	The lack of, or failure to, eject sperm.
Azoospermia	Absence of sperm in the semen.
Balanitis	Inflammation of the skin covering the glans penis.
Benign prostatic hypertrophy	Enlargement of the prostate gland commonly seen in males over 50.
Carcinoma of the testes	Cancer of one or both testes.
Cryptorchidism	Failure of the testes to descend into the scrotal sac before birth. Generally, the testes will descend permanently before the boy is one year old. A surgical procedure called an orchidopecy may be required to bring the testes down into the scrotum permanently and secure them permanently. Failure of the testes to descend could result in sterility in the male.
Epididymitis	Inflammation of the epididymis which causes pain and swelling in the inguinal area.
Epispadias	Congenital opening of the male urethra on the dorsal surface of the penis.
Hydrocele	Accumulation of fluid within the testes.
Hypospadias	Congenital opening of the male urethra on the underside of the penis.
Impotent	Inability to copulate due to inability to maintain an erection or to achieve orgasm.
Perineum	In the male, the external region between the scrotum and the anus.
Phimosis	Narrowing of the foreskin over the glans penis which results in difficulty with hygiene. The condition can lead to infection or difficulty with urination. The condition is treated with circumcision, the surgical removal of the foreskin.
Prostate cancer	A slow-growing cancer that affects a large number of males after 50. The PSA (prostate-specific antigen) test is used to assist in early detection of this disease.
Prostatic hyperplasia	Abnormal cell growth within the prostate.
Prostatitis	An inflamed condition of the prostate gland which may be the result of infection.
Varicocele	Enlargement of the veins of the spermatic cord which commonly occurs on the left side of adolescent males. This seldom needs treatment.

TABLE 25 Procedures and Diagnostic Tests Relating to the Male Reproductive System

Procedure/Test	Description
Castration	Excision of the testicles in the male or the ovaries in the female.
Cauterization	Destruction of tissue with an electric current, a caustic agent, hot iron, or by freezing.
Circumcision	Surgical removal of the end of the prepuce or foreskin of the penis. Generally performed on the newborn male at the request of the parents. The primary reason is for ease of hygiene. Circumcision is also a ritual practiced in some religions.
Orchidopexy	Surgical fixation to move undescended testes into the scrotum, and attaching them to prevent retraction.
Prostatectomy	Surgical removal of the prostate gland.
Sterilization	Process of rendering a male or female sterile or unable to conceive children.
Transurethral resection of the prostate (TUR)	Surgical removal of the prostate gland by inserting a device through the urethra and removing prostate tissue.
Vasectomy	Removal of a segment or all of the vas deferens to prevent sperm from leaving the male body. Used for contraception purposes. A bilateral vasectomy would render the male sterile.
Semen analysis	This procedure is used when performing a fertility workup to determine if the male is able to produce sperm. Sperm is collected by the patient after abstaining from sexual intercourse for a period of three to five days. Also used to determine if a vasectomy has been successful. After a period of six weeks, no further sperm should be present in a sample from the patient.

TABLE 26 Sexually Transmitted Diseases

Disease	Description
Acquired immune deficiency syndrome (AIDS)	The final stage of infection from the human immunodeficiency virus (HIV). At present there is no cure.
Candidiasis	A yeastlike infection of the skin and mucous membranes which can result in white plaques on the tongue and vagina.
Chancroid	Highly infectious nonsyphilitic ulcer.
Chlamydial infection	Parasitic microorganism causing genital infections in males and females. Can lead to pelvic inflammatory disease (PID) in females and eventual infertility.
Genital herpes	Growths and elevations of warts on the genitalia of both males and females which can lead to cancer of the cervix in females. These painful vesicles on the skin and mucosa erupt periodically and can be transmitted through the placenta or at birth.
Genital warts	Growths and elevations of warts on the genitalia of both males and females which can lead to cancer of the cervix in females. There is currently no cure.
Gonorrhea	Sexually transmitted inflammation of the mucous membranes of either sex. Can be passed on to an infant during the birth process.
Hepatitis	Infectious, inflammatory disease of the liver. Hepatitis B and C types are spread by contact with blood and bodily fluids of an infected person.
Syphilis	Infectious, chronic, venereal disease that can involve any organ. May exist for years without symptoms.
Trichomoniasis	Genitourinary infection that is usually without symptoms (asymptomatic) in both males and females. In women the disease can produce itching and/or burning, a foul-smelling discharge, and results in vaginitis.

TABLE 27 Genetic Disorders

Disorder	Description
Alopecia	Baldness in particular patterns, especially on the head.
Cooley's anemia	A rare form of anemia or a reduction of red blood cells which is found in some people of Mediterranean origin.
Cystic fibrosis	A disorder of the exocrine glands which causes these glands to produce abnormally thick secretions of mucus. The disease affects many organs, including the pancreas and the respiratory system. One reliable diagnostic test in children is the sweat test, which will show elevated sodium and potassium levels. There is presently no known cure for the disease, which can shorten the life span.
Down syndrome	A disorder which produces moderate-to-severe mental retardation and multiple defects. The physical characteristics of a child with this disorder are a sloping forehead, flat nose or absent bridge to the nose, low-set eyes, and a general dwarfed physical growth. The disorder occurs more commonly when the mother is over 40. Also called Trisomy 21.
Duchene muscular dystrophy	A muscular disorder in which there is progressive wasting away of various muscles, including leg, pelvic, and shoulder muscles. Children with this disorder have difficulty climbing stairs and running. They may eventually be confined to a wheelchair. Other complications relating to the heart and respiratory system can be present. It is caused by a recessive gene and is more common in males. This disorder often results in a shortened life-span.

(continued)

TABLE 27   (continued)

Disorder	Description
Hemophilia	A bleeding disorder in which there is a deficiency in one of the factors necessary for blood to clot. There is an abnormal tendency to bleed, and victims of this disorder may require frequent blood transfusions. The female (mother) carries this recessive gene and it is passed on to males. Therefore, it is found almost exclusively in boys.
Huntington's chorea	A rare condition characterized by bizarre involuntary movements called chorea. The patient may have progressive mental and physical disturbances, which generally begin around 40.
Retinitis pigmentosa	Chronic progressive disease that begins in early childhood and is characterized by degeneration of the retina. This can lead to blindness by middle age.
Sickle cell anemia	Severe, chronic, incurable disorder that results in anemia and causes joint pain, chronic weakness, and infections. Occurs more commonly in people of Mediterranean and African heritage. The blood cell in this disease is sickle shaped.
Spina bifida	A congenital disorder that results in a defect in the walls of the spinal column, causing the membranes of the spinal cord to push through to the outside. It may be associated with other defects, such as hydrocephalus, which is an enlarged head as a result of the accumulation of fluid on the brain.
Tay-Sachs disease	A disorder caused by a deficiency of an enzyme, which can result in mental and physical retardation and blindness. It is transferred by a recessive trait and is most commonly found in families of Eastern European Jewish decent. Death generally occurs before the age of 4.

TABLE 28   Respiratory Disorders and Pathology

Disorder/Pathology	Description
Asthma	Disease caused by various conditions, such as allergens, and resulting in constriction of the bronchial airways and labored respirations. It can cause violent spasms of the bronchi (bronchospasms) but is not generally life-threatening. Medication can be very effective.
Atelectasis	A condition in which the lung tissue collapses, which prevents the respiratory exchange of oxygen and carbon dioxide. It can be caused by a variety of conditions, including pressure upon the lung from a tumor or other object.
Bronchiectasis	An abnormal stretching of the bronchi which results from a dilation of a bronchus or the bronchi that can be the result of an infection. The major symptom is a large amount of purulent (pus-filled) sputum. Rales (bubbling chest sounds) and hemoptysis (spitting up blood) may be present. This can be irreversible and may result in destruction of the bronchial walls.
Bronchitis	Inflammation of the mucous membranes of the bronchial tubes which results in a typical barking cough, fever, and **malaise** or discomfort.
Bronchogenic carcinoma	Malignant lung tumor that originates in the bronchi. It is usually associated with a history of cigarette smoking.
Chronic obstructive pulmonary disease (COPD)	Progressive, chronic, and usually irreversible condition in which the lungs have a diminished capacity for inspiration (inhalation) and expiration (exhalation). The patient may have difficulty breathing upon exertion (dyspnea) and a cough. Also called chronic obstructive lung disease.
Croup	An acute respiratory condition found in infants and children which is characterized by a barking type of cough or stridor.
Emphysema	Pulmonary condition that can occur as a result of long-term heavy smoking. Air pollution also worsens this disease. The patient may not be able to breath except in a sitting or standing position.
Empyema	Pus within the plural space, usually the result of infection.
Epistaxis	Nosebleed.
Histoplasmosis	A pulmonary disease from dust in the droppings of pigeons and chickens.
Hyaline membrane disease	Condition seen in premature infants whose lungs have not had time to develop properly. The lungs are not able to expand fully and a membrane (hyaline membrane) actually forms which causes extreme difficulty in breathing and may result in death. It is also known as infant respiratory distress syndrome (IRDS).
Laryngitis	Inflammation of the larynx (voicebox) causing difficulty in speaking.
Legionnaires' disease	Severe, often fatal disease characterized by pneumonia and gastrointestinal symptoms. It is caused by a gram-negative bacillus and named after people who came down with it at an American Legion Convention in 1976.
Paroxysmal nocturnal dyspnea	Attacks of shortness of breath (SOB) which occur only at night and awaken the patient.
Pertussis	Commonly called whooping cough, due to the "whoop" sound made when coughing. It is an infectious disease which children receive immunization against as part of their DPT shots.
Pleural effusion	The abnormal presence of fluid or gas in the pleural cavity. Physicians can detect the presence of fluid by tapping the chest (percussion) or listening with a stethoscope (auscultation).
Pleurisy	Inflammation of the pleura surrounding the lungs. The patient will experience pain upon inspiration due to friction caused by a rubbing of the pleural lining.
Pneumonia	Inflammatory condition of the lung which can be caused by bacterial and viral infections, diseases, and chemicals.
Pneumoconiosis	A condition that occurs as a result of inhaling environmental particles that become toxic. Can be the result of inhaling coal dust (anthracosis), or asbestos (asbestosis).
Pneumonomycosis	A disease of the lungs caused by a fungus.
Pneumothorax	Collection of air or gas in the pleural cavity which may result in collapse of the lung.
Pulmonary edema	Condition in which lung tissue retains an excessive amount of fluid. This results in labored breathing.

(continued)

TABLE 28   *(continued)*

Disorder/Pathology	Description
Pulmonary embolism	Blood clot or air bubble that moves to the pulmonary artery or one of its branches.
Respiratory distress syndrome (RDS)	Impairment of the respiratory function in premature infants due to immaturity.
Silicosis	A form of respiratory disease resulting from the inhalation of silica (quartz) dust. It is considered an occupational disease.
Sudden infant death syndrome (SIDS)	Unexpected and unexplained death of an apparently well infant.
Tracheostenosis	A narrowing and stenosis of the lumen or opening into the trachea.
Tuberculosis	An infectious disease caused by the tubercle bacillus, Mycobacterium tuberculosis. It most commonly affects the respiratory system and causes inflammation and calcification of the system. Tuberculosis is again on the uprise and is seen in many patients who have an impaired immune system, such as in AIDS.

TABLE 29   Procedures and Tests Relating to the Respiratory System

Procedure/Test	Description
Arterial blood gases	Testing for the gases present in the blood. This test is generally used to assist in determining the levels of oxygen (O_2) and carbon dioxide (CO_2) in the blood.
Bronchography	X-ray of the lung after a radiopaque substance has been inserted into the trachea or bronchial tube.
Bronchoplasty	The surgical repair of a bronchial defect.
Bronchoscopy	Using an instrument, the bronchoscope, to visualize the bronchi. During this procedure, tissue can be obtained for biopsy and foreign bodies can be removed.
Bronchotomy	A surgical incision of a bronchus, larynx, or trachea.
Cardiopulmonary resuscitation (CPR)	Emergency treatment provided by persons trained in CPR given to patients when their respirations and heart stop. CPR provides oxygen to the brain, heart, and other vital organs until medical treatment can restore a normal heart and pulmonary function. See an illustration of adult and infant CPR in Chapter 35.
Chest x-ray	Taking a radiographic picture of the lungs and heart from the back and front of the patient.
Endotracheal intubation	Placing a tube through the mouth to create an airway.
Heimlich maneuver	A technique for removing a foreign body from the trachea or pharynx by exerting diaphragmatic pressure.
Hyperbaric oxygen therapy	The use of oxygen under greater than normal pressure to treat cases of smoke inhalation, carbon monoxide poisoning, and other conditions. In some cases, the patient is placed in a hyperbaric oxygen chamber for this treatment.
Intermittent positive pressure breathing (IPPB)	A method for assisting the breathing of patients with a mask that is connected to a machine that produces an increased pressure.
Laryngectomy	The surgical removal of the larynx. This procedure is most frequently performed for excision of cancer.
Laryngoplasty	Surgical repair of the larynx.
Laryngoscopy	Examination of the interior of the larynx with a lighted instrument.
Lobectomy	Surgical removal of a lobe of the lung. Often the treatment of choice for lung cancer.
Pneumonectomy	The surgical removal of lung tissue.
Postural drainage	Drainage of secretions from the bronchi by placing the patient in a position that uses gravity to promote drainage. It is used for the treatment of cystic fibrosis, bronchiectasis, and before lobectomy surgery. May be combined with clapping and vibrating maneuvers to dislodge secretions.
Pulmonary angiography	Injecting dye into a blood vessel for the purpose of taking an x-ray of the arteries and veins of the lungs.
Pulmonary function test (PFT)	Breathing equipment used to determine respiratory function and measure lung volumes and gas exchange. Also called spirometry.
Rhinoplasty	Plastic surgery of the nose performed for cosmetic reasons and to facilitate breathing.
Sinus x-ray	An x-ray view of the sinus cavities from the front of the head.
Spirometry	Using a device to measure the breathing capacity of the lungs.
Sputum culture and sensitivity (CS)	Testing sputum by placing it on a culture medium and observing any bacterial growth. The specimen is then tested to determine antibiotic effectiveness.
Sputum cytology	Testing for malignant cells in sputum.
Throat culture	Removing a small sample of tissue or material from the pharynx and placing it upon a culture medium to determine bacterial growth.
Thoracentesis	The surgical puncture of the chest wall for the removal of fluids.
Thoracostomy	An insertion of a tube into the chest for the purpose of draining off fluid or air.
Tracheotomy	Surgical incision into the trachea to provide an airway. This is generally performed as an emergency procedure to provide oxygen.
Tuberculin skin tests (TB test)	Applying a chemical agent (Tine or Mantoux tests) under the surface of the skin to determine if the patient has been exposed to tuberculosis.

TABLE 30   Disorders and Diseases of the Urinary System

Disorder/Disease	Description
Anuria	No urine formed by the kidneys and a complete lack of urine excretion.
Bladder neck obstruction	Blockage of the bladder outlet.
Dysuria	Abnormal secretion of large amounts of urine.
Enuresis	Involuntary discharge of urine after the age by which bladder control should have been established. This usually occurs by the age of 5. Also called bed-wetting at night.
Glomerulonephritis	Inflammation of the kidney (primarily of the glomerulus). Since the glomerular membrane is inflamed, it becomes more permeable and this results in protein (proteinuria) and blood (hematuria) in the urine.
Hematuria	A condition of blood in the urine. This is a symptom of disease process.
Hypospadius	A congenital opening of the male urethra on the underside of the penis.
Interstitial cystitis	Disease of an unknown cause in which there is inflammation and irritation of the bladder. It is most commonly seen in middle-aged women.
Lithotomy	Surgical incision to remove kidney stones.
Meatotomy	A surgical enlargement of the urinary opening (meatus).
Nocturia	Excessive urination during the night. This may or may not be abnormal.
Pyelitis	Inflammation of the renal pelvis.
Pyelonephritis	Inflammation of the renal pelvis and the kidney. This is one of the most common types of kidney disease. It may be the result of a lower urinary tract infection that moved up to the kidney via the ureters. There may be large quantities of white blood cells and bacteria in the urine. Hematuria may also be present. This condition can occur whenever there is an untreated or persistent case of cystitis.
Pyuria	Presence of pus in the urine.
Renal colic	Pain caused by a kidney stone. This type of pain can be excruciating and generally requires medical treatment.

TABLE 31   Procedures and Tests Relating to the Urinary System

Procedure/Test	Description
Catheterization	The insertion of a sterile tube through the urethra and into the urinary bladder for the purpose of withdrawing urine. This procedure is used to obtain a sterile urine specimen and also to relieve distension when the patient is unable to void on their own. See Chapter 26 for procedure.
Cystography	The process of instilling a contrast material or dye into the bladder by catheter to visualize the urinary bladder.
Cystoscopy	Visual examination of the urinary bladder using an instrument called a cystoscope. The patient may receive a general anesthetic for this procedure.
Dialysis	The artificial filtration of waste material from the blood. It is used when the kidneys fail to function.
Excretory urography	Injection of dye into the bloodstream followed by taking an x-ray to trace the action of the kidney as it excretes the dye.
Hemodialysis	Use of an artificial kidney that filters the blood of a person to remove waste products. Use of this technique in patients who have defective kidneys is lifesaving.
Intravenous pyelogram (IVP)	An x-ray examination of the kidneys, ureters, and bladder by injecting a radiopaque dye into the circulatory system and tracing its route as it is excreted.
Lithotripsy	Destroying or crushing kidney stones in the bladder or urethra with a device called a lithotriptor.
Peritoneal dialysis	The removal of toxic waste substances from the body by placing warm chemically balanced solutions into the peritoneal cavity. This is used in treating renal failure and in certain types of poisonings.
Renal transplant	Surgical placement of a donor kidney.
Urinalysis	A laboratory test that consists of the physical, chemical, and microscopic examination of urine.
Urography	The use of a contrast medium to provide an x-ray of the urinary tract.

INDEX